Diagnostic Atlas of Renal Pathology, Second Edition

A Companion to Brenner & Rector's
The Kidney, 9th edition

Agnes B. Fogo, MD

John L. Shapiro Professor of Pathology
Professor of Medicine and Pediatrics
Director, Renal/Electron Microscopy Laboratory
Department of Pathology
Vanderbilt University Medical Center
Nashville, Tennessee

Michael Kashgarian, MD

Professor Emeritus of Pathology and
    Molecular, Cellular, and Developmental Biology
Department of Pathology
Yale University
New Haven, Connecticut

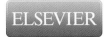

1600 John F. Kennedy Blvd.
Ste 1800
Philadelphia, PA 19103-2899

DIAGNOSTIC ATLAS OF RENAL PATHOLOGY, SECOND EDITION 978-1-4377-0427-3

Notice

Knowledge and best practice in this field are constantly changing. As new research and experience broaden our knowledge, changes in practice, treatment and drug therapy may become necessary or appropriate. Readers are advised to check the most current information provided (i) on procedures featured or (ii) by the manufacturer of each product to be administered, to verify the recommended dose or formula, the method and duration of administration, and contraindications. It is the responsibility of the practitioner, relying on their own experience and knowledge of the patient, to make diagnoses, to determine dosages and the best treatment for each individual patient, and to take all appropriate safety precautions. To the fullest extent of the law, neither the Publisher nor the Editors assumes any liability for any injury and/or damage to persons or property arising out of or related to any use of the material contained in this book.

The Publisher

Library of Congress Cataloging-in-Publication Data

Fogo, Agnes B.
  Diagnostic atlas of renal pathology : a companion to Brenner & Rector's the Kidney / Agnes B. Fogo, Michael Kashgarian. – 2nd ed.
    p. ; cm.
  Companion v. to Brenner & Rector's the kidney / edited by Barry M. Brenner. 8th ed. c2008.
  Includes bibliographical references and index.
  ISBN 978-1-4377-0427-3 (hardcover : alk. paper)   1. Kidneys–Diseases–Atlases.   I. Kashgarian, Michael.   II. Brenner & Rector's the kidney.   III. Title.
  [DNLM: 1. Kidney Diseases–diagnosis–Atlases.   2. Kidney Diseases–pathology–Atlases.   WJ 17]
  RC903.F64   2012
  616.6′1–dc23   2011025821

Acquisitions Editor: Kate Dimock
Developmental Editor: Ann Ruzycka Anderson
Publishing Services Manager: Jeff Patterson
Project Manager: Tracey Schriefer
Design Direction: Lou Forgione

Printed in China

Last digit is the print number: 9 8 7 6 5 4 3 2 1

Preface

In the 5 years since our first edition was published, there have been many advances in the genetics, etiology, pathogenesis, and treatment of medical renal diseases. These advances have led to a therapeutic focus on a more specific and personalized approach and, in turn, further emphasized the importance and central role of the renal biopsy in patient management. We have taken these factors into consideration in organizing material for the second edition of this renal pathology companion book to the newest edition of Brenner and Rector's *The Kidney*, edited by Taal et al. The organization of this edition follows that of the first, with each of the sections being expanded and updated to include new classifications of various kidney diseases, both native and transplant related. In addition, we have added a new chapter focusing on an approach to end-stage kidney disease as the prevention of progression of chronic renal disease has become an increasingly important goal in nephrology. Sections on genetics, etiology, and pathogenesis have also been expanded. References have been updated, and continue to be focused, rather than encyclopedic and comprehensive. These selected reading suggestions can act as a key to the greater detail present in the larger comprehensive text, *The Kidney*.

Because this is primarily an atlas, we have added numerous new images. These include illustrations of additional entities and expanded illustrations of the spectrum of lesions present in diseases already included in the previous edition. Two new features are tables of key diagnostic features of each of the entities and summaries of differential diagnoses. Together with the numerous images and focused text, this atlas thus provides in-depth and detailed illustrations of a large spectrum of morphologic lesions encountered in the renal biopsy and an approach to differential diagnosis and key prognostic, pathogenetic, and etiologic information.

Acknowledgments

Renal pathology is an exciting process of integrating complex information, relying on a team of nephrologists, pathologists, and highly skilled laboratory personnel. Similar teamwork has gone into the preparation of this book. The deep satisfaction derived from the first edition of our atlas, along with ongoing advances and realizations that we could further update and enhance our presentation of renal pathology in a usable and concise format, have led to this second edition. The ongoing dedication and partnership with Dr. Michael Kashgarian have been essential to the success of our project. I would also like to thank my renal pathology laboratory team, my fellows and colleagues, who have been essential for both the first edition and this second edition. I continue to be grateful to my past fellows, Drs. Paisit Paueksakon, Xochi Geiger, Patricia Revelo, and Michele Rossini, and my more recent fellows, Drs. Aruna Dash and Huma Fatima, who have searched and hunted for the most instructive and beautiful examples of lesions to expand this atlas. I am also indebted to the expert help of Brent Weedman for imaging and photography assistance.

Lastly, I would like to thank my husband, Byron, and my children, Katherine, Michelle, and Kristin, for their enthusiastic support and encouragement for all of my endeavors.

AGNES B. FOGO

This second edition follows our commitment to present medical renal pathology in a form that is accessible to a wide audience. We have used the lessons learned from the residents, fellows, and colleagues who have commented on our previous work in presenting the expansion of knowledge in this field. As such, it reflects a maturation of our discipline over the past 50 years that began with the contributions of the early pioneers of renal pathology, Robert Heptinstall, Conrad Pirani, Jacob Churg, Ben Spargo, and Robert McCluskey. I am indebted to the many clinical and pathology colleagues that I have had the pleasure of working with during these formative years of renal pathology. I would also like to dedicate this work to those who initially started me on the path of studying the kidney. Franklin Epstein was the first to introduce me to the wonders and complexity of the physiology of the kidney. Karl Ullrich taught me the scientific methods and tools necessary to investigate them. Averill Liebow inspired me to pursue pathology as a career. The field of renal pathology was in its infancy when I began my career, and it was the encouragement of these mentors and early pioneers in the field that kept me focused on this discipline. The expert help of my administrative assistant and the staffs of the Yale Pathology Graphics and Imaging and Histology sections was essential to the preparation of the images and the manuscript. Finally, I would like to thank my wife Jean for her patience and encouragement as I prepared this work.

MICHAEL KASHGARIAN

Contents

CHAPTER 4

Chronic Kidney Disease 465

CHAPTER 5

Renal Transplantation 473

CHAPTER 6

Cystic Diseases of the Kidney 499

CHAPTER 7

Renal Neoplasia 517

Glomerular Diseases

chapter

1

Normal Growth and Maturation

The normal glomerulus consists of a complex branching network of capillaries originating at the afferent arteriole and draining into the efferent arteriole (Figs. 1.1-1.3). The glomerulus contains three resident cell types: mesangial, endothelial, and epithelial. The visceral epithelial cells (also called podocytes) cover the urinary surface of the glomerular basement membrane (GBM) with its foot processes, with intervening slit diaphragms. Endothelial cells are opposed to the inner surface of the GBM and are fenestrated (Figs. 1.4, 1.5). At the stalk of the capillary, the endothelial cell is separated from the mesangial cells by the intervening mesangial matrix. The term *endocapillary* is used to describe proliferation filling up the capillary lumen, contributed to by the proliferation of mesangial, endothelial, and infiltrating inflammatory cells. In contrast, extracapillary proliferation refers to proliferation of the parietal epithelial cells that line Bowman's capsule. Specific lesions are described according to their distribution

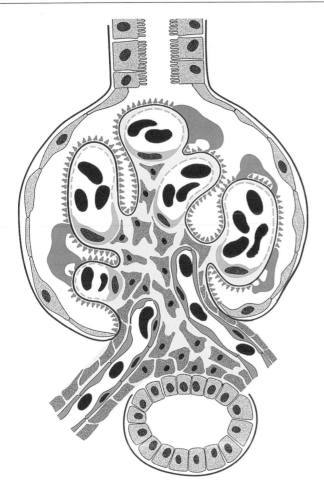

FIG. 1.1 In the normal glomerulus, the capillary loops are open, the mesangial areas have no more than three nuclei each, and foot processes are intact, without any deposits or proliferation.

as being segmental versus global, or diffuse versus focal. Specialized terminology is also used to describe the specific lesions. A list of commonly used terms and their definitions are provided in Table 1.1.

The mesangial cell is a contractile cell that lies embedded in the mesangial matrix in the stalk region of the capillary loops, attached to anchor sites at the ends of the loop by thin extensions of its cytoplasm. Normally up to three mesangial cell nuclei are present per lobule. The GBM consists of three layers distinguished by electron microscopy, the central broadest lamina densa and the less electron-dense zones of lamina rara externa and interna (Figs. 1.4, 1.5).

The glomerulus is surrounded by Bowman's capsule, which is lined by parietal epithelial cells. These are continuous with the proximal tubule, identifiable by its periodic acid Schiff (PAS)–positive brush border. The efferent and afferent arterioles can be distinguished morphologically in favorably oriented sections or by tracing their origins on serial sections. Segmental, interlobular, and arcuate arteries may also be present in the renal biopsy specimen. The cortical biopsy also allows assessment of the tubulointerstitium. Proximal tubules are readily identified by their PAS-positive brush border, lacking in the distal tubules. Collecting ducts show cuboidal, cobblestone-like epithelium. The medulla may also be included in the biopsy.

During fetal maturation, the glomerular capillary tufts are initially covered by large, cuboidal, darkly staining epithelial cells with only small capillary lumina visible (Figs. 1.6-1.8). The cells lining Bowman's space undergo similar change from initial tall columnar to cuboidal to flattened epithelial cells, except for those located at the opening of the proximal tubule, where cells remain taller. Immature nephrons may occasionally be seen in the superficial cortex of children up to 1 year of age (Figs. 1.6-1.11). Glomerular growth continues until adulthood,

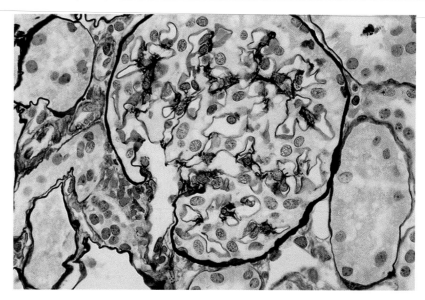

FIG. 1.2 The normal glomerulus has thin, delicate glomerular basement membranes, three or fewer mesangial cell nuclei per mesangial area, and is surrounded by Bowman's capsule. The adjacent tubules show a thin, delicate tubular basement membrane without lamellation or surrounding interstitial fibrosis. The vascular pole shows surrounding extraglomerular mesangial cells. The apparent mesangial cellularity of the glomerulus is highly dependent on the thickness of the section, and it is recommended that renal biopsies be cut at 2 μm thickness. This plastic embedded section is cut at 1 μm (Jones silver stain, ×400).

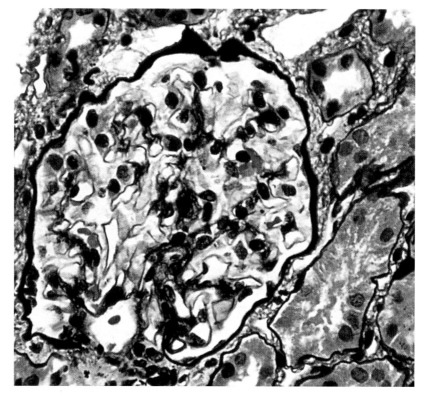

FIG. 1.3 This paraffin-embedded 2-μm section illustrates a normal glomerulus with normal vascular pole with minimal periglomerular interstitial fibrosis and surrounding intact tubules. Mesangial cellularity and matrix are within normal limits (Jones silver stain, ×400).

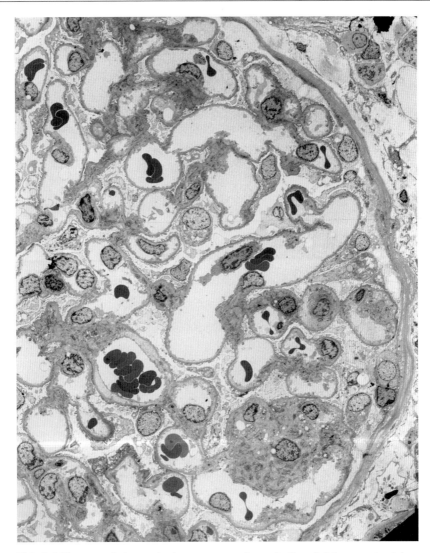

FIG. 1.4 The normal glomerular basement membrane in the adult is approximately 325-375 nm in thickness. Overlying podocytes show intact foot processes with minimal effacement in this case. The mesangial matrix surrounds mesangial cells without expansion or hypercellularity. Endothelial cells show normal fenestration. The parietal cells lining Bowman's capsule are flat and squamous in appearance (transmission electron microscopy, ×1500).

with average normal glomerular diameter approximately 95 μm in a group of patients younger than age 5 years (average age 2.2 years) and 140-160 μm in adulthood. Thickening of the GBM also occurs normally with maturational growth. Normal ranges are from 220 to 260 nm at age 1 year, 280 to 327 nm at age 5 years, 329 to 370 nm at age 10 years, and 358 to 399 nm at age 15 years, the latter similar to adult normal thickness (Figs. 1.4, 1.5). Global glomerulosclerosis may occur without renal disease as a part of normal maturation aging and

Text continued on page 10

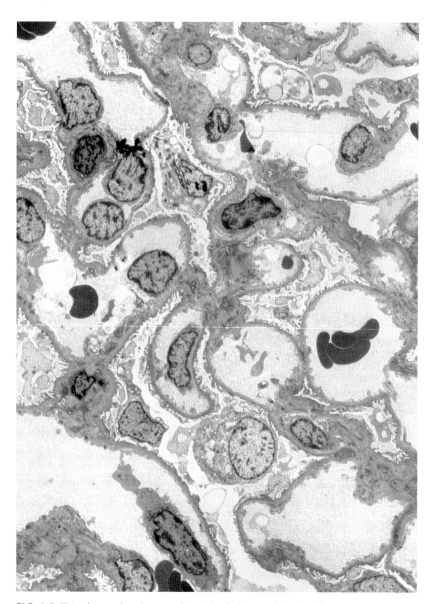

FIG. 1.5 This glomerulus shows only minimal abnormalities by electron microscopy, with rare vacuoles and blebs in the podocytes. The foot processes are largely intact. The glomerular basement membrane is of normal thickness. Red blood cells and rare platelet fragments are found within capillary lumina. The mesangial areas show mesangial cells surrounded by matrix (transmission electron microscopy, ×3000).

TABLE 1-1 Definitions of Common Terms to Describe Morphological Lesions

LIGHT MICROSCOPY

Focal	Involving some glomeruli
Diffuse	Involving all glomeruli
Segmental	Involving part of glomerular tuft
Global	Involving total glomerular tuft
Lobular	Simplified, lobular appearance of capillary loop architecture due to endocapillary proliferation (defined below) (seen in, e.g., MPGN)
Nodular	Relatively acellular areas of mesangial matrix expansion (seen in, e.g., diabetic nephropathy)
Glomerular sclerosis	Obliteration of capillary loop and increased matrix
Crescent	Proliferation of parietal epithelial cells
Spikes	Projections of glomerular basement membrane intervening between subepithelial immune deposits (seen in, e.g., membranous nephropathy)
Endocapillary proliferation	Proliferation of mesangial and/or endothelial cells and infiltrating inflammatory cells, filling up and distending capillary lumens (seen in e.g., proliferative lupus nephritis)
Hyaline	Descriptive of glassy, smooth-appearing material
Hyalinosis	Hyaline-appearing insudation of plasma proteins (seen in e.g., focal segmental glomerulosclerosis)
Mesangial area	Stalk region of capillary loop with mesangial cells surrounded by matrix
Subepithelial	Between podocyte and glomerular basement membrane
Subendothelial	Between endothelial cell and glomerular basement membrane
Tram-track	Double contour of glomerular basement due to deposits and/or circumferential interposition (see EM definitions below)
Wire loop	Thick, rigid appearance of capillary loop due to massive subendothelial deposits
Activity	Description encompassing possible treatment-sensitive lesions, e.g., extent of cellular crescents, cellular infiltrate, necrosis, proliferation
Chronicity	Description of probable irreversible lesions, e.g., extent of tubular atrophy, interstitial fibrosis, fibrous crescents, sclerosis

IMMUNOFLUORESCENCE MICROSCOPY

Granular	Discontinuous flecks of staining producing granular pattern; seen along capillary loop in membranous nephropathy
Linear	Smooth continuous staining, seen along capillary loop in, e.g., anti-GBM antibody–mediated GN, or along TBM in anti-TBM nephritis

ELECTRON MICROSCOPY

Foot process effacement	Flattening of foot processes so that they cover the basement membrane, with loss of slit diaphragms
Microvillous transformation	Small extensions of visceral epithelial cells with villus-like appearance
Circumferential interposition (CIP)	Extension of mesangial cell or infiltrating monocyte cytoplasm with interposition between endothelial cell cytoplasm and basement membrane, often with underlying new basement membrane formation
Reticular aggregates	Organized arrays of membrane particles within endothelial cells (also called tuboloreticular inclusions)
Immunotactoid GP	Large, organized microtubular deposits, >30 nm diameter
Fibrillary GN	Fibrils 14–20 nm diameter without organization

EM, electron microscopy; *GP*, glomerulopathy; *GN*, glomerulonephritis; *GBM*, glomerular basement membrane; *TBM*, tubular basement membrane; *MPGN*, membranoproliferative glomerulonephritis.

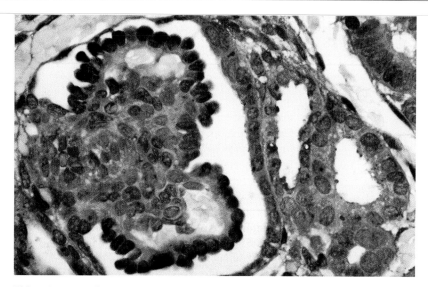

FIG. 1.6 During development, various stages of immature glomeruli may be found at different cortical levels within the kidney. The deep juxtamedullary glomeruli mature first. This immature glomerulus is from the midcortical level of a 28-week-gestation premature baby. There is prominent mesangium and very simple capillary branching with overlying plump, cuboidal glomerular visceral epithelial cells. The parietal epithelial cells lining Bowman's capsule are also more cuboidal than in the mature state (periodic acid Schiff, ×400).

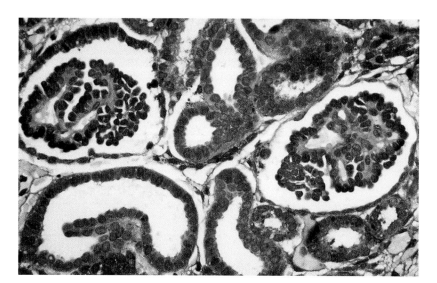

FIG. 1.7 These glomeruli are from the same 28-week-gestation baby as shown in Figure 1.3. They have more complex capillary branching pattern but maintain immature, plump glomerular visceral epithelial cells. In one glomerulus (on the right), the parietal epithelial cells are flattened and more mature in appearance (periodic acid Schiff, ×200).

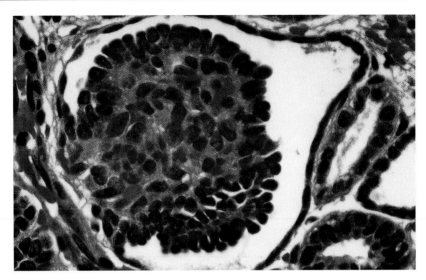

FIG. 1.8 This deep juxtamedullary glomerulus is from the same 28-week-gestation baby as shown in the previous figures. There is a complex capillary branching pattern with overlying plump, still immature glomerular visceral epithelial cells. Bowman's space is pouching out to form a junction with the proximal tubular epithelium on the right (periodic acid Schiff, ×400).

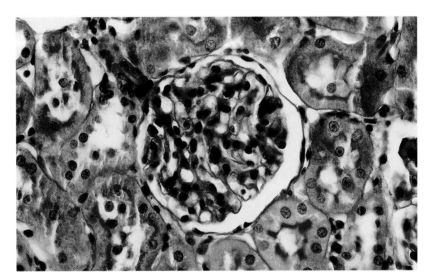

FIG. 1.9 The small but completely mature glomerulus of a normal term baby is illustrated, with complex capillary branching pattern and mature, pale-gray flattened podocytes overlying the capillary loops. The normal vascular pole is seen at the upper left. Normal proximal tubules with PAS-positive brush border with intervening peritubular capillaries are also illustrated. Although glomeruli do not increase in number with maturational growth, they increase in size. Normal glomerular diameter in children less than 5 years old in our biopsy practice is <95 μm. Individual laboratories must establish their own normal parameters because fixation and processing conditions may influence this parameter (periodic acid Schiff, ×100).

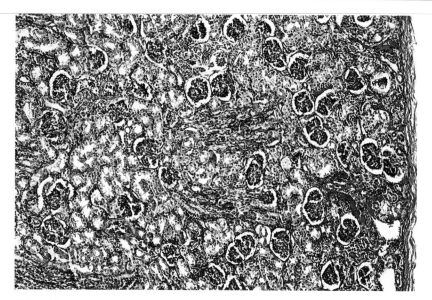

FIG. 1.10 The more superficial glomeruli (right) are less mature than the deeper juxtamedullary glomeruli (left) in this term infant. There is persistence of immature podocytes of the more superficial glomeruli, although capillary branching pattern already is complex (periodic acid Schiff, ×100).

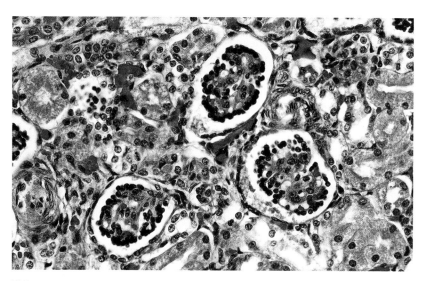

FIG. 1.11 Immature glomeruli from a 3-day-old infant show immature, plump cuboidal podocytes, with moderately complex capillary branching pattern of the glomerulus on the right, and more simple branching pattern of the glomeruli on the left (periodic acid Schiff, ×100).

repair. Less than 5% global glomerulosclerosis is expected in children and young adults, and less than (age divided by 2, minus 10) percent in aged normal individuals.

Selected Reading

Fogo, A., Hawkins, E.P., Berry, P.L., et al., 1990. Glomerular hypertrophy in minimal change disease predicts subsequent progression to focal glomerular sclerosis. Kidney International 38, 115-123.

Fogo, A.B., Kon, V., 2010. The glomerulus—a view from the inside—the endothelial cell. International Journal of Biochemistry and Cell Biology 42, 1388-1397.

Kaplan, C., Pasternack, B., Shah, H., et al., 1975. Age-related incidence of sclerotic glomeruli in human kidneys. American Journal of Pathology 80, 227-234.

Kappel, B., Olsen, S., 1980. Cortical interstitial tissue and sclerosed glomeruli in the normal human kidney, related to age and sex. A quantitative study. Virchows Archiv (Pathological Anatomy) 387, 271-277.

Morita, M., White, R.H.R., Raafat, F., et al., 1988. Glomerular basement membrane thickness in children. A morphometric study. Pediatric Nephrology 2, 190-195.

Shindo, S., Yoshimoto, M., Kuriya, N., et al., 1988. Glomerular basement membrane thickness in recurrent and persistent hematuria and nephrotic syndrome: correlation with sex and age. Pediatric Nephrology 2, 196-199.

Smith, S.M., Hoy, W.E., Cobb, L., 1989. Low incidence of glomerulosclerosis in normal kidneys. Archives of Pathology and Laboratory Medicine 113, 1253-1256.

Primary Glomerular Diseases

Glomerular Diseases That Cause Nephrotic Syndrome: Non–Immune Complex

MINIMAL CHANGE DISEASE AND FOCAL SEGMENTAL GLOMERULOSCLEROSIS: INTRODUCTION

Minimal change disease (MCD) and focal segmental glomerulosclerosis (FSGS) both typically present as the nephrotic syndrome and cannot be readily distinguished based solely on clinical presentation. In children, nephrotic syndrome is presumed to be due to MCD and biopsy is only done if the child is steroid unresponsive or has clinical features suggesting another etiology of the nephrotic syndrome. In adults, MCD accounts for 10-15% of nephrotic syndrome. FSGS has increased in incidence, and in the United States in adults has surpassed membranous nephropathy as a cause of nephrotic syndrome (18.7% incidence), especially in African Americans and in Hispanics. Similar increases have also been reported in children with nephrotic syndrome. Serologic studies, including complement levels, are typically within normal limits in both MCD and FSGS. Renal biopsy is essential to determine the etiology of nephrotic syndrome in adults, and also in children who are not steroid responders. The ultimate prognosis differs dramatically, with complete recovery the rule in MCD, contrasting progressive renal insufficiency in FSGS. Several variants of FSGS have also been investigated for their prognostic significance. A working classification proposal is given in Table 1.2 and the hierarchical relationship of the variants is shown in Figure 1.12. Each of the subtypes will be discussed below.

TABLE 1-2 FSGS Variants	
Type	**Defining Feature**
FSGS, not otherwise specified	Discrete segmental sclerosis
FSGS, perihilar variant	Perihilar sclerosis and hyalinosis
FSGS, cellular variant	Endocapillary hypercellularity
FSGS, tip variant	Sclerosis at tubular pole with adhesion at tubular lumen/neck
FSGS, collapsing variant (Collapsing glomerulopathy)	Segmental or global collapse of tuft and visceral epithelial cell hyperplasia/hypertrophy

FSGS, focal segmental glomerulosclerosis.

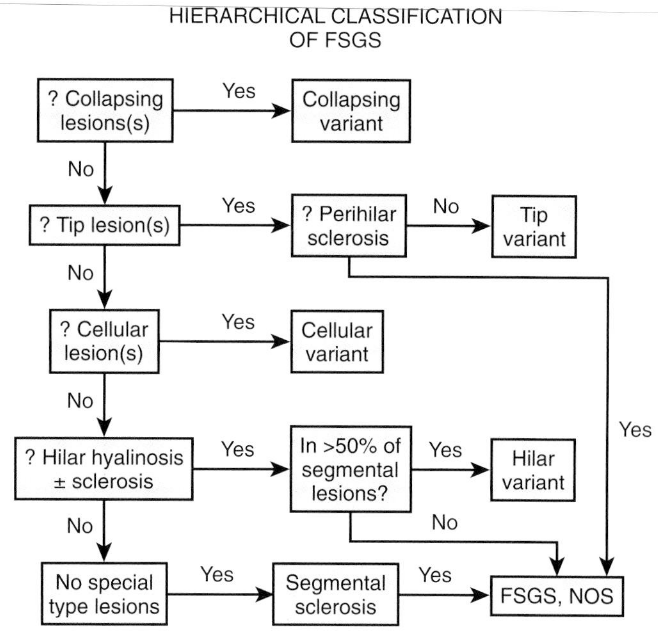

HIERARCHICAL CLASSIFICATION
OF FSGS

```
┌─────────────┐   Yes   ┌─────────────┐
│ ? Collapsing│────────▶│  Collapsing │
│  lesions(s) │         │   variant   │
└─────────────┘         └─────────────┘
       │ No
       ▼
┌─────────────┐   Yes   ┌─────────────┐  No  ┌──────────┐
│ ? Tip lesion(s)│─────▶│ ? Perihilar │─────▶│   Tip    │
│             │         │  sclerosis  │      │ variant  │
└─────────────┘         └─────────────┘      └──────────┘
       │ No
       ▼
┌─────────────┐   Yes   ┌─────────────┐
│ ? Cellular  │────────▶│  Cellular   │
│  lesion(s)  │         │   variant   │
└─────────────┘         └─────────────┘
       │ No
       ▼
┌─────────────┐   Yes   ┌─────────────┐  Yes  ┌──────────┐
│ ? Hilar hyalinosis│──▶│  In >50% of │──────▶│  Hilar   │
│  ± sclerosis│         │  segmental  │       │ variant  │
└─────────────┘         │  lesions?   │       └──────────┘
       │ No             └─────────────┘
       │                       │ No
       ▼                       │
┌─────────────┐   Yes   ┌─────────────┐  Yes  ┌──────────┐
│ No special  │────────▶│  Segmental  │──────▶│FSGS, NOS │
│ type lesions│         │  sclerosis  │       └──────────┘
└─────────────┘         └─────────────┘
```

FIG. 1.12 Hierarchical classification of focal segmental glomerulosclerosis.

MINIMAL CHANGE DISEASE

Minimal change disease (MCD) is named for the apparent structurally normal glomeruli by light microscopy (Figs. 1.13, 1.14). There are no specific vascular or tubulointerstitial lesions in idiopathic MCD. However, MCD may also occur in the middle-aged or older adult who has nonspecific focal areas of tubulointerstitial scarring and mild vascular lesions (arteriosclerosis, arteriolar hyaline related to hypertension, or other unrelated disease). Global glomerulosclerosis, in contrast to the segmental lesion, is not of special diagnostic significance in considering the differential of MCD versus FSGS. Globally sclerotic glomeruli may be normally seen at any age and are thought to result from normal "wear and tear" and not specific disease mechanisms in most cases. Up to 10% of glomeruli may be normally totally sclerosed in people younger than age 40 years. The extent of global sclerosis increases with aging, up to 30% by age 80 years (estimate by calculating half the patient's age, minus 10).

Associated acute interstitial nephritis (AIN), which is characterized by edema and interstitial lymphoplasmacytic infiltrate, often with eosinophils, suggests a drug-induced hypersensitivity reaction. This combined syndrome of MCD and AIN is classically due to nonsteroidal anti-inflammatory drugs (NSAIDs). This condition is usually reversible with discontinuation of the drug.

Immunofluorescence studies are typically negative in MCD. The presence of IgM staining in otherwise apparent MCD biopsies has been a source of previous controversy, with some authors considering this a specific entity, so-called IgM nephropathy (see below).

Electron microscopy shows extensive foot process effacement, vacuolization, and microvillous transformation of podocytes in MCD (Figs. 1.15, 1.16).

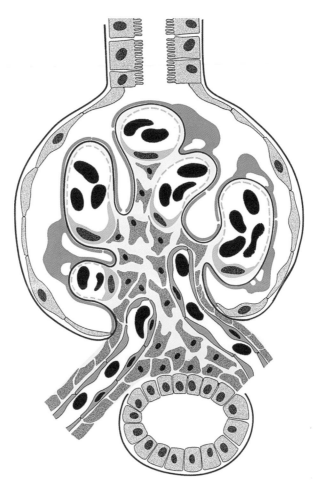

FIG. 1.13 The glomeruli are normal by light microscopy, but with diffuse effacement of foot processes by electron microscopy.

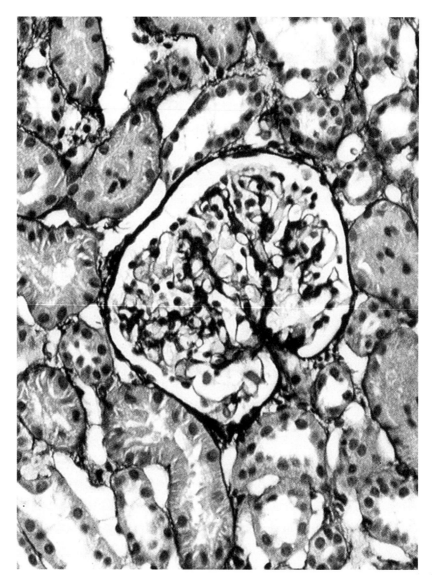

FIG 1.14 Minimal change disease (MCD). Glomeruli appear unremarkable by light microscopy, and in young patients there is no tubulointerstitial fibrosis, as in this patient. In older patients, MCD may occur on a background of nonspecific scarring of the tubulointerstitium (Jones silver stain, ×200).

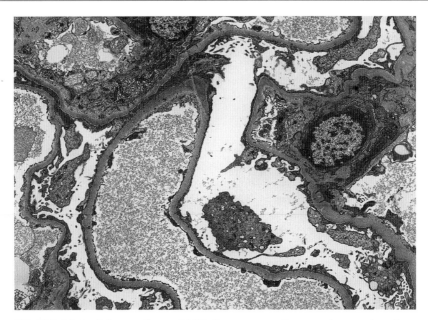

FIG 1.15 Minimal change disease (MCD). Foot process effacement is extensive, often complete, in MCD, although extent of foot process effacement cannot be used as a definitive criterion to differentiate this entity from focal segmental glomerulosclerosis. The glomerular basement membrane is unremarkable, and there are no deposits (transmission electron microscopy, ×3000).

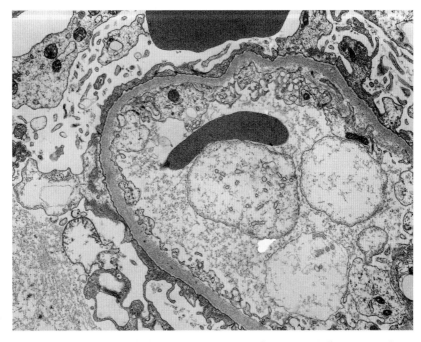

FIG. 1.16 Minimal change disease (MCD). Extensive foot process effacement and microvillous transformation of visceral epithelial cells in MCD. Although the endothelial cells are mildly swollen, the glomerular basement membrane is unremarkable, and there are no deposits (transmission electron microscopy, ×8000).

Selected Reading

Fogo, A., Ichikawa, I., 1996. Focal segmental glomerulosclerosis – a view and review. Pediatric Nephrology 10, 374-391.

Gulati, S., Sharma, A.P., Sharma, R.K., et al., 1999. Changing trends of histopathology in childhood nephrotic syndrome. American Journal of Kidney Disease 3, 646-650.

FOCAL SEGMENTAL GLOMERULOSCLEROSIS

In FSGS of usual type (not otherwise specified, NOS, Table 1.2), sclerosis involves some, but not all, glomeruli (focal), and the sclerosis affects a portion of, but not the entire, glomerular tuft (segmental) (Figs. 1.17, 1.18). The morphologic diagnosis of focal segmental glomerulosclerosis is a light microscopic description of this pattern of scarring, which may occur in many settings. Differentiation of MCD (see above) from FSGS relies on a large enough sample to detect the sclerotic glomeruli, since the detection of even a single glomerulus involved with segmental sclerosis is sufficient to invoke a diagnosis of FSGS rather than MCD. Thus, it is apparent that the distinction of MCD and FSGS may be difficult, especially with the smaller samples obtained with current biopsy guns and smaller needles. A sample of only 10 glomeruli has a 35% probability of missing a focal lesion that affects 10% of the nephrons, decreasing to 12% if 20 glomeruli are sampled. The initial sclerosis is in the juxtamedullary glomeruli, and this region should be included in the sample (Fig. 1.18). Conversely, sampling on one section by definition cannot identify all of the focally and segmentally distributed scars.

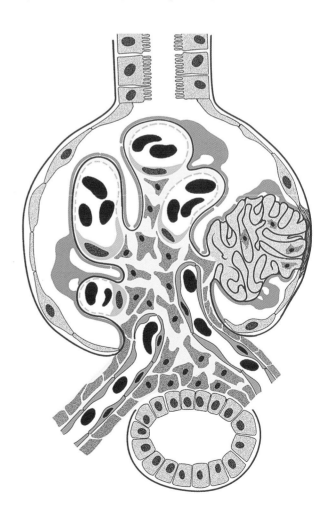

FIG. 1.17 Focal segmental glomerulosclerosis. There is sharply defined segmental sclerosis, defined as obliteration of capillary loops and increased matrix, without deposits and with diffuse foot process effacement by electron microscopy. Adhesions can also be present.

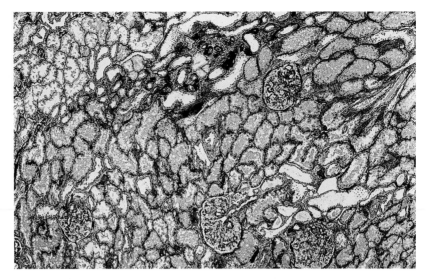

FIG. 1.18 Focal segmental glomerulosclerosis (FSGS). Early in FSGS, lesions are very focal, involving initially the juxtamedullary glomeruli. Tubulointerstitial fibrosis in a given section may be a clue to adjacent early segmental sclerotic lesions, which can be detected by careful serial section examination. In this field, one of four glomeruli (top) shows early segmental sclerosis of usual type, with an adjacent area of tubulointerstitial fibrosis (Jones silver stain, ×100).

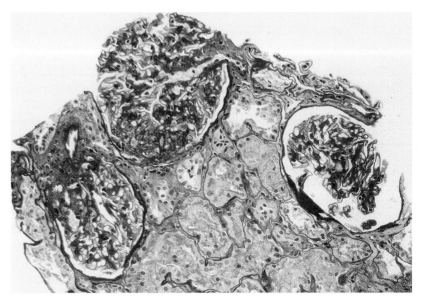

FIG. 1.19 Focal segmental glomerulosclerosis (FSGS). There is early segmental sclerosis that involves the periphery in one glomerulus (top), and the hilar area in another glomerulus (left), but without significant hyalinosis. This mixed pattern of sclerosis is characteristic of FSGS (periodic acid Schiff, ×200).

Three-dimensional studies examining serial sections of glomeruli in cases of idiopathic FSGS have demonstrated that the process indeed is focal, that is, glomeruli without any sclerosis exist even when disease is well established (Figs. 1.19, 1.20).

Because of these limitations in detection of sclerotic lesions, other diagnostic features in glomeruli uninvolved by the sclerotic process have been sought to suspect FSGS even without sclerosed glomeruli. Abnormal glomerular enlargement (see below) appears to be an early

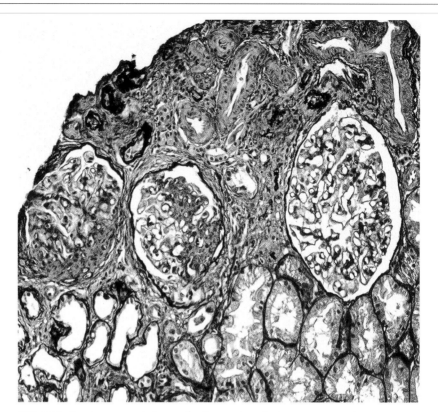

FIG. 1.20 Focal segmental glomerulosclerosis (FSGS). There are more advanced segmental sclerotic lesions affecting two of the three glomeruli in this field, with surrounding proportionate tubulointerstitial fibrosis. The sclerosis is characterized by increased matrix and obliteration of capillary lumens, and is of the usual type of FSGS (Jones silver stain, ×200).

indicator of the sclerotic process even before overt sclerosis can be detected. The presence of marked glomerular enlargement in a biopsy of otherwise apparent MCD would therefore rather suggest an early, incipient stage of FSGS. Dystroglycan, a component of normal GBM that contributes to podocyte–matrix interaction, is generally maintained in nonsclerotic segments in FSGS, and decreased in MCD (but also in collapsing type FSGS). This marker, or other emerging biomarkers from molecular and proteomic studies, while not completely sensitive or specific, may be of aid in favoring unsampled FSGS versus MCD in a biopsy with extensive foot process effacement and no defining segmental lesion. Diffuse mesangial hypercellularity may be a morphological feature superimposed on changes of either MCD or FSGS, with or without IgM deposits, without defined prognostic significance (see below).

The PAS-positive acellular material in the segmental sclerotic lesions of the glomerulus may have different composition depending on the diverse pathophysiologic mechanisms discussed below. The sclerotic process is defined by glomerular capillary obliteration with increase in matrix, and varies from small, early lesions to near global sclerosis (Figs. 1.21-1.24). The segmental sclerosis lesions are discrete and may be located in perihilar and/or peripheral portions of the glomerulus. There may be associated global glomerulosclerosis, which has no specific diagnostic significance. Uninvolved glomeruli show no apparent lesions by light microscopy, but may appear enlarged, as do glomeruli with early-stage segmental sclerosis. The glomerulosclerosis may be associated with hyalinosis, resulting from insudation of plasma proteins, producing a smooth, glassy (hyaline) appearance (Fig. 1.25). This occurs particularly in the axial, vascular pole region. Of note, arteriolar hyalinosis may occur with hypertensive injury and should not be taken per se as evidence of a sclerotic lesion (see hilar-type FSGS

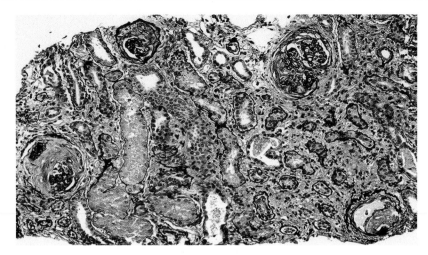

FIG. 1.21 Focal segmental glomerulosclerosis (FSGS). Near end-stage FSGS is present, with global or near global sclerosis of all glomeruli and extensive tubulointerstitial fibrosis and vascular thickening (Jones silver stain, ×200).

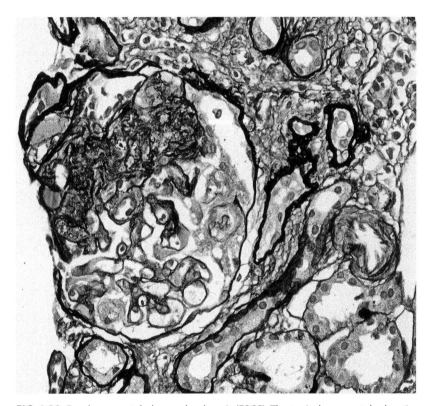

FIG. 1.22 Focal segmental glomerulosclerosis (FSGS). The typical segmental sclerotic lesion in FSGS is characterized by increased matrix and obliteration of capillary lumina, frequently with hyalinosis and adhesions, as illustrated here. There is surrounding tubulointerstitial fibrosis. The uninvolved segment of the glomerulus appears unremarkable (Jones silver stain, ×200).

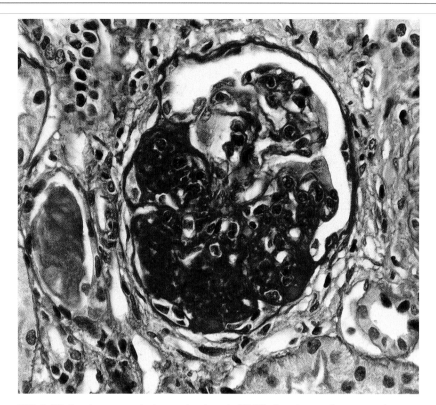

FIG. 1.23 Focal segmental glomerulosclerosis (FSGS). An advanced segmental sclerotic lesion of FSGS is shown, with only minimal hyaline droplets. There is increased mesangial matrix and obliteration of capillary lumina involving the majority of the glomerulus. The uninvolved portion of the glomerulus has mild increase in mesangial matrix. The adjacent tubule shows atrophy and a proteinaceous cast (periodic acid Schiff, ×400).

Key Diagnostic Features of FSGS

- Extensive foot process effacement
- Absence of immune complexes
- Diagnostic segmental lesions

Note: Segmental lesions vary, and define the subtype of focal segmental glomerulosclerosis (FSGS).

---

below). Vascular thickening may be prominent late in the course of FSGS. Adhesion of the podocyte to Bowman's capsule (synechiae) can be an early manifestation of sclerosis (Fig. 1.26). The glomerulosclerosis is accompanied by tubular atrophy, interstitial fibrosis with interstitial lymphocytes, proportional to the degree of scarring in the glomerulus (Fig. 1.22). Of note, in HIV-associated nephropathy (HIVAN) and collapsing glomerulopathy, tubular lesions are disproportionally severe (see below).

Immunofluorescence may show nonspecific entrapment of IgM and C3 in sclerotic areas or areas where the mesangial matrix is increased (Fig. 1.27).

Electron microscopy shows extensive foot process effacement (Fig. 1.28). Thus, extent of foot process effacement does not allow precise distinction between MCD and FSGS in individual cases. Foot process effacement tends to be more extensive in primary FSGS compared

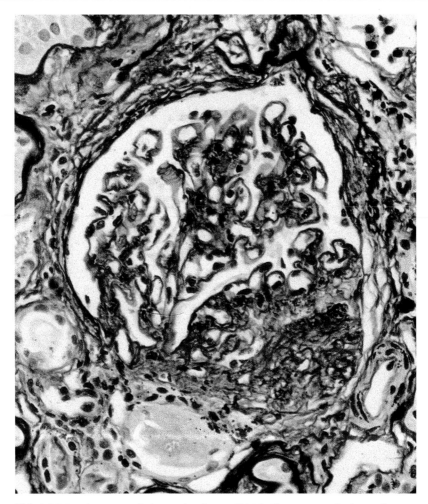

FIG. 1.24 Focal segmental glomerulosclerosis (FSGS). The segmental sclerotic lesion of FSGS is illustrated, with increased mesangial matrix and obliteration of capillary lumina. The remnants of the glomerular basement membrane in the sclerosed segment can be seen as wrinkled lines on this silver stain. The uninvolved portion of the glomerulus shows minimal mesangial matrix increase. Although this sclerotic lesion involves the vascular pole, there is not associated hyalinosis, and the lesion is therefore best classified as FSGS, not otherwise specified (Jones silver stain, ×400).

Differential Diagnosis of Minimal Change Disease versus FSGS

- Global sclerosis may be found in any condition, and does not differentiate between minimal change disease and FSGS.
- Extent of foot process effacement does not distinguish between primary FSGS and minimal change disease: <50% effacement indicates the process is not likely either MCD or primary FSGS.
- Even in the absence of diagnostic segmental lesions (see above), unsampled FSGS may be considered in biopsies with small sample size.
- Surrogate markers of unsampled FSGS include marked glomerulomegaly, interstitial fibrosis in young patients.

FSGS, focal segmental glomerulosclerosis.

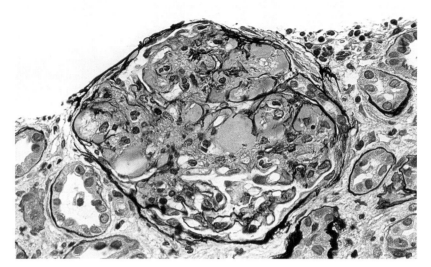

FIG. 1.25 Focal segmental glomerulosclerosis (FSGS). In this case of FSGS, there was extensive hyalinosis in the sclerotic areas, which are characterized by increased mesangial matrix and obliteration of capillary lumina. There are also adhesions of the sclerotic segments to Bowman's capsule, with thickened and disrupted Bowman's capsule. The hyalinosis represents an insudation of plasma proteins, reflecting endothelial injury (Jones silver stain, ×400).

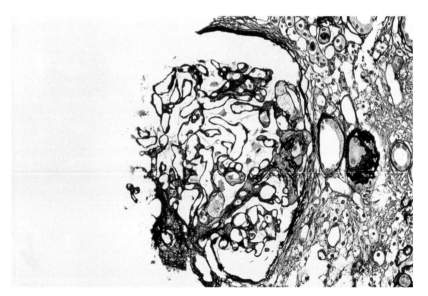

FIG. 1.26 Focal segmental glomerulosclerosis (FSGS). Early lesion of FSGS with adhesion of glomerular tuft to Bowman's capsule and small segmental area of hyalinosis and intracapillary foam cells (Jones silver stain, ×400).

with secondary FSGS; however, the overlap between these two categories does not allow one to use this as a diagnostic feature in individual cases. The absence of significant, that is, >50%, foot process effacement should cast doubt on the diagnosis of primary, idiopathic FSGS. There are no immune deposits in idiopathic FSGS, but mesangial matrix is increased in sclerotic areas (Fig. 1.29). Areas of hyalin may be present in the sclerotic segments and appear dense by electron microscopy, but should be readily recognized as hyalin by correlating with scout

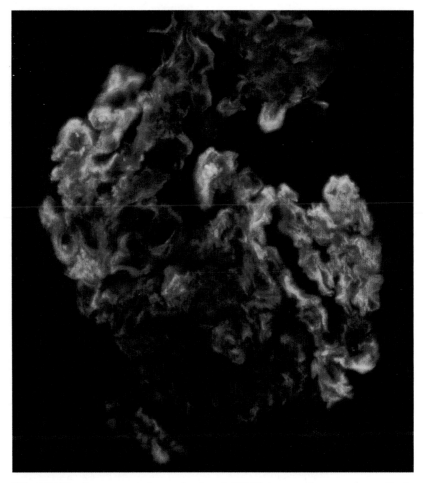

FIG. 1.27 Focal segmental glomerulosclerosis (FSGS). Immunofluorescence studies in FSGS do not show immune complexes, but may show IgM in sclerotic areas or in areas of mesangial expansion (anti-IgM antibody immunofluorescence, ×400).

Differential Diagnosis of Primary versus Secondary FSGS Lesions

- Subtotal (i.e., <50%) foot process effacement strongly favors secondary FSGS.
- Extensive foot process effacement may, however, occasionally occur even in secondary FSGS.
- Key differential features:
  - Arterionephrosclerosis: extensive vascular sclerosis, periglomerular fibrosis around non-sclerotic glomeruli, increased lamina rara interna.
  - Chronic pyelonephritis/reflux nephropathy: sharply delineated, geographic pattern of scarring and thyroidization of tubules, periglomerular fibrosis, occasionally increased lamina rara interna and subtotal foot process effacement.
- Secondary collapsing glomerulopathy causes:
  - HIV-associated nephropathy; numerous reticular aggregates suggest HIV-associated nephropathy (or possibly systemic lupus erythematosus [SLE]).
  - Other secondary causes of collapsing lesions usually with less extensive foot process effacement: pamidronate toxicity, severe ischemia (such as that seen with cyclosporin, cocaine), SLE, and possibly parvovirus. Clinical correlation is essential.

FSGS, focal segmental glomerulosclerosis.

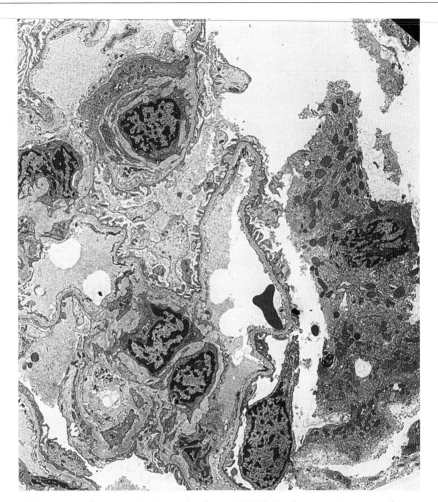

FIG. 1.28 Focal segmental glomerulosclerosis (FSGS). By electron microscopy, there is extensive foot process effacement in FSGS. However, it may not be complete, as illustrated here. If there is less than approximately 50% foot process effacement, the diagnosis of primary FSGS is in doubt. There is also mesangial matrix expansion, without immune deposits (transmission electron microscopy, ×3000).

section light microscopic appearance (Fig. 1.30). The presence of numerous reticular aggregates in endothelial cells in the setting of segmental glomerulosclerosis with collapsing features suggests possible HIVAN (see below).

Diagnosis of Recurrence of FSGS in the Transplant

Most recurrences occur within the first months after transplantation, although proteinuria may recur immediately after the graft is implanted. Foot process effacement is present at time of recurrence of proteinuria and precedes the development of sclerosis, typically by weeks to months. Glomerular enlargement at this stage of recurrent FSGS is prominent in children, who otherwise do not undergo glomerular enlargement when receiving an adult kidney. (In contrast, an adult recipient of a single kidney will normally have marked renal and glomerular growth to provide adequate glomerular filtration rate [GFR]). Overt sclerosis is not noted until weeks to even months after recurrence of nephrotic syndrome. Thus, during this time interval in the setting of the FSGS patient with nephrotic syndrome in the transplant, foot process effacement alone, even without detectable segmental sclerosis, is evidence of recurrent FSGS.

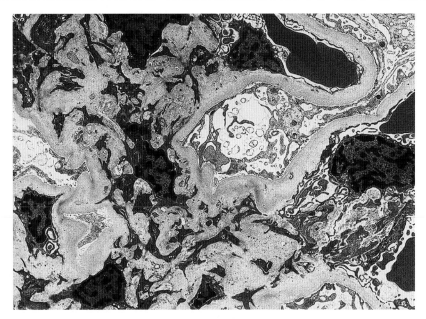

FIG. 1.29 Focal segmental glomerulosclerosis (FSGS). Segmental increase in matrix with obliterated capillary lumens is apparent in this case of FSGS. The overlying visceral epithelial cells show vacuolization, microvillous transformation, and extensive foot process effacement. The corrugated, collapsed glomerular basement membrane is evident. There are no immune deposits (transmission electron microscopy, ×5000).

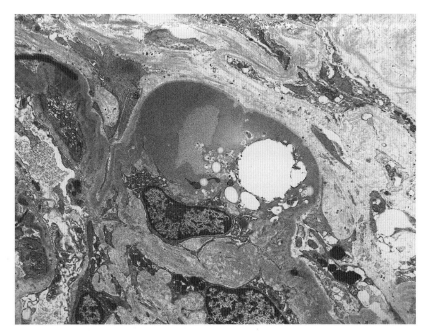

FIG. 1.30 Focal segmental glomerulosclerosis (FSGS). Hyaline deposit within a segmentally sclerotic area in FSGS. Hyaline is smooth, homogeneous, usually located in areas of sclerosis, and frequently contains lipid (clear, round areas). The sclerotic segment is characterized by increased matrix and obliteration of the capillary lumen, with dense adhesion to the overlying fibrotic Bowman's capsule (transmission electron microscopy, ×3000).

Differential Diagnosis of MCD vs. FSGS

Some investigators have felt that the common clinical presentation and similar findings in intact glomeruli indicate that MCD and FSGS are two manifestations of the same disease. Our data and those from others rather support differences even at the earliest time points. Much evidence has pointed to the participation of abnormal glomerular adaptation and growth factors in the pathogenesis of glomerulosclerosis. Several studies have shown that glomerular enlargement precedes overt glomerulosclerosis, both in pediatric and adult patients who otherwise had apparent MCD initially. Patients with abnormal glomerular growth, even on initial biopsies that did not show overt sclerotic lesions, subsequently developed overt glomerulosclerosis, as documented in later biopsies. A cut-off of >50% larger glomerular area than normal for age was a sensitive indicator of increased risk for progression in one series of children with nephrotic syndrome. Of note, glomeruli grow in size until approximately age 18 years, although no new glomeruli are formed after birth, so age-matched controls must be used in the pediatric population to assess normal glomerular size.

The finding of mesangial hypercellularity (>80% of glomeruli with >3 cells per mesangial region) has been proposed to indicate a subgroup of patients with poorer prognosis and increased risk for development of FSGS. However, several series have failed to confirm a definite clinical correlation of this morphologic variant. Thus, in several series, patients with this manifestation on renal biopsies that otherwise show apparent MCD despite decreased initial response to steroids ultimately had good prognosis. Lack of uniform application of criteria for morphologic definition of mesangial hypercellularity makes it difficult to assess the impact of this feature on prognosis. Children with FSGS and mesangial hypercellularity did not show worse prognosis than those with typical FSGS. Thus, diffuse mesangial hypercellularity does not appear to impart a specific prognostic significance in either MCD or FSGS, nor does it differentiate between apparent MCD and unsampled FSGS.

IgM deposits by immunofluorescence in association with mesangial hypercellularity may indicate a poorer response to steroids, and some patients have shown histological FSGS on second biopsy after an initial biopsy showed IgM nephropathy. However, the significance of IgM deposits by immunofluorescence in the setting of normal glomeruli by light microscopy has been difficult to assess. Again, series of biopsies from children with FSGS and nephrotic syndrome have failed to show a specific predictive value of the IgM staining with or without diffuse mesangial hypercellularity. If deposits are present by electron microscopy as well as by immunofluorescence, a mesangiopathic immune complex glomerulonephritis should be diagnosed.

In summary, the diagnosis of FSGS cannot be completely excluded when segmental sclerotic lesions are not detected, even with an adequate-size biopsy. It is therefore best to include the possibility of unsampled FSGS in biopsies from patients with nephrotic syndrome, no immune complexes and foot process effacement, especially when glomerular number is less than 25, or other morphologic findings indicative of probability of undersampled FSGS are present. These include glomerular enlargement and interstitial fibrosis (in young patients), and possibly preserved dystroglycan staining.

Etiology/Pathogenesis

The pathogenesis of MCD appears related to abnormal cytokines that only affect glomerular permeability, and do not promote sclerogenic mechanisms. Recent data point to increased urinary CD80 in MCD but not FSGS patients. MCD has been associated with drug-induced hypersensitivity reactions. MCD also has been associated with Hodgkin's disease, bee stings, and other venom exposure, implicating immune dysfunction as an initiating factor.

Primary FSGS is thought to result from an undefined circulating factor or factors, which mediate abnormal glomerular permeability and ultimately sclerosis. Recent studies have pointed to podocyte injury and dedifferentiation of its phenotype in the pathogenesis of nephrotic syndrome.

New studies of the molecular biology of the podocyte and identification of genes mutated in rare familial forms of FSGS (e.g., *ACTN4*, *NPHS2*, which encodes podocin, *TRPC-6*, *PLCE1*, *INF-2*, *WT1*, *CD2AP*, *LAMB2*), or in congenital nephrotic syndrome of Finnish type (nephrin, coded by the *NPHS1* gene), have given important new insights into the mechanisms of progressive glomerulosclerosis and nephrotic syndrome. We will only briefly discuss some of these genetic forms of FSGS. Nephrin localizes to the slit diaphragm of the podocyte and is tightly associated with CD2-associated protein (CD2AP). Nephrin functions as a zona occludens-type junction protein, and along with CD2AP provides a crucial role in receptor patterning, cytoskeletal polarity, and signaling. Mice engineered to be deficient in CD2AP develop congenital nephrotic syndrome, similar to congenital nephrotic syndrome of Finnish type. Autosomal dominant FSGS is caused by mutation in α-actinin 4 (ACTN4). This is hypothesized to cause altered actin cytoskeleton interaction, perhaps causing FSGS through a gain-of-function mechanism, contrasting the loss-of-function mechanism implicated for disease caused by the nephrin mutation mice with either knockout or knocking of mutated ACTN4 develop FSGS lesions. Thus, balance of α-actinin 4 is crucial for the podocyte. Patients with α-actinin 4 mutation progress to end stage by age 30 years, with rare recurrence in the transplant. Transient receptor potential cation channel-6 (TRPC-6) is a channel molecule expressed in the podocyte, and when mutated, a gain of function altered calcium flux occurs. FSGS develops in adulthood with variable penetrance. Podocin, another podocyte-specific gene (*NPHS2*), is mutated in autosomal recessive FSGS that has an early onset in childhood with rapid progression to end stage with frequent steroid resistance. Podocin is an integral stomatin protein family member and interacts with the CD2AP–nephrin complex, indicating that podocin could serve in the structural organization of the slit diaphragm. In contrast to the steroid resistance of the above, some patients with PLCE1 mutations may respond to steroids. Acquired disruption of some of these complexly interacting podocyte molecules has been demonstrated in experimental models and in human proteinuric diseases. Recently, a variant of apolipoprotein L1 that is protective against trypanosomal disease has been linked to increased FSGS in African Americans, although mechanisms for renal disease susceptibility remain unknown. Thus, it is possible that novel molecular and immunostaining techniques to detect abnormalities in these genes will become of diagnostic and prognostic utility, although there currently are no specific morphologic findings recognized to distinguish the FSGS cases due to mutations in these genes from other types of FSGS.

Selected Reading

General

Braden, G.L., Mulhern, J.G., O'Shea, M.H., et al., 2000. Changing incidence of glomerular diseases in adults. American Journal of Kidney Disease 35, 878-883.

Corwin, H.L., Schwartz, M.M., Lewis, E.J., 1988. The importance of sample size in the interpretation of the renal biopsy. American Journal of Nephrology 8, 85-89.

D'Agati, V., 1994. The many masks of focal segmental glomerulosclerosis. Kidney International 46, 1223-1241.

D'Agati, V.D., Fogo, A.B., Bruijn, J.A., et al., 2004. Pathologic classification of focal segmental glomerulosclerosis: a working proposal. American Journal of Kidney Disease 43, 368-382.

Deegens, J.K., Dijkman, H.B., Borm, G.F., et al., 2008. Podocyte foot process effacement as a diagnostic tool in focal segmental glomerulosclerosis. Kidney International 74, 1568-1576.

Fogo, A., Hawkins, E.P., Berry, P.L., et al., 1990. Glomerular hypertrophy in minimal change disease predicts subsequent progression to focal glomerular sclerosis. Kidney International 38, 115-123.

Fogo, A., Ichikawa, I., 1996. Focal segmental glomerulosclerosis – a view and review. Pediatric Nephrology 10, 374-391.

Garin, E.H., Mu, W., Arthur, J.M., et al., 2010. Urinary CD80 is elevated in minimal change disease but not in focal segmental glomerulosclerosis. Kidney International 78, 296-302.

Gulati, S., Sharma, A.P., Sharma, R.K., et al., 1999. Changing trends of histopathology in childhood nephrotic syndrome. American Journal of Kidney Disease 3, 646-650.

Haas, M., Spargo, B., Coventry, S., 1995. Increasing incidence of focal-segmental glomerulosclerosis among adult nephropathies: A 20-year renal biopsy study. American Journal of Kidney Disease 26, 740-750.

Ijpelaar, D.H., Farris, A.B., Goemaere, N., et al., 2008. Fidelity and evolution of recurrent FSGS in renal allografts. Journal of the American Society of Nephrology 19, 2219-2224.

Smith, S.M., Hoy, W.E., Cobb, L., 1989. Low incidence of glomerulosclerosis in normal kidneys. Archives of Pathology and Laboratory Medicine 113, 1253-1256.

Genetics

Boute, N., Gribouval, O., Roselli, S., et al., 2000. NPHS2, encoding the glomerular protein podocin, is mutated in autosomal recessive steroid-resistant nephrotic syndrome. Nature Genetics 24, 349-354.

Brown, E.J., Schlöndorff, J.S., Becker, D.J., et al., 2010. Mutations in the formin gene INF2 cause focal segmental glomerulosclerosis. Nature Genetics 42, 72-76.

Genovese, G., Friedman, D.J., Ross, M.D., et al., 2010. Association of trypanolytic ApoL1 variants with kidney disease in African Americans. Science 329, 841-845.

Hildebrandt, F., Heeringa, S.F., 2009. Specific podocin mutations determine age of onset of nephrotic syndrome all the way into adult life. Kidney International 75, 669-771.

Kaplan, J.M., Kim, S.H., North, K.N., et al., 2000. Mutations in ACTN4, encoding alpha-actinin-4, cause familial focal segmental glomerulosclerosis. Nature Genetics 24, 251-256.

Karle, S.M., Uetz, B., Ronner, V., et al., 2002. Novel mutations in NPHS2 detected in both familial and sporadic steroid-resistant nephrotic syndrome. Journal of the American Society of Nephrology 13, 388-393.

Ruf, R.G., Lichtenberger, A., Karle, S.M., et al., 2004. Arbeitsgemeinschaft Für Pädiatrische Nephrologie Study Group: Patients with mutations in NPHS2 (podocin) do not respond to standard steroid treatment of nephrotic syndrome. Journal of the American Society of Nephrology 15, 722-732.

Winn, M.P., Conlon, P.J., Lynn, K.L., et al., 2005. A mutation in the TRPC6 cation channel causes familial focal segmental glomerulosclerosis. Science 308, 1801-1804.

COLLAPSING GLOMERULOPATHY

Collapsing glomerulopathy has a poor prognosis, with marked proteinuria, rapid loss of renal function, and virtually no responsiveness to corticosteroids alone. This lesion occurs in both Caucasians and in African Americans, with strong African American preponderance. The incidence of this lesion varies in different geographic regions. In New York, the incidence has increased from 11% of all cases of idiopathic FSGS from 1979 to 1985, to 20% of this group from 1986 to 1989, and to 24% of idiopathic FSGS from 1990 to 1993. In a large renal biopsy practice centered in Chicago, the collapsing variant accounted for only 4.7% of FSGS biopsies.

By light microscopy, there is glomerular tuft collapse (segmental or global) and overlying podocyte hyperplasia and hypertrophy (Fig. 1.31). Collapsing lesions are more often global than segmental (Table 1.2, Figs. 1.32, 1.33). Segmental lesions may involve perihilar and/or peripheral portions of the glomerulus (Fig. 1.34). There are frequent marked protein droplets in the hypertrophied visceral epithelial cells (Fig. 1.35). Adhesions and hyalinosis are uncommon in the early stage of the lesion, as are mesangial hypercellularity and glomerulomegaly. Involvement of even a single glomerulus with this collapsing lesion is proposed to warrant classification as collapsing glomerulopathy, with its attendant poor prognosis (Fig. 1.36).

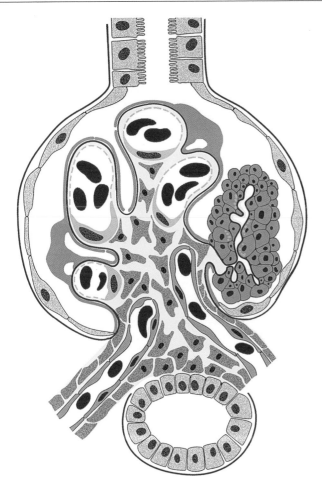

FIG. 1.31 Collapsing glomerulopathy. There is segmental or global collapse of the capillary tuft with overlying visceral epithelial cell hyperplasia, without deposits.

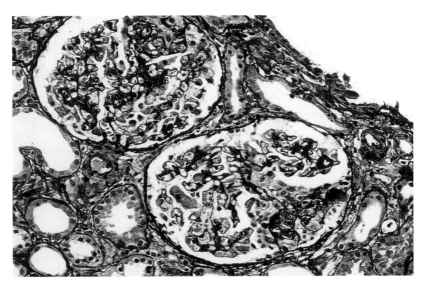

FIG. 1.32 Collapsing glomerulopathy. Collapsing glomerulopathy is characterized by collapse of the glomerular tuft with marked proliferation of overlying visceral epithelial cells, often with prominent protein droplets. The collapse may be global, or more segmental (Jones silver stain, ×400).

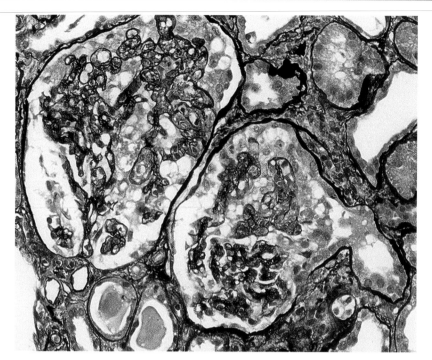

FIG. 1.33 Collapsing glomerulopathy. Extensive collapse with marked visceral epithelial cell hyperplasia in collapsing glomerulopathy (Jones silver stain, ×400).

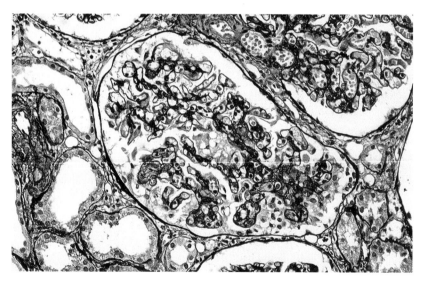

FIG. 1.34 Collapsing glomerulopathy. Occasionally the collapse may be quite segmental, with the remainder of the glomerular capillary tuft showing no alterations. There is marked segmental collapse with overlying visceral epithelial cell hyperplasia in this case of collapsing glomerulopathy (Jones silver stain, ×200).

Other types of segmental sclerosis (Table 1.2) may coexist. Differentiation of cellular or collapsing-type FSGS from usual, NOS FSGS, may be difficult in some cases (Fig. 1.37). Vessels do not show specific lesions. Tubules show injury disproportionate to the sclerosis with microcystic change (Fig. 1.38), and there is interstitial inflammation.

Immunofluorescence may show IgM and C3 in sclerotic segments. Electron microscopy shows the wrinkled, collapsed glomerular basement membrane (GBM) and overlying visceral

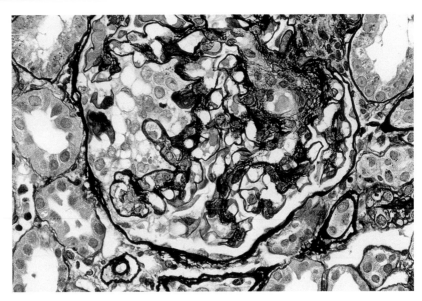

FIG. 1.35 Collapsing glomerulopathy. There is collapse of the glomerular tuft and overlying hyperplasia of the visceral epithelial cells, with prominent protein reabsorption droplets (Jones silver stain, ×400).

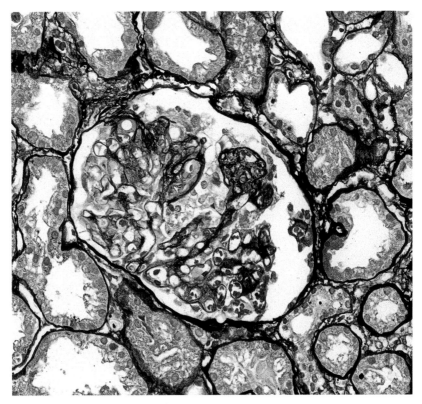

FIG. 1.36 Collapsing glomerulopathy. There are some overlap features between the cellular type of focal segmental glomerulosclerosis and collapsing glomerulopathy, as illustrated here. There is collapse in areas, and segmental endocapillary hypercellularity, with occasional neutrophils and foam cells, with overlying visceral epithelial cell hyperplasia. However, the endocapillary hypercellularity is not quite prominent enough to classify as a cellular lesion, and this lesion would best be classified as collapsing glomerulopathy (Jones silver stain, ×400).

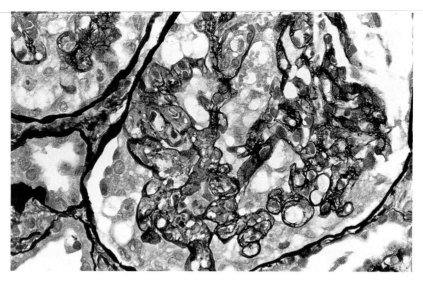

FIG. 1.37 Complex focal segmental glomerulosclerosis (FSGS). This glomerulus shows an early, complex sclerosing lesion with varying features. There is a segmental area of adhesion with hyalinosis (left), with mild overlying visceral epithelial cell hypertrophy/hyperplasia. In the adjacent lobule, there is an early cellular lesion with mild endocapillary hypercellularity, but without the typical foam cells of FSGS, cellular variant. There is not well-established collapse, and the cellular lesion occupies only a very small portion of the tuft. This is therefore best classified as FSGS, not otherwise specified, although it shows some overlapping features with both the cellular and collapsing variants of FSGS (endocapillary hypercellularity and visceral epithelial cell hypertrophy/hyperplasia). This most likely represents an early sclerosing lesion (Jones silver stain, ×400).

epithelial cell hypertrophy/hyperplasia with frequent vacuoles and protein droplets. No immune complexes are present (Fig. 1.39). Reticular aggregates are not present in idiopathic collapsing glomerulopathy.

Etiology/Pathogenesis

Mature podocytes do not usually proliferate because of high expression of cyclin-dependent kinase inhibitor p27kip1. In collapsing glomerulopathy and HIVAN, p27kip1 expression is lost in areas of collapse, with proliferation and dedifferentiation. These observations point to a dysregulated phenotype of these epithelial cells in the pathogenesis of these disorders. Parietal epithelial cells likely contribute to this hyperplasia, and may also migrate along the GBM to replace injured podocytes. The etiology of collapsing glomerulopathy has not yet been defined; however, a possible viral agent has been proposed. Evidence of parvovirus infection was more frequent in patients with collapsing glomerulopathy compared with controls, usual-type FSGS, or HIVAN, suggesting an association. Treatment with pamidronate also has been linked to development of collapsing glomerulopathy. Recurrence in the transplant has been reported. De novo collapsing glomerulopathy has also been noted in the transplant, linked to calcineurin inhibitor toxicity. Collapsing glomerular lesions also occur in native kidneys in a zonal distribution associated with severe vascular injury. Interferon therapy has also been associated with collapsing glomerulopathy lesions. In rare cases, collapsing glomerulopathy has been observed in patients with SLE. The excess incidence of this lesion in African Americans has been linked to a mutant variant of an apolipoprotein, ApoL1. This ApoL1 confers protection against a strain of trypanosomiasis. How ApoL1 might predispose to podocyte damage and collapsing glomerulopathy is unknown.

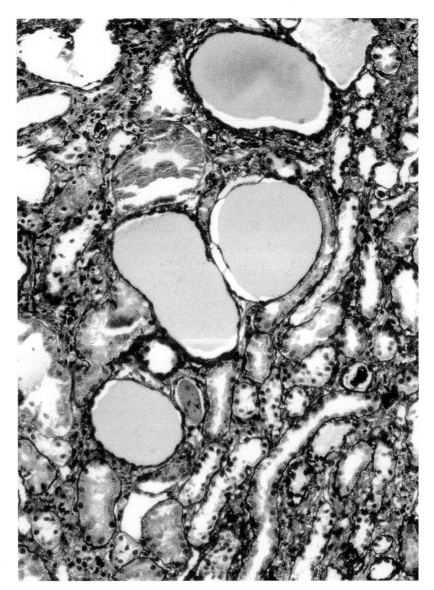

FIG. 1.38 Collapsing glomerulopathy. Collapsing glomerulopathy is often associated with disproportionate tubulointerstitial injury with microcystic change with proteinaceous casts, as shown here (Jones silver stain, ×200).

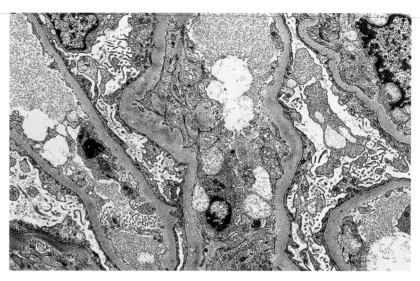

FIG. 1.39 Collapsing glomerulopathy. There is corrugation of the glomerular basement membrane with segmental areas of collapse by electron microscopy, without any deposits. Podocytes show extensive foot process effacement, vacuolization, and microvillous transformation as illustrated here. In idiopathic collapsing glomerulopathy, there are no reticular aggregates, in contrast to HIV-associated nephropathy, where they are frequent (transmission electron microscopy, ×7000).

Selected Reading

Barisoni, L., Kriz, W., Mundel, P., et al., 1999. The dysregulated podocyte phenotype: a novel concept in the pathogenesis of collapsing idiopathic focal segmental glomerulosclerosis and HIV-associated nephropathy. Journal of the American Society of Nephrology 10, 51-56.

Detwiler, R.K., Falk, R.F., Hogan, S.L., et al., 1994. Collapsing glomerulopathy: A clinically and pathologically distinct variant of focal segmental glomerulosclerosis. Kidney International 45, 1416-1424.

Genovese, G., Friedman, D.J., Ross, M.D., et al., 2010. Association of trypanolytic ApoL1 variants with kidney disease in African Americans. Science 329, 841-845.

Lasagni, L., Romagnani, P., 2010. Glomerular epithelial stem cells: the good, the bad, and the ugly. Journal of the American Society of Nephrology 21, 1612-1619.

Laurinavicius, A., Hurwitz, S., Rennke, H.G., 1999. Collapsing glomerulopathy in HIV and non-HIV patients: a clinicopathological and follow-up study. Kidney International 56, 2203-2213.

Markowitz, G.S., Appel, G.B., Fine, P.L., et al., 2001. Collapsing focal segmental glomerulosclerosis following treatment with high-dose pamidronate. Journal of the American Society of Nephrology 12, 1164-1172.

Markowitz, G.S., Nasr, S.H., Stokes, M.B., et al., 2010. Treatment with IFN-α, -β, or -γ is associated with collapsing focal segmental glomerulosclerosis. Clinical Journal of the American Society of Nephrology 5, 607-615.

Moudgil, A., Nast, C.C., Bagga, A., et al., 2001. Association of parvovirus B19 infection with idiopathic collapsing glomerulopathy. Kidney International 59, 2126-2133.

Valeri, A., Barisoni, L., Appel, G.B., et al., 1996. Idiopathic collapsing focal segmental glomerulosclerosis: a clinicopathologic study. Kidney International 50, 1734-1746.

TIP LESION VARIANT OF FSGS

Patients with tip lesion variant of FSGS present with nephrotic syndrome. This lesion was proposed to represent an early lesion with good prognosis similar to MCD. However, later follow-up has revealed a less than benign prognosis in some patients.

The tip lesion is defined as glomerulosclerosis involving only the tubular pole of the glomerulus (Fig. 1.40). The collapsing glomerulopathy variant must be excluded to diagnose tip variant FSGS (Table 1.2). It is defined as the presence of at least one segmental lesion involving the outer 25% of the glomerulus next to the proximal tubule pole with adhesion between the tuft and Bowman's capsule at the tubule lumen or neck (Figs. 1.41, 1.42). Thus, the proximal tubule pole must be identified in order to recognize and diagnose the lesion. The segmental lesion may be characterized by either endocapillary hypercellularity (involving <50% of the tuft) or sclerosis (involving <25% of the tuft). Foam cells are common, but hyalinosis is variable. The involved area often shows podocyte hypertrophy/hyperplasia. Mesangial hypercellularity, glomerulomegaly, and arteriolar hyalinosis are variable. Other glomeruli may show usual segmental lesions or cellular lesions according to the Columbia classification. So-called pure tip lesion, as originally defined, that is, when this is the only segmental lesion present, may have even better prognosis. Immunofluorescence and electron microscopy findings are as in usual-type FSGS.

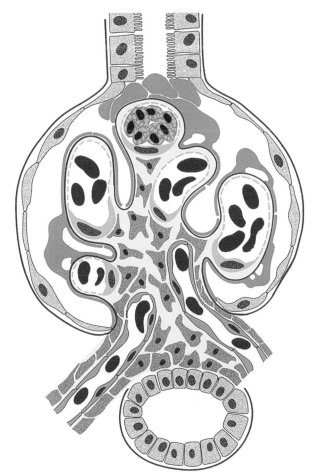

FIG. 1.40 Focal segmental glomerulosclerosis, tip lesion. Segmental sclerosis is confined to the proximal tubular pole and often has endocapillary proliferation with foam cells and overlying visceral epithelial cell hyperplasia. Foot processes are diffusely effaced, without deposits.

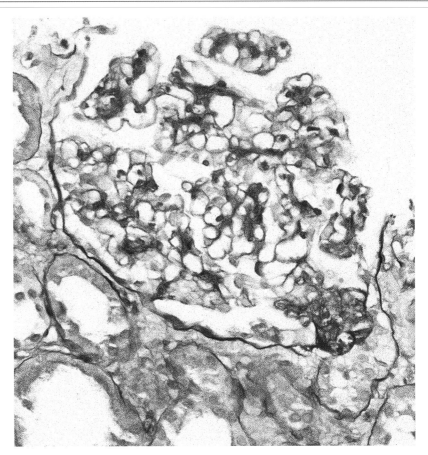

FIG. 1.41 Focal segmental glomerulosclerosis (FSGS), tip lesion. The localized sclerotic lesion that only involves the proximal tubular pole of the glomerulus is classified as the tip variant of FSGS (periodic acid Schiff, ×100).

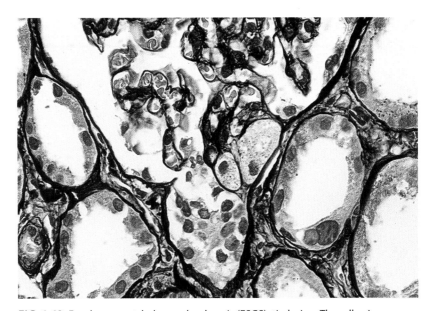

FIG. 1.42 Focal segmental glomerulosclerosis (FSGS), tip lesion. The adhesion between the glomerular tuft and the neck of the proximal tubule with intracapillary foam cells is evident in this tip lesion variant of FSGS (Jones silver stain, ×400).

Etiology/Pathogenesis

The etiology and pathogenesis are unknown. Hypotheses include increased turbulence at the tubular outflow causing podocyte injury. Tip lesions may also be seen incidentally at autopsy and superimposed in other glomerular diseases.

Selected Reading

Howie, A.J., Brewer, D.B., 1985. Further studies on the glomerular tip lesion: Early and late stages and life table analysis. Journal of Pathology 147, 245-255.

Howie, A.J., Pankhurst, T., Sarioglu, S., et al., 2005. Evolution of nephrotic-associated focal segmental glomerulosclerosis and relation to the glomerular tip lesion. Kidney International 67, 987-1001.

Stokes, M.B., Markowitz, G.S., Lin, J., et al., 2004. Glomerular tip lesion: a distinct entity within the minimal change disease/focal segmental glomerulosclerosis spectrum. Kidney International 65, 1690-1702.

Thomas, D.B., Franceschini, N., Hogan, S.L., et al., 2006. Clinical and pathologic characteristics of focal segmental glomerulosclerosis pathologic variants. Kidney International 69, 920-926.

CELLULAR VARIANT OF FSGS

Patients with the cellular variant of FSGS present with abrupt onset of nephrotic syndrome. This lesion is the rarest of the idiopathic FSGS subtypes. To diagnose the cellular variant of FSGS, the FSGS working classification proposes that tip lesion and collapsing glomerulopathy must be excluded (Table 1.2). The cellular variant of FSGS is then defined as at least one glomerulus with endocapillary proliferation involving at least 25% of the tuft and occluding the lumen (Figs. 1.43, 1.44). The endocapillary cells typically include foam cells, macrophages,

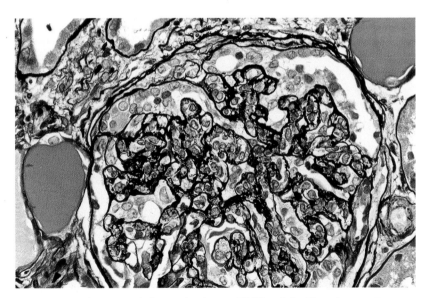

FIG. 1.43 Focal segmental glomerulosclerosis (FSGS), cellular. There is extensive endocapillary hypercellularity with frequent mononuclear cells and multifocal, early adhesions of the tuft to Bowman's capsule in this cellular variant of FSGS. There is mild prominence of the overlying podocytes, but not frank hyperplasia, and no collapse of the glomerular tuft to indicate collapsing glomerulopathy. Immune complexes were excluded by immunofluorescence and electron microscopy (Jones silver stain, ×400).

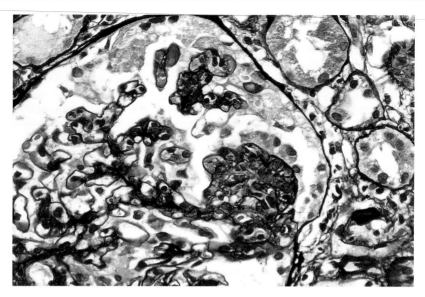

FIG. 1.44 Focal segmental glomerulosclerosis (FSGS), cellular. There is only a segmental area of endocapillary hypercellularity with hypertrophy of overlying podocytes in this cellular variant of FSGS. Immune complexes were excluded by immunofluorescence and electron microscopy (Jones silver stain, ×400).

and endothelial cells. Neutrophils and lymphocytes may also be present. There may be podocyte hyperplasia/hypertrophy overlying this lesion, but unlike in collapsing glomerulopathy, this is not a required feature. These lesions may develop into progressively less cellular, more sclerotic lesions, becoming indistinguishable clinically and morphologically from classical FSGS (Fig. 1.37). Thus, other glomeruli in the biopsy may contain usual type of segmental or global glomerulosclerosis. Immunofluorescence and electron microscopy findings are as in usual-type FSGS.

Etiology/Pathogenesis

This cellular lesion may be an early abnormality seen by light microscopy when FSGS recurs in the transplant. Thus, this morphologic variant is postulated to represent an early, active FSGS lesion. The cellular lesion has also been seen more commonly in children with FSGS than in adults. Cellular variant FSGS showed intermediate prognosis compared to collapsing glomerulopathy and tip variant of FSGS.

Selected Reading

Schwartz, M.M., Evans, J., Bain, R., et al., 1999. Focal segmental glomerulosclerosis: prognostic implications of the cellular lesion. Journal of the American Society of Nephrology 10, 1900-1907.

Silverstein, D.M., Craver, R., 2007. Presenting features and short-term outcome according to pathologic variant in childhood primary focal segmental glomerulosclerosis. Clinical Journal of the American Society of Nephrology 2, 700-707.

Stokes, M.B., Valeri, A.M., Markowitz, G.S., et al., 2006. Cellular focal segmental glomerulosclerosis: Clinical and pathologic features. Kidney International 70, 1783-1792.

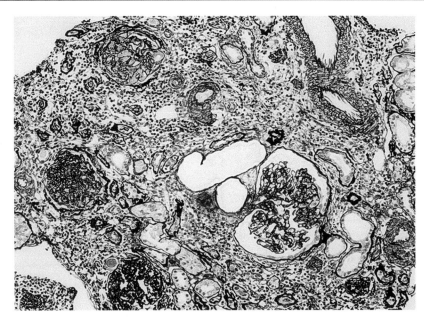

FIG. 1.45 Secondary focal segmental glomerulosclerosis (FSGS). Segmental sclerosis may also be seen secondary to other conditions, or be associated with hypertensive arterionephrosclerosis, as in this case. The diagnosis of primary FSGS was excluded by very limited foot process effacement, disproportionate vascular sclerosis, extensive global sclerosis, and most importantly, the clinical course with long-standing hypertension preceding any evidence of renal dysfunction (Jones silver stain, ×100).

PERIHILAR VARIANT OF FSGS

Patients present with proteinuria. Patients may have hypertension or other underlying conditions linked to renal scarring (Fig. 1.45). To diagnose this type, cellular, tip variants of FSGS and collapsing glomerulopathy must first be excluded (Table 1.2). Perihilar-type FSGS is defined by perihilar sclerosis and hyalinosis involving >50% of involved glomeruli. Glomerulomegaly and adhesions are common. There is often arteriolar hyalinosis, but arteriolar hyalin alone is insufficient for diagnosis (Figs. 1.46, 1.47). Mesangial hypercellularity is usually absent, and podocytes do not typically show hyperplasia/hypertrophy. Immunofluorescence and electron microscopy findings are as in usual-type FSGS.

Etiology/Pathogenesis—Secondary Forms of FSGS

Predominantly perihilar lesions of sclerosis are proposed to represent a response to reduced renal mass. This variant may occur in idiopathic FSGS but is also common in patients with secondary forms of FSGS related to adaptive responses to reduced nephron mass and/or glomerular hypertension. Many insults to the kidney may result in secondary FSGS, either as the sole manifestation of injury, or superimposed on other renal disease manifestations. Lesions of FSGS may be seen in association with diseases with abnormal, maladaptive responses of glomerular growth and pressures, for example, in diabetes, obesity, heroin abuse, cyanotic heart disease, or sickle cell disease. Thus, secondary sclerosis occurs in the chronic stage of many immune complex or proliferative diseases. In some of these settings, the morphologic appearance of sclerosis can indicate the nature of the initial insult: Obesity-associated FSGS shows mild changes related to glucose intolerance (mesangial expansion, GBM thickening), subtotal foot process effacement, and marked glomerulomegaly. The course is more indolent than for idiopathic FSGS, with less frequent nephrotic syndrome. Anabolic steroid use has also been linked to FSGS, with some patients showing hilar lesions. In FSGS

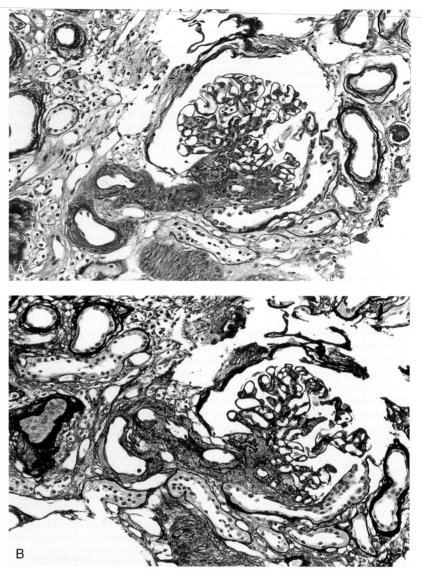

FIG. 1.46 Focal segmental glomerulosclerosis (FSGS), perihilar. The perihilar type of FSGS shows vascular pole sclerosis with hyalinosis, often with hyalin extending into the arteriolar pole, as seen on these adjacent sections of a glomerulus with perihilar variant of FSGS. This may often be secondary to other conditions or associated with arterionephrosclerosis, or be idiopathic (a, periodic acid Schiff; b, Jones silver stain, ×200).

secondary to reflux nephropathy, there is frequently prominent periglomerular fibrosis and thickening of Bowman's capsule and patchy, "geographic"-pattern interstitial scarring, in addition to the heterogeneous glomerulosclerosis. FSGS associated with heroin use does not show pathognomonic features, although global glomerulosclerosis, epithelial cell changes, interstitial fibrosis, and tubular injury tend to be more prominent than in idiopathic cases of FSGS. FSGS also can develop in association with decreased renal mass. The best example is oligomeganephronia, where nephron number is greatly reduced, with resulting marked enlargement of the remaining glomeruli, and occurrence of FSGS. Patients with unilateral renal agenesis show apparent higher risk of FSGS than the general population. Loss of one kidney later in life does not elicit the same degree of growth response in the remaining kidney as in

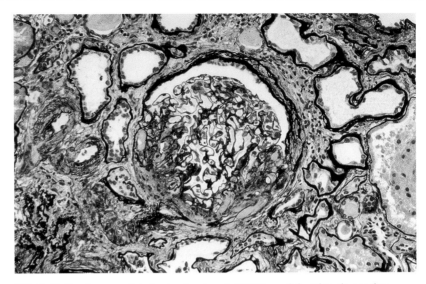

FIG. 1.47 Focal segmental glomerulosclerosis (FSGS), perihilar. This glomerulus shows a more extensive perihilar lesion of FSGS, associated with hyalinosis and periglomerular fibrosis. In this case, the lesion was likely due to arterionephrosclerosis associated with hypertension (Jones silver stain, ×400).

Key Diagnostic Features of Subtypes of FSGS

- Collapsing lesion (even in only one glomerulus) → collapsing glomerulopathy
- Tip lesion in the absence of collapsing lesion or hilar lesion → tip lesion variant of FSGS
- Cellular lesion in the absence of tip and collapsing features → cellular variant
- Hilar lesion in the absence of above, involving most of the segmentally affected → hilar variant FSGS
- Segmental lesions that do not fit in to any of the above categories, or the standard segmental sclerosis lesion → FSGS, NOS

FSGS, focal segmental glomerulosclerosis; *NOS,* not otherwise specified.

---

the young and has a lesser association with scarring in the remaining kidney. However, when one kidney and a portion of the other are lost in the adult, patients appear to have increased risk of developing FSGS. Similarly, low birth weight has been associated with fewer nephrons, presumed to contribute to the linkage with chronic kidney disease and hypertension. FSGS has been reported in some of these patients as well.

Selected Reading

Herlitz, L.C., Markowitz, G.S., Farris, A.B, et al., 2010. Development of focal segmental glomerulosclerosis after anabolic steroid abuse. Journal of the American Society of Nephrology 21, 163-172.

Hodgin, J.B., Rasoulpour, M., Markowitz, G.S., et al., 2009. Very low birth weight is a risk factor for secondary focal segmental glomerulosclerosis. Clinical Journal of the American Society of Nephrology 4, 71-76.

Kambham, N., Markowitz, G.S., Valeri, A.M., et al., 2001. Obesity-related glomerulopathy: an emerging epidemic. Kidney International 59, 1498-1509.

Rennke, H.G., Klein, P.S., 1989. Pathogenesis and significance of nonprimary focal and segmental glomerulosclerosis. American Journal of Kidney Disease 13, 443-456.

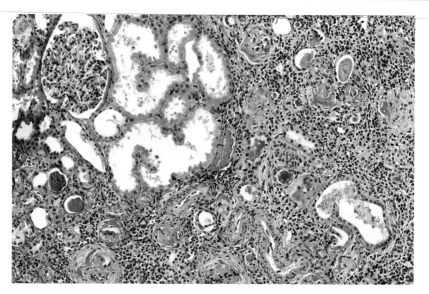

FIG. 1.48 Congenital nephrotic syndrome of Finnish type. Glomeruli do not show specific lesions but may have varying mesangial hypercellularity. There is microcystic dilatation of proximal tubules, here associated with global glomerulosclerosis and interstitial fibrosis (hematoxylin and eosin, ×100).

CONGENITAL NEPHROTIC SYNDROME OF FINNISH TYPE

Congenital nephrotic syndrome of Finnish type (CNF) is an inherited autosomal recessive disease caused by mutation of the nephrin gene (NPHS1), located on chromosome 19. The disease is not exclusive to the Finnish population. Nephrotic syndrome manifests at birth or usually by age 3 months, and usually results in death from complications secondary to nephrotic syndrome by age 1 year unless treated with renal transplantation. Microscopic hematuria is often present.

Glomeruli may be immature, more so than expected for term birth, but this may in part reflect the usual premature birth of affected infants. Mature glomeruli have variable mesangial increase and nonspecific sclerosis and occasional proliferation (Fig. 1.48). Occasional crescents may be present, but without necrosis. Glomeruli may also be unremarkable by light microscopy. The proximal tubules are dilated (Figs 1.49-1.51). Tubules may show atrophy and Bowman's capsule may be dilated in some cases, although collecting ducts are not typically dilated. Of note, these typical tubular lesions may be absent in early biopsies. Glomerulosclerosis develops late in the course (Fig. 1.52).

There are no deposits by immunofluorescence. By electron microscopy, there is widespread effacement of foot processes. The GBM may be focally attenuated.

Etiology/Pathogenesis

The nephrin gene is mutated in CNF. The nephrin gene is a prominent component of the slit diaphragm of the foot processes of the podocyte. Studies in knock-out mice reveal that intact nephrin is required for maintaining normal capillary permselectivity. Mutation of a protein tightly associated with nephrin, CD2-associated protein (CD2AP), in mice has demonstrated that mutation of other components of the slit diaphragm or its anchoring proteins also lead to nephrotic syndrome, with clinical characteristics mirroring many of those of congenital nephrotic syndrome of Finnish type. Approximately one quarter of patients

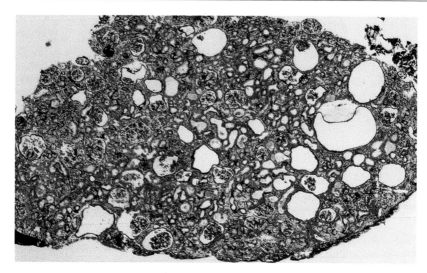

FIG. 1.49 Congenital nephrotic syndrome of Finnish type. Glomeruli are unremarkable and microcystic dilatation of proximal tubules is widespread (Jones silver stain, ×100).

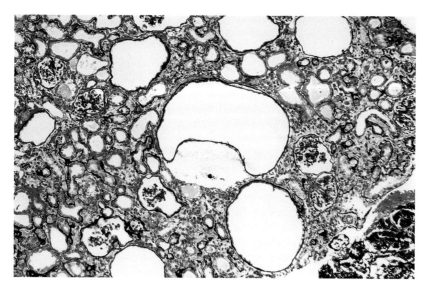

FIG. 1.50 Congenital nephrotic syndrome of Finnish type. Proximal tubules are microcystically dilated. Glomeruli show normal maturity for age in this newborn (Jones silver stain, ×200).

transplanted develop recurrent nephrotic syndrome. Renal biopsies of the transplant performed from 3 days to 2 weeks after onset of recurrent nephrotic syndrome showed glomerular capillary endothelial cell swelling and extensive foot process effacement. These recurrences typically develop in patients with the Fin-major/Fin-major genotype, resulting in completely absent nephrin. Some of these patients had detectable anti-nephrin antibodies after transplant, supporting immune injury to the normal nephrin-bearing podocytes in the graft, although usual immune complexes are not observed.

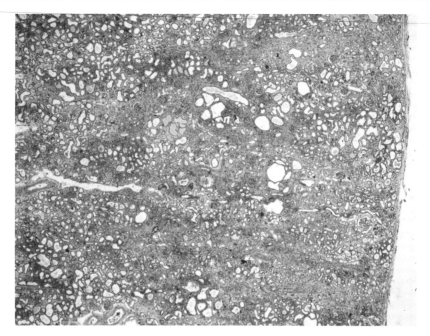

FIG. 1.51 Congenital nephrotic syndrome of Finnish type. This low-power view demonstrates the disproportional tubular dilatation with mild interstitial fibrosis without specific glomerular lesions early in the course of congenital nephrotic syndrome of Finnish type (periodic acid Schiff, ×40).

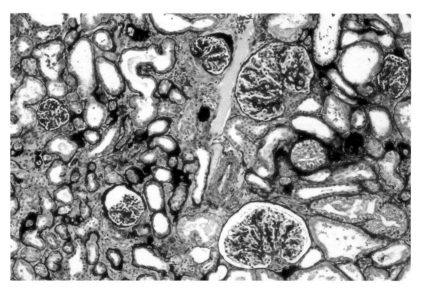

FIG. 1.52 Congenital nephrotic syndrome of Finnish type. The glomeruli show mild mesangial proliferation, and there is focal tubular dilation with very mild interstitial fibrosis (Jones silver stain, ×200).

Selected Reading

Rapola, J., 1987. Congenital nephrotic syndrome. Pediatric Nephrology 1, 441-446.

Huttunen, N.P., Rapola, J., Wilska, J., et al., 1980. Renal pathology in congenital nephrotic syndrome of Finnish type: A quantitative light microscopic study on 50 patients. International Journal of Pediatric Nephrology 1, 10.

Ruotsalainen, V., Ljungberg, P., Wartiovaara, J., et al., 1999. Nephrin is specifically located at the slit diaphragm of glomerular podocytes. Proceedings of the National Academy of Sciences of the United States of America 96, 7962-7967.

Patrakka, J., Ruotsalainen, V., Reponen, P., et al., 2002. Recurrence of nephrotic syndrome in kidney grafts of patients with congenital nephrotic syndrome of the Finnish type: role of nephrin. Transplantation 73, 394-403.

DIFFUSE MESANGIAL SCLEROSIS

Diffuse mesangial sclerosis may occur as an isolated lesion manifesting as nephrotic syndrome, or be part of Denys–Drash syndrome. Mutations in the Wilms tumor gene (WT1) occur both in isolated diffuse mesangial sclerosis and in patients with Denys–Drash syndrome. Onset is typically congenital or in the first years of life. Patients may have renal failure at presentation, and typically progress to end-stage kidney disease before age 4 years. Clinically, patients with Denys–Drash syndrome are usually 46XY and have ambiguous external genitalia or male pseudohermaphroditism with female external genitalia with streak gonads or abnormal testes and are at risk for Wilms tumor. Occasional patients are 46XX with nephropathy and Wilms tumor without abnormal genitalia.

The earliest renal lesions are characterized by an increase in mesangial matrix and hypertrophic podocytes, followed by increase in mesangial matrix that initially appears delicate and loosely woven, culminating in further mesangial increase and sclerosis with obliteration of the capillary lumens (Figs. 1.53-1.55). There is no increase in mesangial cellularity, and a dense core of disorganized collagen is present in the sclerotic glomeruli. The overlying podocytes typically are hypertrophic and may appear immature, dense, and cobblestone-like. Occasional epithelial cell proliferation may be present (Fig. 1.56). In contrast to idiopathic FSGS, the deeper corticomedullary glomeruli are less affected. Interstitial fibrosis and tubular atrophy is proportional to the glomerulosclerosis (Fig. 1.57). Although tubules may be dilated, this is not a prominent or early feature as in congenital nephrotic syndrome of Finnish type (see above).

There are no immune complex deposits by immunofluorescence, although variable trapping of IgM, C1q, and C3 may be present in the sclerotic mesangial areas. By electron microscopy, the GBM is somewhat thickened and foot processes are effaced.

Frasier Syndrome

Patients with Frasier syndrome also have WT1 mutations, but do not have early-onset disease with diffuse mesangial sclerosis. Onset of proteinuria and renal failure is in late childhood and late adolescence. Patients show complete male pseudohermaphroditism with complete gonadal dysgenesis and thus appear externally female but do not undergo menarche at puberty. Patients have increased risk of gonadoblastoma developing in the abnormal gonads, but do not develop Wilms tumor.

Renal biopsy demonstrates focal segmental glomerulosclerosis lesions of NOS type by light microscopy without immune deposits (Fig. 1.58). By electron microscopy, some patients with Frasier syndrome may show lamellation and basket-weaving appearance that resembles Alport syndrome, although there are no mutations in type IV collagen alpha chains (Fig. 1.59).

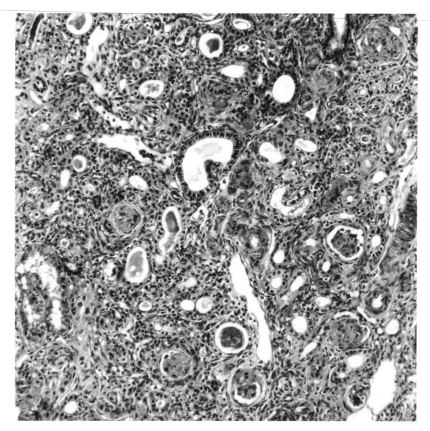

FIG. 1.53 Diffuse mesangial sclerosis. Glomeruli show extensive sclerosis, with small, shrunken appearance and dense expansion of mesangial matrix, blue on trichrome stain, with little increase in mesangial cellularity. There is associated proportional tubular atrophy and interstitial fibrosis. Occasional dilated tubules may be present (Masson trichrome stain, ×100).

Etiology/Pathogenesis

WT1 is crucial for development of the kidney and genitalia. In the mature kidney, WT1 is expressed in podocytes and controls slit diaphragm proteins and differentiation.

Various WT1 mutations contribute to the spectrum of diffuse mesangial sclerosis, Denys–Drash syndrome, and Frasier syndrome. Denys–Drash syndrome typically is caused by mutations in the Wilms tumor in the WT1 gene. Isolated diffuse mesangial sclerosis has also occasionally been associated with WT1 mutations. Diffuse mesangial sclerosis is rarely caused by mutations in phospholipase C epsilon, but without the associated syndrome abnormalities seen in Denys–Drash syndrome.

Effects of altered WT1 on podocyte differentiation have been suggested. This gene encodes a transcription factor of the zinc finger family, with four transcripts of WT1 resulting from alternative splicing. Various mutations have been reported. When WT1 point mutations in the donor splice site in intron 9 occurs, Frasier syndrome results, with focal segmental glomerulosclerosis lesions.

Transplantation has resulted in a good outcome, without reports of recurrence in the transplant of nephrotic syndrome or glomerular lesions in patients with diffuse mesangial sclerosis or Denys–Drash syndrome or Frasier syndrome.

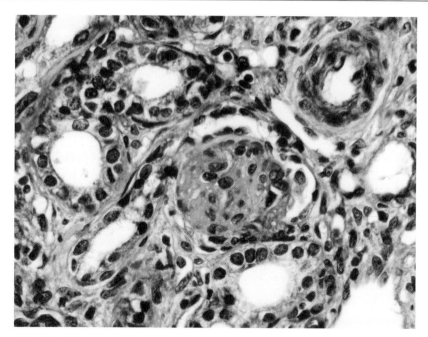

FIG. 1.54 Diffuse mesangial sclerosis with typical appearance of dense expansion of collagenous material within mesangium with minimal increase in mesangial cellularity. There is associated tubular atrophy and interstitial fibrosis (Masson trichrome stain, ×400).

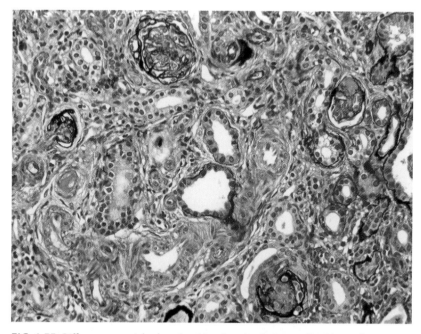

FIG. 1.55 Diffuse mesangial sclerosis with sclerosis of glomeruli, with small, shrunken appearance, with dense sclerosis obliterating the tuft and associated tubular atrophy and interstitial fibrosis. Occasional tubules show mild dilatation (Jones silver stain, ×200).

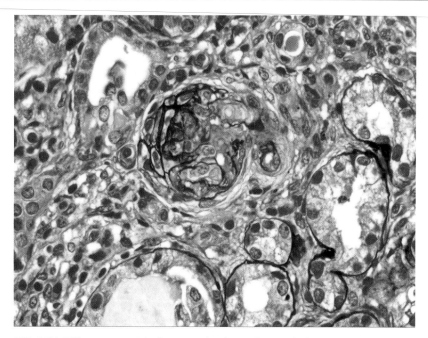

FIG. 1.56 Diffuse mesangial sclerosis with sclerosed expanded mesangial matrix and a fibrocellular crescent, but without glomerular basement membrane breaks or fibrinoid necrosis. This type of epithelial cell proliferation may be seen in aggressive sclerosing conditions and is not indicative of a primary necrotizing crescentic process (Jones silver stain, ×400).

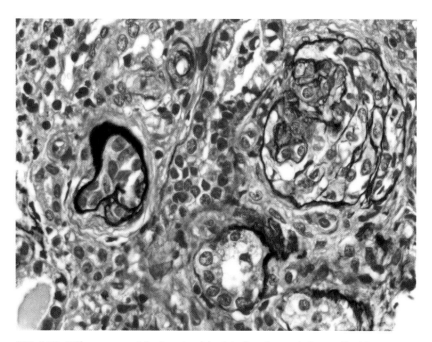

FIG. 1.57 Diffuse mesangial sclerosis with globally sclerosed glomeruli with expansion of mesangial matrix and fibrocellular crescent (right) on Jones silver stain and surrounding tubular atrophy and interstitial fibrosis (Jones silver stain, ×400).

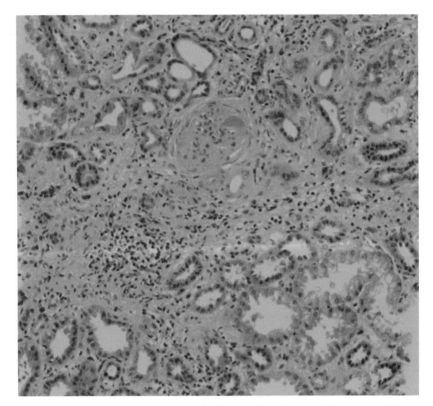

FIG. 1.58 Frasier syndrome. Segmental sclerosis of usual type with proportional tubular atrophy and interstitial fibrosis are present (periodic acid Schiff, ×200). (Case kindly shared by Dr. Susan Rigdon and Dr. Patrick O'Donnell, Guy's Hospital, London, United Kingdom.)

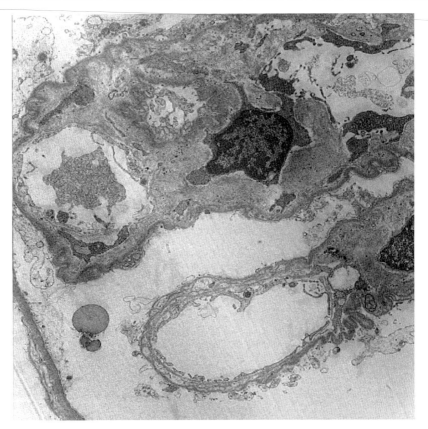

FIG. 1.59 Frasier syndrome. By electron microscopy, irregular, scalloped appearance of the glomerular basement membrane is evident, with no immune complex deposits. Foot processes are effaced (transmission electron microscopy, ×5000). (Case kindly shared by Dr. Susan Rigdon and Dr. Patrick O'Donnell, Guy's Hospital, London, United Kingdom.)

Selected Reading

Barbaux, S., Niaudet, P., Gubler, M.C., et al., 1997. Donor splice-site mutations in the WT1 gene are responsible for Frasier syndrome. Nature Genetics 17, 467-469.

Habib, R., 1993. Nephrotic syndrome in the 1st year of life. Pediatric Nephrology 7, 347-353.

Salomon, R., Gubler, M.C., Niaudet, P., 2000. Genetics of the nephrotic syndrome. Current Opinion in Pediatrics 12, 129-134.

Glomerular Diseases That Cause Nephrotic/Nephritic Syndrome: Complement Related

C1Q NEPHROPATHY

C1q nephropathy appears to represent a variable pattern of glomerular injury with abnormality in complement, defined by the presence of mesangial and occasional capillary wall immunoglobulin and complement deposits, with C1q immunofluorescence staining intensity being greater than or equal to that of other components. C1q nephropathy occurs primarily in children and young adults. Patients typically present with nephrotic syndrome, especially if biopsy showed sclerosing or minimal change–type lesions, and may have an active urinary

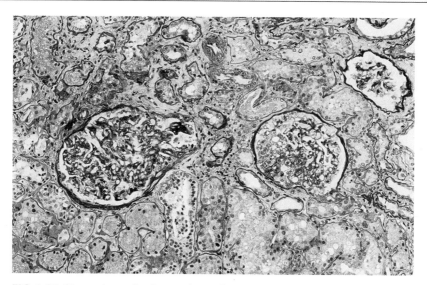

FIG. 1.60 C1q nephropathy. C1q nephropathy may show a variety of lesions by light microscopy, from nearly normal, to mesangial or focal proliferative or segmental sclerosis. The glomerulus on the left shows a small area of segmental sclerosis with adhesion at proximal tubular pole, whereas the glomerulus on the right shows segmental proliferation. There is associated mild tubulointerstitial fibrosis (periodic acid Schiff, ×200).

Key Diagnostic Features of C1q Nephropathy

- Extensive foot process effacement
- Absence of morphologic features of lupus nephritis (i.e., absence of clinical history of systemic lupus erythematosus, no reticular aggregates or full house staining by immunofluorescence).

Note: The light microscopic features are variable, from minimal change–type lesions to segmental sclerosis or proliferative lesions.

---

sediment when proliferative changes are present but do not have SLE clinically. About a third of patients with sclerosis at time of biopsy developed end-stage kidney disease. In contrast, complete remission of the nephrotic syndrome occurred in 77% of those with a minimal change–like lesion. Renal disease remained stable in just over half of those with proliferative glomerulonephritis at time of biopsy.

By light microscopy, there is a spectrum of possible glomerular alterations, including no histologic abnormalities, mesangial proliferation, focal or diffuse proliferative glomerulonephritis, or focal segmental glomerulosclerosis with or without associated mesangial proliferation (Figs. 1.60, 1.61).

Immunofluorescence microscopy typically shows predominant C1q, along with C3 and immunoglobulins (Fig. 1.62), which by definition is not more than C1q.

Electron microscopy typically shows foot process effacement and deposits confined to the mesangium. In cases with proliferation, deposits often extend to subendothelial areas. In cases without proliferation, foot process effacement is quite extensive and deposits are confined to the mesangium. Notably, reticular aggregates, a common feature in patients with lupus nephritis, are absent (Fig. 1.63).

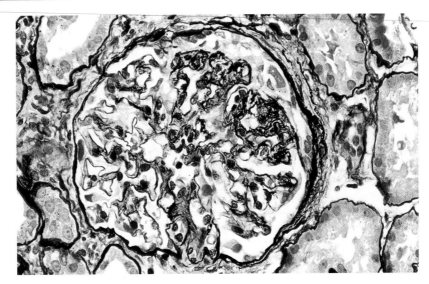

FIG. 1.61 C1q nephropathy. There is mild mesangial proliferation and early sclerosis of portions of the tuft, with mild periglomerular fibrosis (Jones silver stain, ×400).

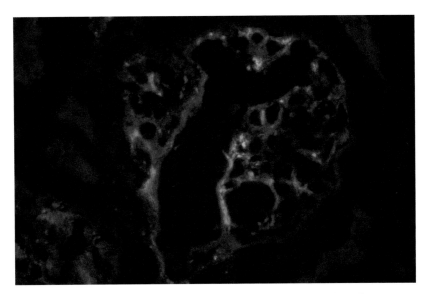

FIG. 1.62 C1q nephropathy. The defining feature of C1q nephropathy is dominant C1q staining by immunofluorescence, typically in a mesangial pattern. Focal peripheral capillary loop extension may also be present (anti-C1q antibody immunofluorescence, ×400).

Etiology/Pathogenesis

The etiology and pathogenesis are unknown. In our opinion, C1q nephropathy without proliferation may be viewed as an unusual lesion related to MCD-FSGS, whereas those patients with proliferative lesions behave more like immune complex disease. The deposition of C1q suggests an abnormality of complement regulation.

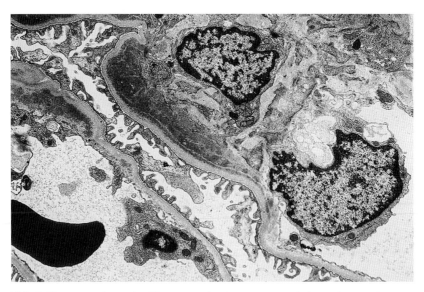

FIG. 1.63 C1q nephropathy. There is predominant mesangial dense deposits by electron microscopy. There may be variable foot process effacement, as in this case. Importantly, reticular aggregates, a characteristic feature of lupus nephritis, are not present in C1q nephropathy (transmission electron microscopy, ×5000).

Selected Reading

Jennette, J.C., Hipp, C.G., 1985. C1q nephropathy: A distinct pathologic entity usually causing nephrotic syndrome. American Journal of Kidney Disease 6, 103-110.

Markowitz, G.S., Schwimmer, J.A., Stokes, M.B., et al., 2003. C1q nephropathy: a variant of focal segmental glomerulosclerosis. Kidney International 64, 1232-1240.

Vizjak, A., Ferluga, D., Rozic, M., et al., 2008. Pathology, clinical presentations, and outcomes of C1q nephropathy. Journal of the American Society of Nephrology 19, 2237-2244.

DENSE DEPOSIT DISEASE

Dense deposit disease (DDD) is a separate disease entity from membranoproliferative glomerulonephritis (MPGN) type I, but because of its similar light microscopic appearance, it has also been called MPGN type II (Fig. 1.64). DDD is much more rare than type I MPGN, accounting for 15-35% of total MPGN type I and DDD cases. Patients with DDD typically present with features of nephritic/nephrotic syndrome and decreased complements, particularly C3, hypertension, and elevated serum creatinine. Early components of the classic pathway, that is, C1q and C4, usually show normal serum levels. Some patients have partial lipodystrophy associated with DDD. Most patients in earlier series were children or young adults; boys were affected slightly more than girls. In another recent series of DDD, slightly more than half of patients were adults, with more than a third of adults older than age 60 years, with nearly twice as many females as males. These patients typically presented with renal insufficiency, and nearly all had hematuria, with nephrotic syndrome present in a third of patients. Children were more likely to have reduced C3 and had less incidence of renal insufficiency than adults in this series. On follow-up, a quarter of patients had complete response to immunosuppression with or without renin angiotensin system blockade, about half had persistent renal dysfunction, and a quarter had end-stage renal disease. Thus, progressive renal failure is common, occurring in the majority of patients, usually developing within 10 years. Rare cases of spontaneous improvement of the disease have been reported. More rapid progression was associated with crescents, and worse prognosis was associated with hump-type

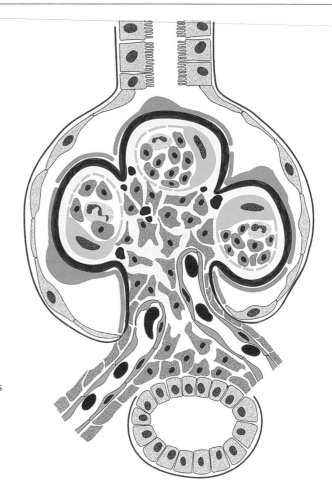

FIG. 1.64 Dense deposit disease. The glomerulus shows a membranoproliferative pattern, with endocapillary proliferation and glomerular basement membrane double contours. The glomerular basement membrane is altered by dense deposits in a ribbon-like pattern, with mesangial dense material as well.

Key Diagnostic Features of Dense Deposit Disease

- Membranoproliferative or mesangial proliferative features by light microscopy
- C3 by immunofluorescence
- Dense transformation of glomerular basement membranes with round, nodular deposits in mesangium by electron microscopy

---

deposits. Predictors of end-stage renal disease were older age and higher creatinine at biopsy and the presence of subepithelial humps.

By light microscopy, mesangial proliferation is the pattern most commonly observed, followed by endocapillary proliferation, often with polymorphonuclear leukocyte (PMN) infiltrate in glomeruli in early stages (Figs. 1.65, 1.66). There may be focal segmental necrotizing proliferative lesions with crescents. The GBMs are thickened and highly refractile and eosinophilic. The involved areas of the GBM resemble a "string of sausages." The deposits are PAS positive and stain brown with silver stain (Figs. 1.67-1.69). The thioflavin T stain also highlights the deposits, as does the toluidine blue stain (Fig. 1.69). Thickening also affects tubular basement membranes and Bowman's capsule.

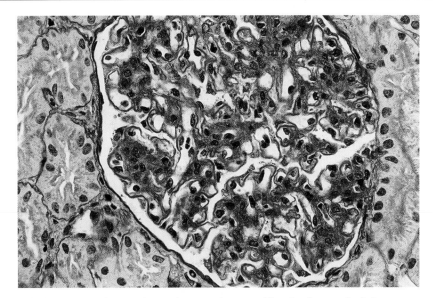

FIG. 1.65 Dense deposit disease has membranoproliferative features by light microscopy, with diffuse, global mesangial and often endocapillary proliferation, and frequent glomerular basement membrane reduplication. The glomerular basement membrane may in some cases appear more refractile than in idiopathic type I membranoproliferative glomerulonephritis (hematoxylin and eosin, ×400).

Immunofluorescence in DDD shows C3 staining irregularly along the capillary wall, in a smooth, granular, or discontinuous pattern (Fig. 1.70). Mesangial bright staining in a distinct globular pattern within the central mesangial area can be present. Immunoglobulin is usually not detected, indicating the dense deposits are not classic antigen–antibody immune complexes. However, segmental IgM or less often IgG and very rarely IgA have been reported.

By electron microscopy, the lamina densa of the basement membrane in DDD shows a very dense transformation without discrete immune complex–type deposits (Figs. 1.71, 1.72). Similar dense globular deposits are often found in the mesangial areas in addition to increased matrix. Increased mesangial cellularity or mesangial interposition are far less common than in MPGN type I. Podocytes show varying degrees of reactive changes, from vacuolization, microvillous transformation to foot process effacement. Tubular basement membranes and Bowman's capsule may show similar densities as in the GBM.

Etiology/Pathogenesis

The precise nature of the dense material is not established. Recent studies have shown that glomeruli in DDD contain components of the alternate and terminal complement pathways.

The pathogenesis of DDD is unknown, but recent advances point to abnormalities in regulation of the alternative complement pathway with uncontrolled activation of C3 convertase. DDD may thus be grouped in the broader category of C3 glomerulopathy (see below). C3 nephritic factor (C3NeF) stabilizes the C3 convertase C3bBb, resulting in alternate pathway-mediated C3 breakdown. DDD sometimes occurs in association with partial lipodystrophy, a condition with loss of adipose tissue, decreased complement, and presence of C3NeF. Further, a porcine model of factor H deficiency has similarities to DDD. Factor H inactivates factor C3bBb. Inadequate factor H, either due to deficiency or antibody to Factor H, has been observed in some patients with DDD. These associations have suggested that

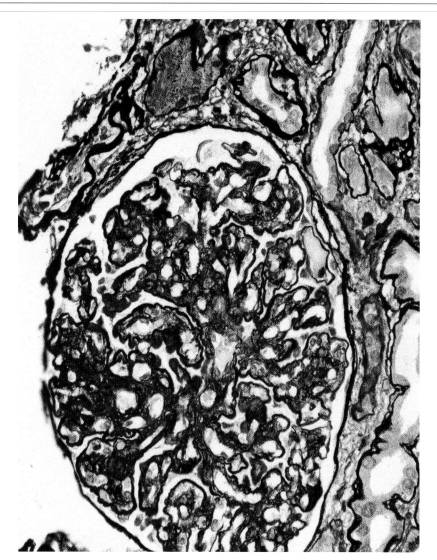

FIG. 1.66 Dense deposit disease. There is moderate mesangial proliferation and endocapillary proliferation and segmental glomerular basement membrane reduplication with interposition. There are no large eosinophilic subendothelial deposits as typically seen in membranoproliferative glomerulonephritis type I (Jones silver stain, ×200).

abnormal complement regulation predisposes to DDD. However, clinical measures of complement, C3NeF, or presence of partial lipodystrophy did not predict clinical outcome among patients with DDD, and some patients with MPGN type I also have C3NeF. Some patients with partial lipodystrophy and C3NeF do not have DDD, further indication that complement abnormalities alone are insufficient to produce the disease.

Crescents or PMNs in capillary loops were associated with worse prognosis, whereas focal segmental glomerulonephritic lesions were less frequently associated with progressive renal disease. DDD invariably recurs morphologically in the transplant, although it does not usually cause graft loss.

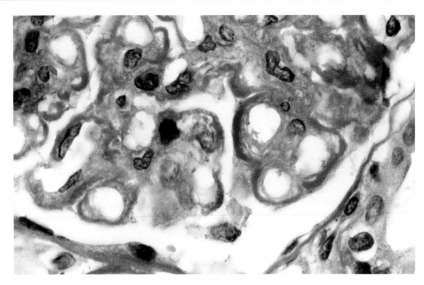

FIG. 1.67 Dense deposit disease. The refractile, dense appearance of the glomerular basement membrane is evident, along with mesangial and endocapillary proliferation. Note that the density is within the basement membrane itself and not in a subendothelial location (periodic acid Schiff, ×1000).

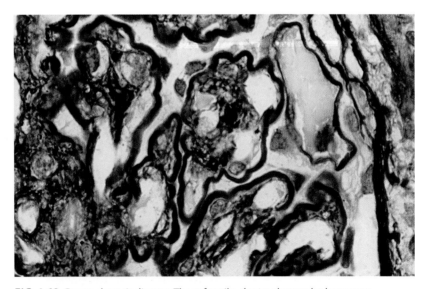

FIG. 1.68 Dense deposit disease. The refractile, dense glomerular basement membrane of dense deposit disease is apparent. The basement membrane appears ribbon-like. There is associated mesangial and segmental endocapillary proliferation with occasional, segmental interposition (Jones silver stain, ×1000).

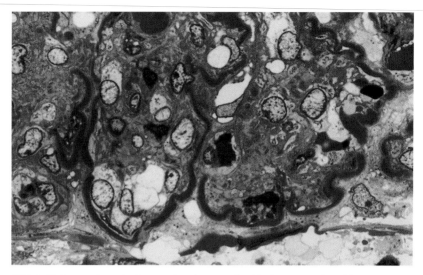

FIG. 1.69 Dense deposit disease. On plastic-embedded sections, the ribbon-like dense transformation of the entire glomerular basement membrane is apparent. There is associated mesangial and endocapillary proliferation (toluidine blue stain, ×1000).

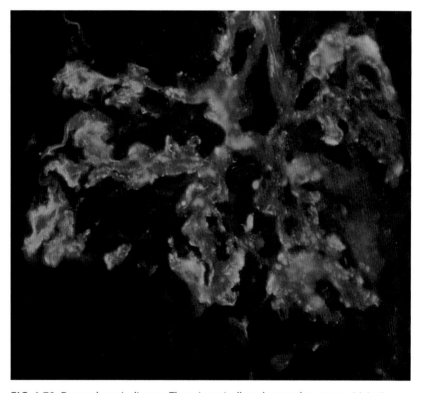

FIG. 1.70 Dense deposit disease. There is typically only complement positivity in dense deposit disease, with chunky mesangial and coarse, irregular capillary loop positivity. Immunoglobulin staining is typically absent, indicating that there are no true immune complex–type (i.e., antibody–antigen) deposits (anti-C3 immunofluorescence, ×400).

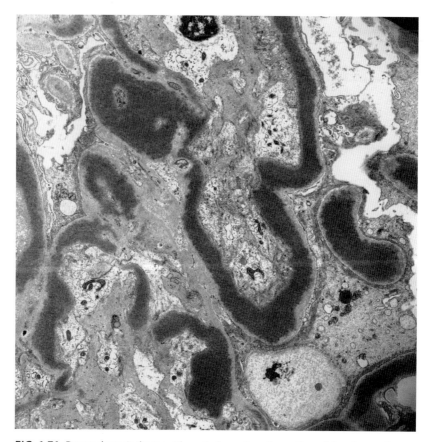

FIG. 1.71 Dense deposit disease. There is dense transformation of the glomerular basement membrane, with associated endocapillary and mesangial proliferation and occasional large, globular mesangial densities (transmission electron microscopy, ×8000).

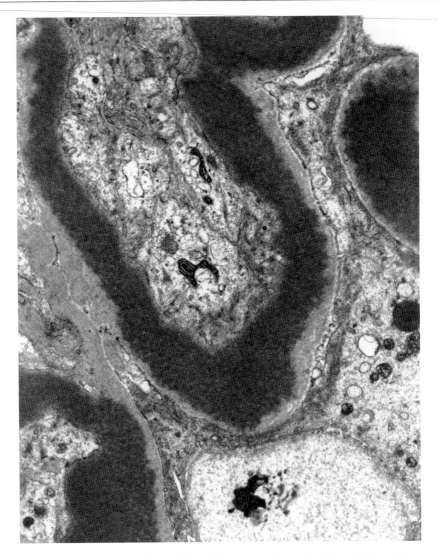

FIG. 1.72 Dense deposit disease. There is dense transformation of nearly the entire thickness of the glomerular basement membrane, with associated endocapillary proliferation. Overlying foot processes are extensively effaced. The transformed material contains complement components (transmission electron microscopy, ×20,250).

Selected Reading

Anders, D., Agricola, B., Sippel, M., et al., 1977. Basement membrane changes in membra-noproliferative glomerulonephritis. II. Characterization of a third type by silver impregnation of ultra thin sections. Virchows Archiv (Pathology and Anatomy) 376, 1-19.

Andresdottir, M.B., Assmann, K.J., Hoitsma, A.J., et al., 1999. Renal transplantation in patients with dense deposit disease: morphological characteristics of recurrent disease and clinical outcome. Nephrology, Dialysis and Transplantation 14 (7), 1723-1731.

Bennett, W.M., Fassett, R.G., Walker, R.G., et al., 1989. Mesangiocapillary glomerulonephritis type II (dense-deposit disease): clinical features of progressive disease. American Journal of Kidney Disease 13 (6), 469-476.

Berger, J., Galle, P., 1963. Dépôts denses au sein des membranes basales du rein: étude en microscopies optique et électronique. Presse Medicale 71, 2351-2354.

Cameron, J.S., Turner, D.R., Heaton, J., et al., 1983. Idiopathic mesangiocapillary glomeru-lonephritis. Comparison of types I and II in children and adults and long-term prognosis. American Journal of Medicine 74, 175-192.

Churg, J., Duffy, J.L., Bernstein, J., 1979. Identification of dense deposit disease. Archives of Pathology 103, 67-72.

Habib, R., Gubler, M.C., Loirat, C., et al., 1975. Dense deposit disease: a variant of mem-branoproliferative glomerulonephritis. Kidney International 7, 204-215.

McEnery, P.T., McAdams, A.J., 1988. Regression of membranoproliferative glomerulonephri-tis type II (dense deposit disease): observations in six children. American Journal of Kidney Disease 12, 138-146.

Nasr, S.H., Valeri, A.M., Appel, G.B, et al., 2009. Dense deposit disease: clinicopathologic study of 32 pediatric and adult patients. Clinical Journal of the American Society of Nephrology 4, 22-32.

Sethi, S., Gamez, J.D., Vrana, J.A., et al., 2009. Glomeruli of dense deposit disease contain components of the alternative and terminal complement pathway. Kidney International 75, 952-960.

Walker, P.D., 2007. Dense deposit disease: new insights. Current Opinion in Nephrology and Hypertension 16, 204-212.

Walker, P.D., Ferrario, F., Joh, K., et al., 2007. Dense deposit disease is not a membranopro-liferative glomerulonephritis. Modern Pathology 20, 605-616.

C3 GLOMERULONEPHRITIS

C3 glomerulonephritis, part of the C3 glomerulopathy, is an uncommon disorder, with an average age of onset of around 30 years, but with a wide reported range, from 7 to 70 years. Patients typically have subnephrotic proteinuria, and most have microhematuria, with nephrotic syndrome present in about 15%. About half of patients presented with hypertension and slightly more than half had evidence of impaired GFR at presentation. About half of these patients maintained normal renal function, with up to 15% progressing to end-stage renal disease.

Light microscopic findings were variable, with two thirds of patients showing a membranoproliferative-type appearance by light microscopy with mesangial proliferation and subendothelial and mesangial and less frequently subepithelial deposits, with reduplication of GBMs (Figs. 1.73, 1.74). About 20% of cases show a nodular appearance. In a third of cases, deposits showed a mesangial and subepithelial distribution without subendothelial deposits or mesangial proliferation. Immunofluorescence microscopy showed isolated C3 deposits without C1q or IgG (Figs. 1.75, 1.76). Deposits mirrored the light microscopic pattern, with mesangial and scattered capillary loop deposits. By electron microscopy, mesangial, subendo-thelial and occasional subepithelial deposits, including occasional humps, were present, without dense transformation of the GBMs (Fig. 1.77).

Etiology/Pathogenesis

C3 glomerulopathy encompasses a group of disorders with isolated C3 deposition in glo-meruli, and includes DDD (see above), C3 glomerulonephritis, and complement factor H-related (CFHR5) nephropathy. Abnormalities of complement regulatory proteins,

---

Key Diagnostic Findings in C3 Glomerulonephritis

- Dominance of C3 staining
- Absent or scanty immunoglobulin deposition in glomeruli

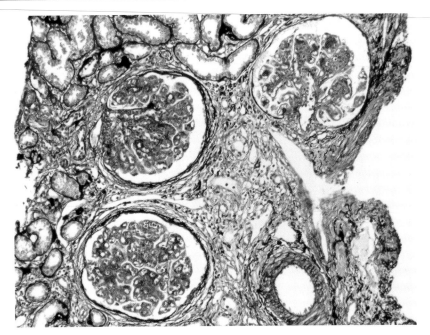

FIG. 1.73 C3 glomerulopathy. In this case of C3 glomerulonephritis, there is frequently a membranoproliferative appearance as shown here, with endocapillary proliferation and occasional double contours of glomerular basement membranes. There is also proportional interstitial fibrosis and tubular atrophy (Jones silver stain, ×200).

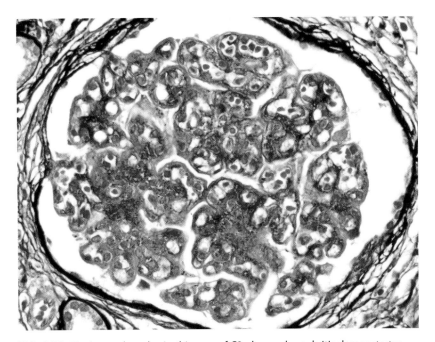

FIG. 1.74 C3 glomerulopathy. In this case of C3 glomerulonephritis demonstrates mesangial proliferation and variable endocapillary proliferation with double contours demonstrated on Jones silver stain. Small adhesions are also present (Jones silver stain, ×400).

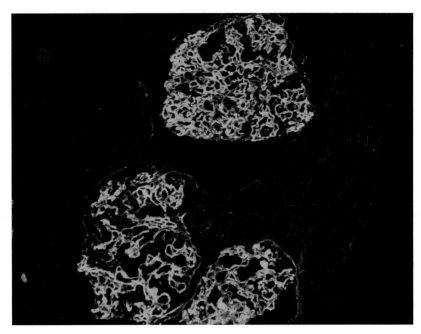

FIG. 1.75 C3 glomerulopathy. In cases of C3 glomerulopathy, there is by definition intense C3 by immunofluorescence, in a mesangial and chunky, irregular capillary loop pattern, with minimal or no immunoglobulin staining (anti-C3 immunofluorescence, ×200).

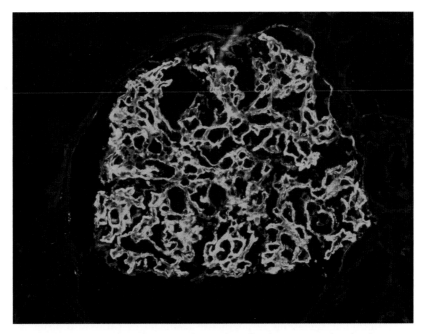

FIG. 1.76 C3 glomerulopathy. In C3 glomerulopathy, there is irregular, chunky to granular capillary loop and mesangial staining evident with C3 with minimal or no staining by immunoglobulin (anti-C3 immunofluorescence, ×400).

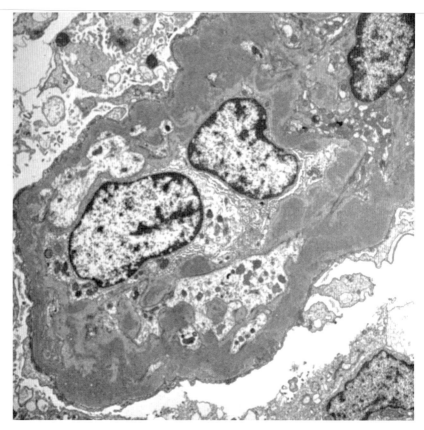

FIG. 1.77 C3 Glomerulopathy. In C3 glomerulopathy, mesangial and subendothelial deposits are apparent by electron microscopy. These differ from dense deposit disease (DDD) in that they are not replacing the lamina densa or do not have the unusual dense appearance of DDD (transmission electron microscopy, ×5000).

Differential Diagnosis of C3 Glomerulopathy

- Dense deposit disease: Characteristic dense transformation of glomerular basement membrane and dense deposits in mesangium
- C3 glomerulonephritis: C3 without immunoglobulin deposits, exclusion of postinfectious glomerulonephritis (often with complement regulatory protein mutation, e.g., factor H or I)
- Familial membranoproliferative glomerulonephritis type III: Dominant C3, frequent subepithelial, occasional hump-type deposits, positive family history
- CFHR5 nephropathy (familial C3 glomerulonephritis associated with heterozygous mutation in CFHR5): Isolated C3 deposits, subendothelial deposits by electron microscopy

---

including mutations in alternative complement pathway proteins and C3NeF have been detected in patients with C3 glomerulonephritis. Occasional families with glomerular disease with an MPGN type III pattern (i.e., with numerous subepithelial deposits), have shown linkage to chromosome 1, a region that also includes complement alternative pathway regulatory protein factor H. In two Cypriot families with inherited renal disease, there were marked unusual subendothelial deposits of C3 without immunoglobulin. In these patients, a mutation in complement factor H–related protein 5 was detected.

Selected Reading

Fakhouri, F., Frémeaux-Bacchi, V., Noël, L.H., et al., 2010. C3 glomerulopathy: a new classification. Nature Review Nephrology 6, 494-499.

Pickering, M., Cook, H.T., 2011. Complement and glomerular disease: new insights. Current Opinion in Nephrology and Hypertension 20, 271-277.

Servais, A., Frémeaux-Bacchi, V., Lequintrec, M., et al., 2007. Primary glomerulonephritis with isolated C3 deposits: a new entity which shares common genetic risk factors with haemolytic uraemic syndrome. Journal of Medical Genetics 44, 193-199.

Glomerular Diseases That Cause Nephrotic Syndrome: Immune Complex

MEMBRANOUS NEPHROPATHY

Membranous nephropathy was until recently the most common cause of nephrotic syndrome in adults in the United States, recently surpassed by focal segmental glomerulosclerosis. The peak incidence is in the fourth and fifth decades, with men affected more commonly than women. Approximately one third of patients may develop slowly progressive renal disease.

Membranous nephropathy is due to diffuse, global subepithelial deposits (Fig. 1.78). At an early time point, these may be only evident by light microscopy by a more rigid-appearing

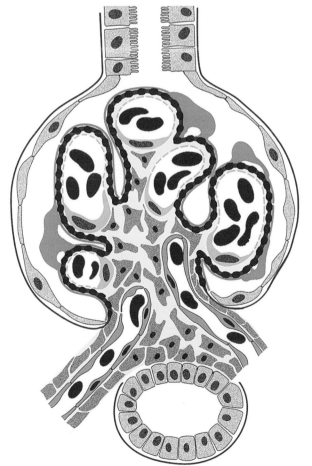

FIG. 1.78 Membranous nephropathy. There is no evident proliferation by light microscopy, with global subepithelial deposits, which may be visualized by light microscopy by the glomerular basement membrane spike reaction on silver stain. At earlier stages, the deposits that do not stain with silver may be seen in tangential sections as holes, producing a corkboard appearance. In advanced stages, the basement membrane reaction may encircle the deposits, with ensuing double contours.

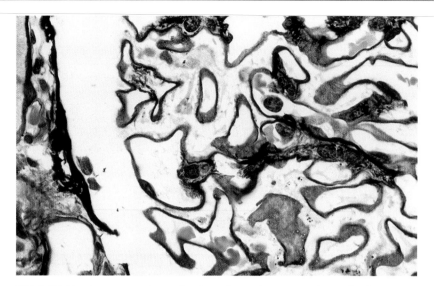

FIG. 1.79 Membranous nephropathy. Stage 1 membranous nephropathy does not show evident spikes by light microscopy. Only rare holes are evident, with a slightly more rigid appearance of the glomerular basement membrane (Jones silver stain, ×400).

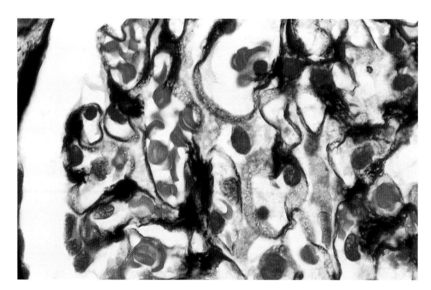

FIG. 1.80 Membranous nephropathy. In some cases of stage 1 membranous nephropathy, holes may be seen in tangential sections, since the deposits do not stain with Jones stain. This gives a corkboard, bubbly type appearance (Jones silver stain, ×1000).

capillary wall without visible deposits (Fig. 1.79). In favorable tangential sections, small areas of lucency seen on Jones silver stain may be detected, representing the lack of silver staining of the deposits (Fig. 1.80). These so-called holes are the earliest manifestation of membranous nephropathy by light microscopy. As deposits persist, the GBM matrix reaction produces small spike-like protrusions visualized by silver stain (Figs. 1.81-1.83). With progressive basement membrane reaction, the matrix encircles the deposits resulting in a lace-like splitting or

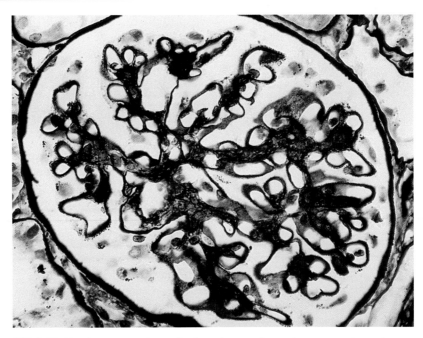

FIG. 1.81 Membranous nephropathy. In early stage 2 membranous nephropathy, small, stubby spike-like projections are seen, representing the basement membrane reaction to the subepithelial deposits. This gives a thick, "fuzzy rope" appearance to the glomerular basement membrane (Jones silver stain, ×400).

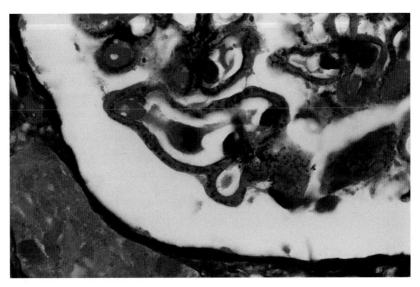

FIG. 1.82 Membranous nephropathy. There are well-developed spikes and "holes" in tangential sections in stage 2 membranous nephropathy (Jones silver stain, ×1000).

laddering appearance of the GBM on silver stain (Fig. 1.84). The morphologic findings related to these subepithelial deposits have been divided into stages (see below).

Additional lesions may be present, ranging from crescents to sclerosis. Segmental sclerosis, interstitial fibrosis, and tubular atrophy are associated with worse prognosis (Figs. 1.85, 1.86). Rarely, crescents may be found in cases of apparent idiopathic membranous nephropathy, but are more common with lupus-associated lesions (Fig. 1.87). Crescents in membranous

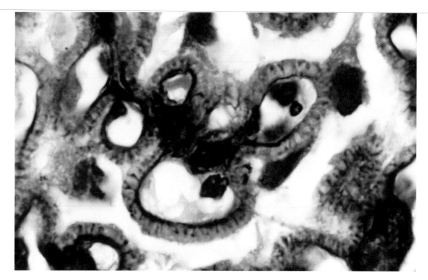

FIG. 1.83 Membranous nephropathy. In late stage 2 membranous nephropathy, the glomerular basement membrane is markedly thickened because of extensive basement membrane spike reaction around the deposits (Jones silver stain, ×1000).

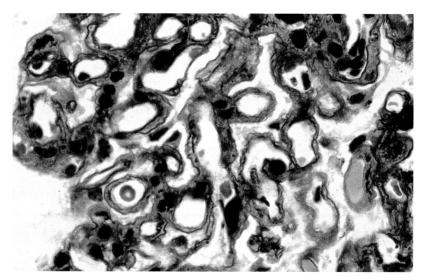

FIG. 1.84 Membranous nephropathy. In stage 3 membranous nephropathy, the basement membrane reaction encircles the deposits, giving rise to a bubbly, double contour appearance of the GBM. This can readily be distinguished from membranoproliferative glomerulonephritis because of the lack of associated endocapillary proliferation. Further, the subepithelial/transmembranous/intramembranous location of the deposits is resolved by immunofluorescence and electron microscopy (Jones silver stain, ×400). *GBM*, glomerular basement membrane.

Key Diagnostic Features of Membranous Nephropathy

- Extensive subepithelial deposits, evidenced as "holes" (i.e., areas of lucency on silver stain) or spikes, granular capillary loop staining by immunofluorescence
- Extensive subepithelial/intramembranous deposits by electron microscopy

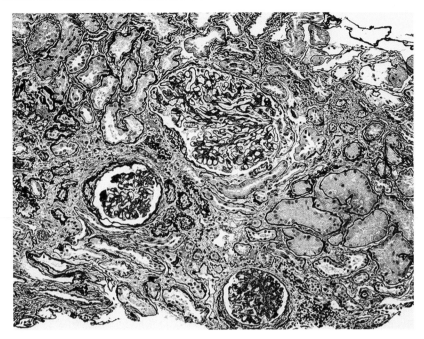

FIG. 1.85 Membranous nephropathy. There may be associated sclerosis with tubulointerstitial fibrosis in more advanced membranous nephropathy, as shown here (Jones silver stain, ×100).

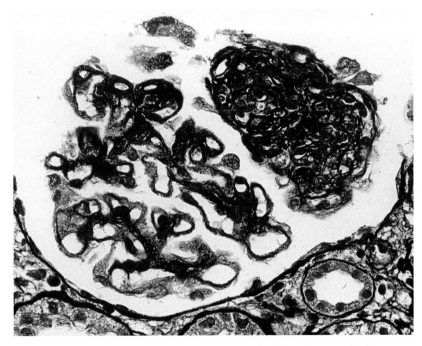

FIG. 1.86 Membranous nephropathy. Membranous nephropathy may also have associated segmental sclerosis as it becomes more chronic. This is not indicative of a second idiopathic sclerosing process but rather is thought to reflect the ongoing chronic injury, and it is associated with worse prognosis. By light microscopy, the small spikes and thickened glomerular basement membrane are evident, with the diagnosis of membranous nephropathy confirmed by immunofluorescence and electron microscopy (Jones silver stain, ×400).

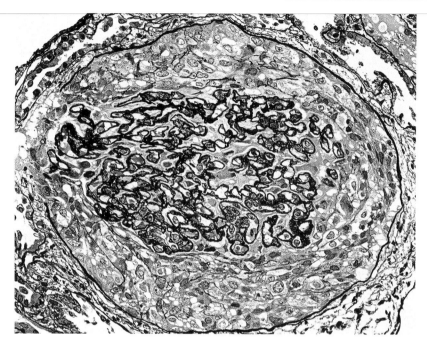

FIG. 1.87 Membranous nephropathy. Idiopathic membranous nephropathy may rarely be associated with crescents. Crescents are more commonly seen with secondary causes of membranous nephropathy, particularly due to systemic lupus erythematosus. The thickened glomerular basement membrane was shown to contain subepithelial deposits by immunofluorescence and electron microscopy (Jones silver stain, ×400).

nephropathy in patients without evidence of SLE should thus raise suspicion of a separate additional disease process, notably anti-GBM antibody–mediated glomerulonephritis.

By immunofluorescence, the subepithelial deposits are visualized as diffuse, global granular positivity along the capillary wall (Figs. 1.88-1.90). Immunofluorescence microscopy is more sensitive than either light microscopy or electron microscopy for detection of deposits and is very finely granular in Stage 1, and coarsely granular with more advanced stages. IgG is typically the predominant immunoglobulin, and C3 is most often also present. In addition, mesangial deposits are typically present in secondary membranous glomerulopathy and are absent in most cases of idiopathic membranous nephropathy. When IgA, IgM, and C1q are also present in addition to mesangial deposits, the possibility of secondary membranous nephropathy due to SLE should be considered. Although IgG4 is dominant in idiopathic membranous nephropathy, versus IgG1 in lupus membranous nephritis and IgG1 and IgG4 in membranous nephropathy associated with malignancy, these IgG subtypes are not sensitive in discerning primary membranous nephropathy versus malignancy-associated cases.

By electron microscopy, deposits corresponding to the stage of membranous glomerulopathy are visualized, with varying surrounding GBM reaction. In early stage 1 membranous nephropathy, deposits may be extremely small and inconspicuous with no surrounding GBM reaction, corresponding to the lack of spikes evident by light microscopy (Figs. 1.91, 1.92). In stage 2 membranous nephropathy, well-formed spike reaction is present (Figs. 1.93, 1.94). In stage 3 membranous nephropathy, the deposits are encircled by the GBM reaction (Figs. 1.95, 1.96). In stage 4 membranous nephropathy, the deposits are resorbed, leaving behind

Text continued on page 75

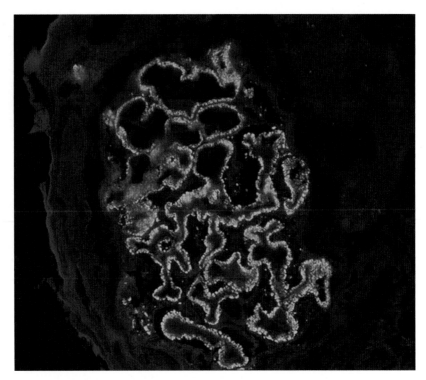

FIG. 1.88 Membranous nephropathy. There is an evenly distributed granular capillary loop pattern of positivity in membranous nephropathy, corresponding to the evenly distributed subepithelial deposits. Deposits in idiopathic membranous nephropathy stain predominately with IgG, with lesser amounts of C3 (anti-IgG immunofluorescence, ×400).

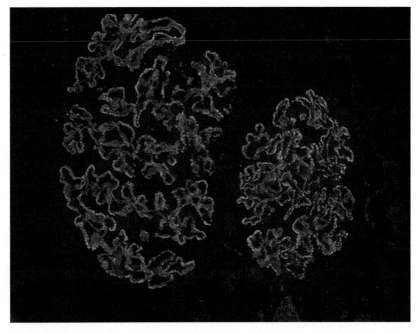

FIG. 1.89 Membranous nephropathy. In secondary membranous nephropathy, there is often associated mesangial staining, along with a granular capillary loop staining (anti-IgG immunofluorescence, ×200).

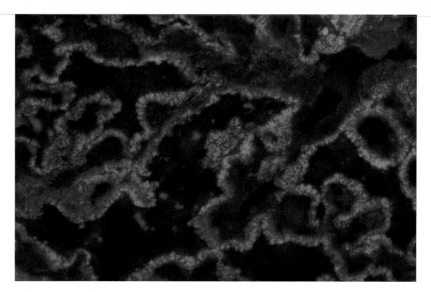

FIG. 1.90 Membranous nephropathy. The granularity of the capillary loop deposits characteristic of membranous nephropathy is evident (anti-IgG immunofluorescence, ×400).

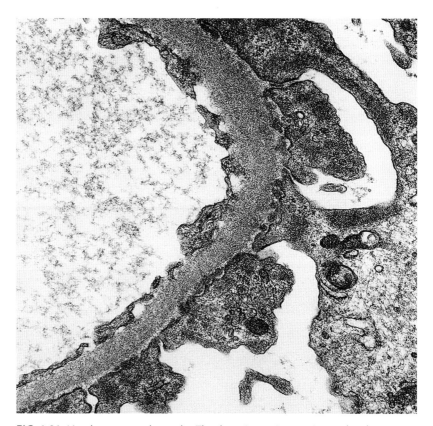

FIG. 1.91 Membranous nephropathy. The deposits are inconspicuous by electron microscopy in stage 1 membranous nephropathy, with blunting and partial effacement of overlying foot processes. There is no surrounding basement reaction (transmission electron microscopy, ×8000).

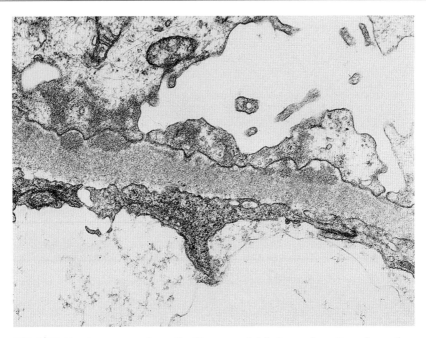

FIG. 1.92 Membranous nephropathy. There are slightly larger deposits underneath the podocyte, without surrounding spike reaction in this stage 1 membranous nephropathy (transmission electron microscopy, ×9000).

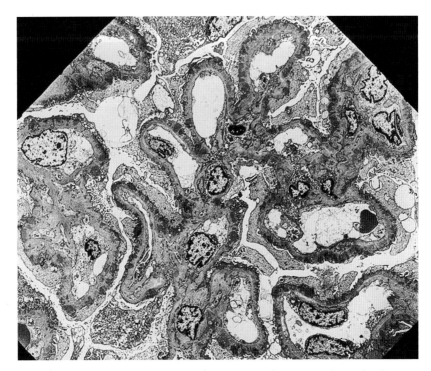

FIG. 1.93 Membranous nephropathy. In stage 2 membranous nephropathy, there are well-developed basement membrane reactions surrounding the evenly distributed subepithelial deposits (transmission electron microscopy, ×1200).

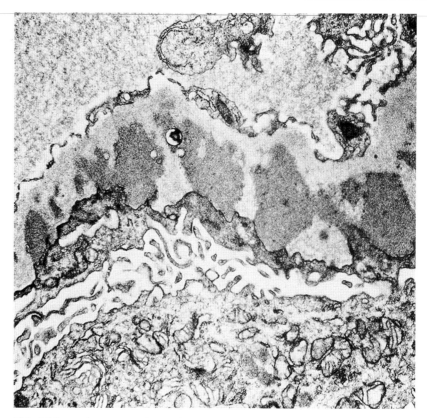

FIG. 1.94 Membranous nephropathy. The well-developed basement membrane reaction surrounding the deposits is evident in stage 2 membranous nephropathy, with overlying foot process effacement (transmission electron microscopy, ×8000).

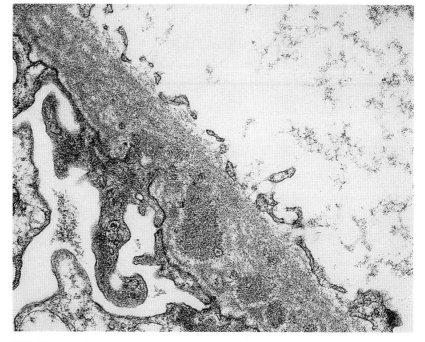

FIG. 1.95 Membranous nephropathy. In early stage 3 membranous nephropathy, the basement membrane reaction encircles the deposits, and there is early resorption. Overlying foot processes are largely effaced (transmission electron microscopy, ×8000).

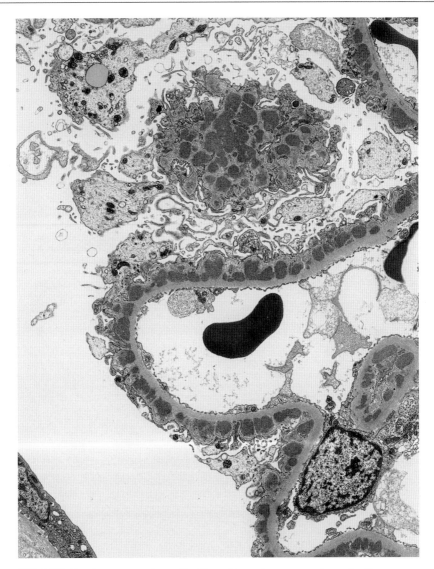

FIG. 1.96 Membranous nephropathy. Stage 3 membranous nephropathy is illustrated, with early resorption and basement membrane reaction overlying the deposits. The tangential section of basement membrane corresponds to the holes seen by light microscopy, since the electron-dense deposits do not stain by Jones stain, whereas the surrounding basement membrane does (transmission electron microscopy, ×8000).

rarefied, lucent areas (Figs. 1.97, 1.98). Varying depths of deposits with transmembranous and deep deposits has been linked to worse prognosis.

The podocytes show diffuse effacement of foot processes. When mesangial deposits are present, the possibility of a secondary etiology of membranous nephropathy should be considered (Figs. 1.99, 1.100). If reticular aggregates are present in endothelial cell cytoplasm, the possibility of lupus-associated membranous nephropathy (ISN/RPS Class V) should be considered.

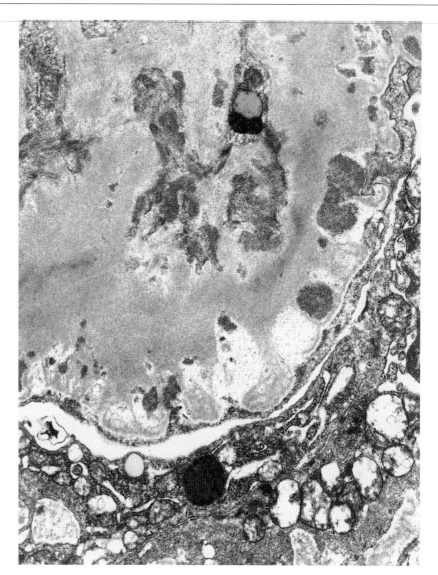

FIG. 1.97 Membranous nephropathy. In stage 4 membranous nephropathy, there is resorption of deposits. Some deposits still remain with surrounding halo or resorption, and the basement membrane reaction encircles the deposits in this largely sclerosed segment (transmission electron microscopy, ×20,250).

Differential Diagnosis of Membranous Nephropathy

- A granular capillary loop pattern may occasionally be seen in fibrillary glomerulonephritis, which has typical fibrillary deposits by electron microscopy and smudgy appearance of deposits by immunofluorescence, and mesangial deposits.
- Mesangial deposits are typically present in secondary membranous nephropathy.
- Mesangial deposits and the additional presence of reticular aggregates and/or full house staining suggest membranous lupus nephritis.

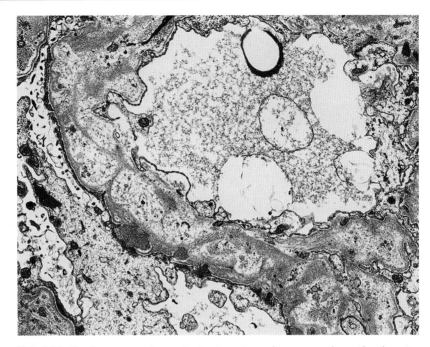

FIG. 1.98 Membranous nephropathy. In stage 4 membranous nephropathy, deposits are largely resorbed, with small electron-dense subepithelial deposits overlying the resorbed areas, indicating ongoing active immune complex deposition (transmission electron microscopy, ×4400).

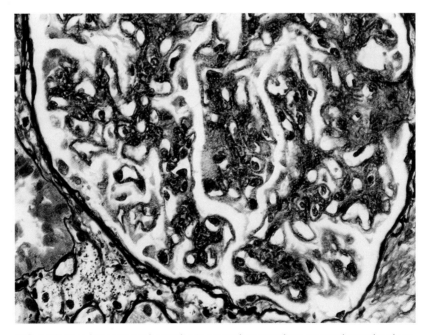

FIG. 1.99 Membranous nephropathy. In secondary membranous nephropathy, there is mesangial expansion, associated with mesangial deposits, in addition to the peripheral loop subepithelial deposits. This patient's disease was related to hepatitis B infection (Jones silver stain, ×400).

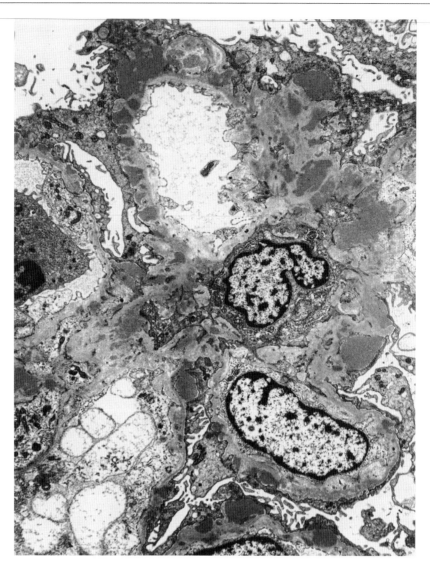

FIG. 1.100 Membranous nephropathy. In this case of secondary membranous nephropathy, advanced stage 2, there are also associated mesangial deposits, indicating a secondary etiology (transmission electron microscopy, ×8000).

Etiology/Pathogenesis

Most cases of previously termed "idiopathic" membranous nephropathy are caused by antibodies to the phospholipase A2 receptor (PLA2R), which is expressed on the podocyte. The subepithelial deposits are then thought to arise from in situ immune complex formation. Infectious agents, including bacterial, viral, or parasitic drugs or thyroglobulin may also be the antigen in secondary membranous nephropathy. Numerous entities have been associated with membranous nephropathy, but causality has only been established for some, including hepatitis B, Hashimoto thyroiditis, SLE, syphilis, penicillamine, gold (Fig. 1.101), mercuric chloride, and Sjögren syndrome. Recently, cationic bovine serum albumin from cow's milk was found to cause membranous nephropathy in some children. Malignancies, in particular some carcinomas, sarcomas, and leukemias, have been linked to membranous nephropathy, but definitive proof of causal linkage, that is, circulating antibody–antigen immune complexes and tumor antigen within the deposits, is lacking in most instances. Interstitial fibrosis and segmental sclerosis are associated with worse prognosis.

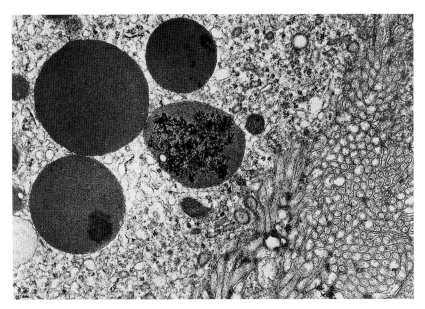

FIG. 1.101 Membranous nephropathy. In rare cases of secondary membranous nephropathy, the etiology may be definitively determined. In this case, rare gold particles were found within lysosomes in tubules, providing a causal etiology for this patient's secondary membranous nephropathy (transmission electron microscopy, ×14,000).

Selected Reading

Beck Jr., L.H., Bonegio, R.G., Lambeau, G., et al., 2009. M-type phospholipase A2 receptor as target antigen in idiopathic membranous nephropathy. New England Journal of Medicine 361, 11-21.

Couser, W.G., Baker, P.J., Adler, S., 1985. Complement and the direct mediation of immune glomerular injury: a new perspective. Kidney International 28, 879-890.

Debiec, H., Lefeu, F., Kemper, M.J., et al., 2011. Early-childhood membranous nephropathy due to cationic bovine serum albumin. New England Journal of Medicine 364, 2101-2110.

Dumoulin, A., Hill, G.S., Montseny, J.J., et al., 2003. Clinical and morphological prognostic factors in membranous nephropathy: significance of focal segmental glomerulosclerosis. American Journal of Kidney Disease 41, 38-48.

Ehrenreich, T., Churg, J., 1968. Pathology of membranous nephropathy. In: Sommers, S.C. (Ed.), Pathology Annual. Appleton-Century-Crofts, New York, 3, pp. 145-154.

Fogo, A.B., 2011. Milk and membranous nephropathy. New England Journal of Medicine 364, 2158-2159.

Gonzalo, A., Mampaso, F., Barcena, R., et al., 1999. Membranous nephropathy associated with hepatitis B virus infection: long-term clinical and histological outcome. Nephrology, Dialysis and Transplantation 14, 416-418.

Jennette, J.C., Iskandar, S.S., Dalldorf, F.G., 1983. Pathologic differentiation between lupus and nonlupus membranous glomerulopathy. Kidney International 24, 377-385.

Kerjaschki, D., 1990. The pathogenesis of membranous glomerulonephritis: From morphology to molecules. Virchows Archiv [B] 58, 253-271.

Lee, H.S., Koh, H.I., 1993. Nature of progressive glomerulosclerosis in human membranous nephropathy. Clinical Nephrology 39, 7-16.

Toth, T., Takebayashi, S., 1992. Idiopathic membranous glomerulonephritis: a clinicopathologic and quantitative morphometric study. Clinical Nephrology 38, 14-19.

Van Damme, B., Tardanico, R., Vanrenterghem, Y., et al., 1990. Adhesions, focal sclerosis, protein crescents, and capsular lesions in membranous nephropathy. Journal of Pathology 161, 47-56.

Wakai, S., Magil, A.B., 1992. Focal glomerulosclerosis in idiopathic membranous glomerulonephritis. Kidney International 41, 428-434.

Wasserstein, A.G., 1997. Membranous glomerulonephritis. Journal of the American Society of Nephrology 8, 664-674.

Yoshimoto, K., Yokoyama, H., Wada, T., et al., 2004. Pathologic findings of initial biopsies reflect the outcomes of membranous nephropathy. Kidney International 65, 148-153.

MEMBRANOPROLIFERATIVE GLOMERULONEPHRITIS, TYPE I

Membranoproliferative glomerulonephritis (MPGN) type I typically presents as combined nephritic/nephrotic syndrome with hypocomplementemia. It occurs mostly in children and young adults, and as a lesion secondary to for instance chronic infections in adults. The incidence of MPGN type I appears to have decreased in children in the past decades, for unknown reasons. Children with MPGN type I tend to be older than children with DDD (also called MPGN type II by some, see Dense Deposit Disease). The presence of the C3 nephritic factor (C3NeF) is more rare, and concurrent partial lipodystrophy is very rare in MPGN type I compared to DDD. Patients typically have progressive renal disease, with about 50% renal survival at age 10 years in children, and similar rates of progression in adults. Many of the patients reaching end stage died of complications of their kidney disease. Clinical indicators of poor prognosis are hypertension, impaired renal function, and nephrotic syndrome. MPGN type I recurs in the transplant in about one third of patients, and may lead to graft loss, particularly if crescents are present. MPGN can also occur de novo in the transplant, related to hepatitis C infection and cryoglobulinemia (see Cryoglobulinemic Glomerulonephritis).

The term *MPGN* describes a light microscopic pattern of injury characterized by diffuse mesangial expansion with increased matrix, mesangial, and infiltrating cells, endocapillary proliferation, and thickened capillary walls, often with a "tram track" appearance (Fig. 1.102). The term *MPGN* is preferably used only when this pattern is caused by immune complex glomerulonephritides. Of note, basement membrane double contours may be seen in other non–immune complex injuries, characterized by chronic endothelial injury with interposition of cells by electron microscopy. These include the organizing phase of thrombotic microangiopathy, radiation nephritis, chronic transplant glomerulopathy, or in sickle cell disease. Although light microscopy may appear similar to MPGN, immunofluorescence findings and electron microscopy readily allow recognition of the immune complexes in MPGN.

MPGN has been divided into three types, all with similar light microscopic appearance. The term *mesangiocapillary glomerulonephritis* has also been used for MPGN type I. There is global, diffuse endocapillary proliferation with increased mesangial cellularity and matrix, and lobular simplification (Figs. 1.103-1.107). Increased mononuclear cells and occasional neutrophils may be present. The proliferation is typically uniform and diffuse in idiopathic MPGN, contrasting the irregular involvement with proliferative lupus nephritis. In some cases, the glomeruli may appear more solid and nodular (Fig. 1.108). The capillary wall is thickened with a double contour by silver stains (Figs. 1.107, 1.109). This appearance results

---

Key Diagnostic Features of Membranoproliferative Glomerulonephritis

- Double contour appearance of glomerular basement membrane by light microscopy
- Endocapillary proliferation
- Chunky, irregular mesangial and capillary loop staining, typical sausage-type deposits underlying basement membrane (IgG or IgM dominant, with complement C3 and C1q)
- Subendothelial and mesangial deposits by electron microscopy

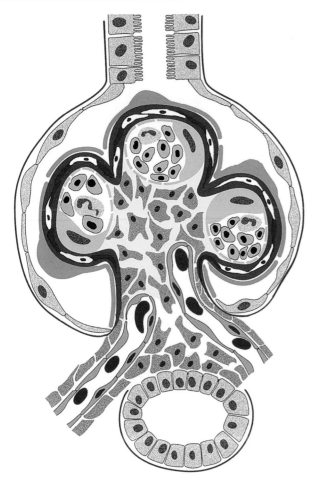

FIG. 1.102 MPGN type 1. There is endocapillary proliferation and glomerular basement membrane double contours, due to mesangial and subendothelial deposits, with resultant interposition and new basement membrane being laid down, causing the "split" appearance. *MPGN,* membranoproliferative glomerulonephritis.

from the presence of subendothelial deposits and so-called circumferential interposition, whereby infiltrating mononuclear cells, occasional mesangial cells, or even portions of endothelial cells interpose themselves between the endothelium and the basement membrane, with new, inner basement membrane being laid down. A circumferential, or partial, double-contour basement membrane results. In secondary forms of MPGN, the injury may be more irregular. Crescents may occur in both idiopathic and secondary forms (Fig. 1.108). Greater than 20% crescents have been associated with worse prognosis. Lesions progress with less cellularity and more pronounced matrix accumulation and sclerosis over time. Tubulointerstitial fibrosis and vascular sclerosis proportional to glomerular scarring are seen late in the course. Tubular atrophy and interstitial fibrosis indicate worse prognosis.

The immunofluorescence findings are variable in MPGN type I. Typically, IgG and IgM and C3 are present in an irregular, chunky capillary and mesangial distribution (Figs. 1.110-1.113). IgA is present in only a small proportion of cases. C3 staining may be dominant, and staining for immunoglobulin may even be lost, especially in secondary MPGN. The peripheral loop deposits typically are sausage-shaped and have a smooth outer edge because they are subendothelial and molded under the GBM (Fig. 1.113).

By electron microscopy, MPGN type I shows numerous deposits in subendothelial and mesangial areas (Figs. 1.114-1.117). The "subendothelial" deposits actually more commonly lie within the GBM, immediately under the original lamina densa, and thus might more precisely be described as "intramembranous" (Fig. 1.117). Vague wormy or microtubular substructure suggests a possible cryoglobulin component (Fig. 1.116). Cellular interposition

Text continued on page 86

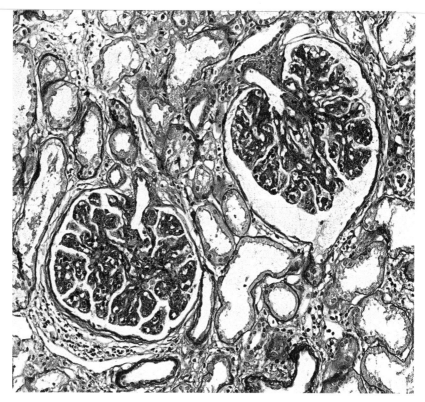

FIG. 1.103 MPGN type I. MPGN is characterized by diffuse endocapillary proliferation, which results in a lobular, uniform appearance of glomeruli (periodic acid Schiff, ×100). *MPGN,* membranoproliferative glomerulonephritis.

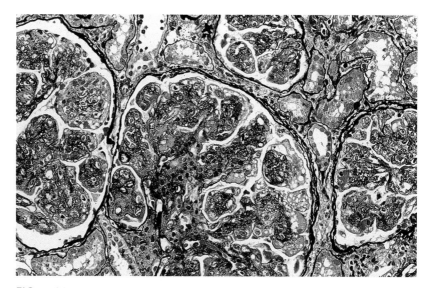

FIG. 1.104 MPGN type I. There is diffuse endocapillary proliferation with extensive duplication of the glomerular basement membrane, with frequent eosinophilic deposits within the capillary wall. There is marked mesangial proliferation, and endocapillary proliferation with a lobular appearance (Jones silver stain, ×200). *MPGN,* membranoproliferative glomerulonephritis.

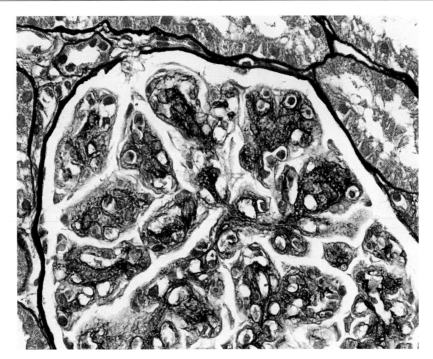

FIG. 1.105 MPGN type I. There is less marked endocapillary proliferation, but still widespread double contours of the glomerular basement membrane, so-called tram tracking (Jones silver stain, ×400). *MPGN, membranoproliferative glomerulonephritis.*

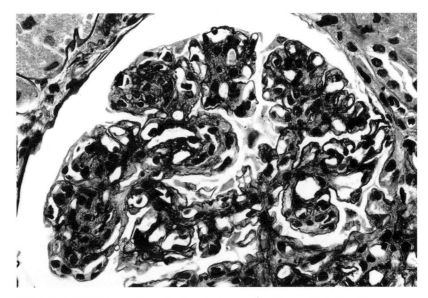

FIG. 1.106 MPGN type I. There is abundant mesangial hypercellularity with proliferation extending to peripheral capillary lumens (endocapillary proliferation), with only segmental glomerular basement membrane double contours in this case. In idiopathic MPGN, the endocapillary proliferation is typically global and diffuse, while in secondary cases, the lesions may be more focal and segmental (Jones silver stain, ×400). *MPGN, membranoproliferative glomerulonephritis.*

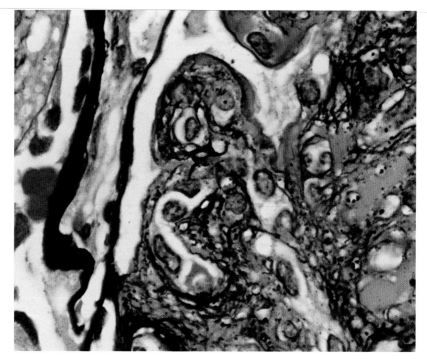

FIG. 1.107 MPGN type I. There is segmental interposition of cells with reduplication of peripheral capillary glomerular basement membrane along with subendothelial deposits (Jones silver stain, ×1000). *MPGN,* membranoproliferative glomerulonephritis.

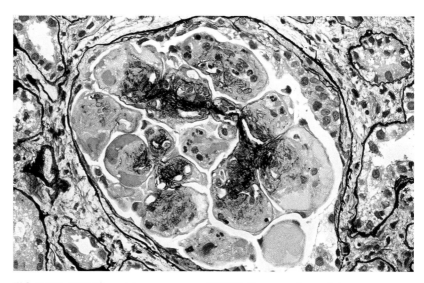

FIG. 1.108 MPGN type I. In some cases of MPGN, there may be nodular glomerulosclerosis and massive deposits. Occasional polymorphonuclear leukocytes are also present, in addition to the mesangial and endocapillary proliferation. A small incipient cellular crescent is present. These morphological features suggest the possibility of a secondary etiology of the MPGN lesion (Jones silver stain, ×400). *MPGN,* membranoproliferative glomerulonephritis.

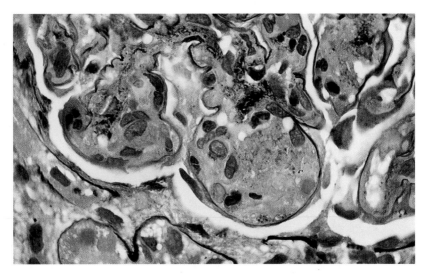

FIG. 1.109 MPGN type I. Large subendothelial deposits and interposed cells are evident, along with endocapillary proliferation. A smaller subendothelial deposit is present at the far right, with small nodular expansion in the middle and left capillary loops (same case as in Fig. 1-108) (Jones silver stain, ×1000). *MPGN,* membranoproliferative glomerulonephritis.

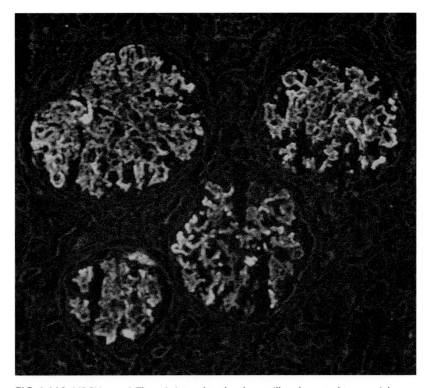

FIG. 1.110 MPGN type I. There is irregular, chunky capillary loop and mesangial staining in MPGN, with coarse, subendothelial deposits with a molded, smooth outer contour (anti-IgG immunofluorescence, ×100). *MPGN,* membranoproliferative glomerulonephritis.

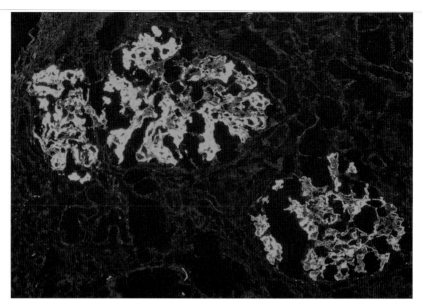

FIG. 1.111 MPGN type I. In addition to IgG, there is often very prominent complement deposition in MPGN, with prominent mesangial and coarse, chunky peripheral loop deposits, corresponding to the subendothelial deposits (anti-C3 immunofluorescence, ×100). *MPGN,* membranoproliferative glomerulonephritis.

Differential Diagnosis of Membranoproliferative-Type Pattern

Double contours or so-called tram-tracking of glomerular basement membranes (GBMs) may occur due to:
- subendothelial immune complexes

    or
- chronic endothelial injury

    or
- unusual deposits with substructure

Notes:
- The term *membranoproliferative glomerulonephritis* should be reserved for disease due to subendothelial immune complex deposits.
- Double contours of GBMs may occur with chronic endothelial injury, where there is no IF positivity for immune complexes. These conditions include chronic thrombotic micrangiopathy, transplant glomerulopathy, radiation nephropathy.
- A membranoproliferative pattern of injury may also be seen without IF positivity in type III collagen glomerulopathy and fibronectin glomerulopathy.

IF, immunofluorescence.

---

is present. This term refers to the interposition of cytoplasmic processes of mesangial or mononuclear cells between the endothelial cell and the basement membrane (Fig. 1.118). Monocyte interposition is particularly common when the MPGN lesion is related to cryo-globulinemia. Reduplication of new basement material is present immediately under the swollen endothelial cells. The overlying podocytes are effaced.

MPGN type III shows, in addition to the subendothelial and mesangial deposits, numerous subepithelial deposits (Fig. 1.119). It may not, however, represent an entity separate from MPGN type I. Although C3 nephritic factor is rarely found in these patients, clinical distinction of this morphology has not been apparent.

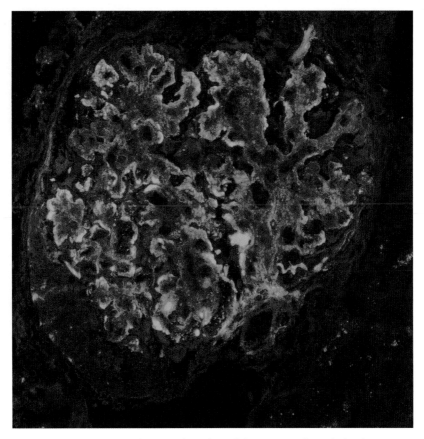

FIG. 1.112 MPGN type I. The smooth outline of the sausage-shaped, chunky peripheral loop deposits is evident along with the scattered mesangial deposits. The smooth outer contour of the peripheral loop deposits reflects their subendothelial location, with molding under the GBM (anti-C3 immunofluorescence, ×200). GBM, glomerular basement membrane; *MPGN,* membranoproliferative glomerulonephritis.

Differential Diagnosis of Membranoproliferative Glomerulonephritis with Deposits

- Fibrillary glomerulonephritis often has membranoproliferative appearance with endocapillary proliferation. EM is diagnostic of the fibrillary nature of the deposits.
- Amyloid may give rise to a nodular appearance of the mesangium and also involve the capillary loops. If due to light chain, IF is positive in a smudgy pattern with clonal staining with a corresponding light chain. EM shows characteristic fibrils, and Congo red stain is positive.
- Monoclonal immunoglobulin deposition disease, including light chain deposition disease, heavy chain deposition disease, and light and heavy chain deposition disease may show variable proliferative appearance. IF is diagnostic in defining the monoclonal component of the deposits.
- Dense deposit disease has a mesangial proliferative or membranoproliferative appearance, typically with only C3 staining. EM is diagnostic of the dense transformation of the basement membranes.

EM, electron microscopy; *IF,* immunofluorescence.

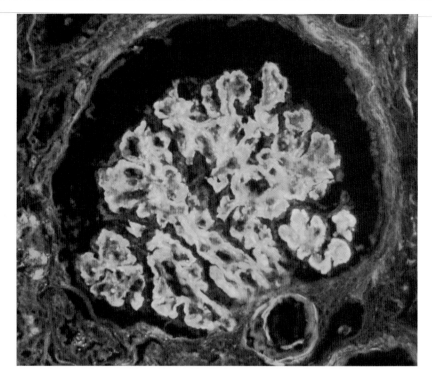

FIG. 1.113 MPGN type I. Both complement pathways are typically activated in MPGN, with frequent C1q positivity in addition to C3. The subendothelial location of the peripheral deposits is evident by their smooth outer contour (anti-C1q immunofluorescence, ×400). *MPGN,* membranoproliferative glomerulonephritis.

Of note, in non–immune complex diseases with GBM double contours seen by light microscopy (e.g., transplant glomerulopathy, chronic thrombotic microangiopathy), electron microscopy shows that the double contour results from widening of the GBM as a result of increased lucency of the lamina rara interna and cellular interposition without immune complexes, with new basement membrane formed underneath the endothelium.

Etiology/Pathogenesis

MPGN-like lesions can occur secondary to a number of chronic infectious processes, including hepatitis B, hepatitis C, subacute bacterial endocarditis, cryoglobulin, syphilis, etc., which are discussed separately. Morphologic features do not allow precise classification of the underlying agent in most cases of MPGN. MPGN-type lesions may rarely occur as a result of inherited deficiency of complement (see above), or partial lipodystrophy. In adults in the United States, many patients with MPGN have associated hepatitis C infection. This association has not been seen in children with MPGN. These hepatitis C–positive cases often show vague substructure of deposits, with short, curved, vaguely fibrillar deposits suggestive of mixed cryoglobulinemia (see Cryoglobulinemic Glomerulonephritis). Features suggestive or even diagnostic of cryoglobulin as an underlying cause of MPGN include strongly PAS-positive cryo-"plugs" in capillary lumina, vasculitis, predominant IgM deposits, sometimes with clonality, and vague substructure of deposits by electron microscopy. Morphologic clues of an underlying chronic bacterial infection causing MPGN-type lesions are the presence of hump-type subepithelial deposits (see Postinfectious Glomerulonephritis).

Text continued on page 93

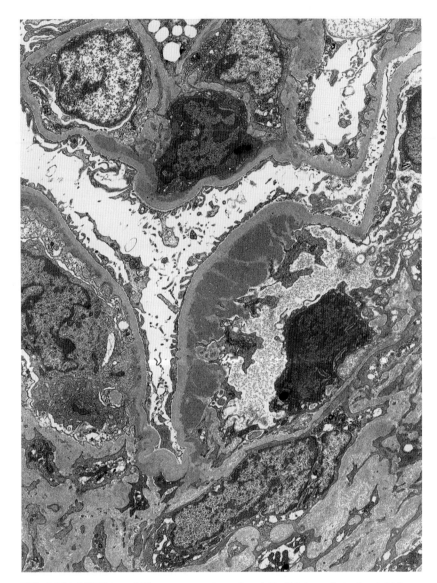

FIG. 1.114 MPGN type I. There are massive subendothelial deposits in the right loop, with minimal endocapillary proliferation, and small, sliver-like deposits on the left and top loops, with associated proliferation. Scattered mesangial deposits are also present. There is subtotal effacement of overlying foot processes. The smooth outer contour of the deposits is also evident by immunofluorescence (see Figs. 1.112, 1.113) (transmission electron microscopy, ×8000). *MPGN,* membranoproliferative glomerulonephritis.

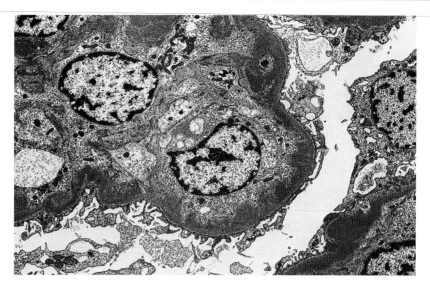

FIG. 1.115 MPGN type I. There is marked endocapillary proliferation, with small subendothelial deposits and a transmembranous deposit (lower right). The endocapillary proliferation is due to a mixture of endothelial cells, mesangial cells, and infiltrating mononuclear cells/macrophages (transmission electron microscopy, ×8000). *MPGN*, membranoproliferative glomerulonephritis.

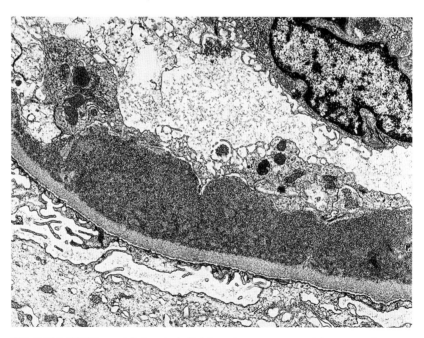

FIG. 1.116 MPGN type I. Subendothelial deposits are present, without attendant proliferation. The mottled, vaguely wormy substructure of the deposits suggests the possibility of a secondary etiology, such as cryoglobulin deposits. Correlation with light microscopy, immunofluorescence, and clinical findings can further support or refute this possibility (transmission electron microscopy, ×11,250). *MPGN*, membranoproliferative glomerulonephritis.

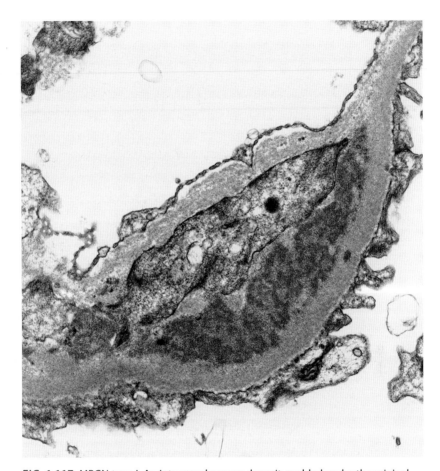

FIG. 1.117 MPGN type I. An intramembranous deposit, molded under the original lamina densa, is associated with an interposed cell and new underlying glomerular basement membrane. Some of the deposit material is subendothelial (far right) (transmission electron microscopy, ×25,625). *MPGN*, membranoproliferative glomerulonephritis.

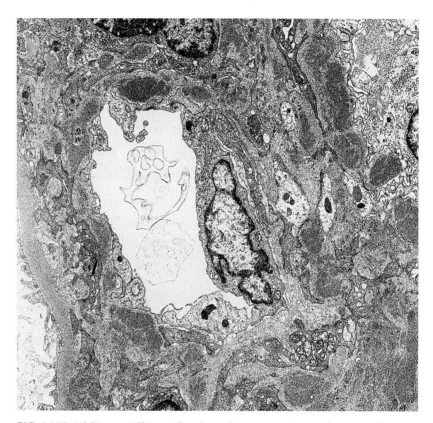

FIG. 1.118 MPGN type I. This capillary loop shows a complex combination of lesions, with interposed cells and intramembranous and subendothelial deposits. Adjacent areas of the glomerulus show mesangial deposits (far right) and mesangial proliferation (transmission electron microscopy, ×14,000). *MPGN,* membranoproliferative glomerulonephritis.

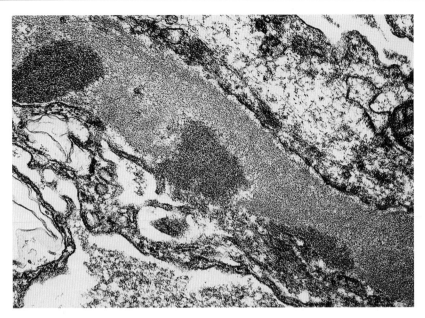

FIG. 1.119 MPGN type I. There may be occasional subepithelial or more frequently transmembranous deposits in cases that otherwise appear as MPGN. These lesions may meet morphologic criteria for MPGN III, which commonly has presence of C3 nephritic factor. Occasional transmembranous deposits may, however, be found in any type of MPGN lesion (transmission electron microscopy, ×17,125). *MPGN,* membranoproliferative glomerulonephritis.

Selected Reading

Alchi, B., Jayne, D., 2010. Membranoproliferative glomerulonephritis. Pediatric Nephrology 25, 1409-1418.

Anders, D., Agricola, B., Sippel, M., et al., 1997. Basement membrane changes in membranoproliferative glomerulonephritis. II. Characterization of a third type by silver impregnation of ultra thin sections. Virchows Archiv (Pathology and Anatomy) 376, 1-19.

Berger, J., Galle, P., 1963. Dépots denses au sein des membranes basales du rein: étude en microscopies optique et électronique. Presse Medicale 71, 2351-2354.

Cameron, J.S., Turner, D.R., Heaton, J., et al., 1983. Idiopathic mesangiocapillary glomerulonephritis. Comparison of types I and II in children and adults and long-term prognosis. American Journal of Medicine 74, 175-192.

D'Amico, G., Ferrario, F., 1992. Mesangiocapillary glomerulonephritis. Journal of the American Society of Nephrology 2 (10 Suppl):S159-166.

Donadio Jr., J.V., Slack, T.K., Holley, K.E., et al., 1979. Idiopathic membranoproliferative (mesangiocapillary) glomerulonephritis: a clinicopathologic study. Mayo Clinic Proceedings 54, 141-150.

Habib, R., Kleinknecht, C., Gubler, M.C., et al., 1973. Idiopathic membranoproliferative glomerulonephritis in children: report of 105 cases. Clinical Nephrology 1, 194-214.

Johnson, R.J., Gretch, D.R., Yamabe, H., et al., 1993. Membranoproliferative glomerulonephritis associated with hepatitis C virus infection. New England Journal of Medicine 328, 465-470.

Katz, S.M., 1981. Reduplication of the glomerular basement membrane: a study of 110 cases. Archives of Pathology and Laboratory Medicine 105, 67-70.

Nowicki, M.J., Welch, T.R., Ahmad, N., et al., 1995. Absence of hepatitis B and C viruses in pediatric idiopathic membranoproliferative glomerulonephritis. Pediatric Nephrology 9, 16-18.

Rennke, H.G., 1995. Nephrology forum: Secondary membranoproliferative glomerulone-phritis. Kidney International 47, 643-656.

Strife, C.F., Jackson, E.C., McAdams, A.J., 1984. Type III membranoproliferative glomeru-lonephritis: long-term clinical and morphological evaluation. Clinical Nephrology 21, 323-334.

Strife, C.F., McEnery, P.T., McAdams, A.J., et al., 1977. Membranoproliferative glomerulo-nephritis with disruption of the glomerular basement membrane. Clinical Nephrology 7, 65-72.

Taguchi, T., Bohle, A., 1989. Evaluation of change with time of glomerular morphology in membranoproliferative glomerulonephritis: a serial biopsy study of 33 cases. Clinical Nephrology 31, 297-306.

FIBRILLARY GLOMERULONEPHRITIS

Fibrillary glomerulonephritis was first reported by Rosenmann and Eliakim as a glomerulopa-thy with material very similar to amyloid that did not stain with Congo red. A distinctly different morphologic form of glomerulopathy with larger, microtubular organized structures has been termed immunotactoid glomerulopathy. The classification of these lesions has been controversial. Some investigators have chosen to use the term immunotactoid glomerulopathy to refer to this entire group of disorders. We prefer to use the term *fibrillary glomerulonephritis* only for the amyloid-like, Congo red–negative form, as this may have implications for prog-nosis and pathogenesis.

Fibrillary glomerulonephritis is a disease of adults, with average age of onset ~50 years. Patients are most often Caucasian, with a slight female predominance. This entity comprises about 1% of diagnoses among adults undergoing native kidney biopsy. Most patients present with nephrotic syndrome and frequently have associated hematuria. Occasional patients had concomitant infection with hepatitis C, although a causal link has not been proven. Rapidly progressive glomerulonephritis clinically was present in approximately one third of patients. The prognosis is one of progression to renal loss in approximately 40% of cases over 5 years, with a median renal survival time of only 24 months from time of biopsy in one large series. Better prognosis was seen in patients younger than age 40 years at presentation. No specific treatment has been described. Patients who progressed to end-stage renal disease generally did so rapidly, reaching end stage within 10 months on average after diagnosis. Elevated serum creatinine at presentation was a clinical sign of poor prognosis. Recurrence in the transplant has been described for fibrillary glomerulonephritis cases in nearly 20% of grafts, with a slower course of loss of GFR in the graft than in the native kidney.

The light microscopic appearance in fibrillary glomerulonephritis most frequently is that of a membranoproliferative, typically lobular, glomerulonephritis, with GBM double contours (Figs. 1.120-1.122). Less frequently, there is a mesangial proliferative or diffuse endocapillary proliferative pattern. Some cases may even appear similar to diabetic nephropathy, with large nodular expansion of mesangial matrix (Fig. 1.120). In rare cases, there are GBM spikes in a membranous pattern, reflecting GBM reaction to the fibrillary deposits in a subepithelial location. Areas of deposits stain weakly PAS and silver positive. Crescents, either cellular or fibrocellular, were present in one third of cases in one series (Fig. 1.123). Crescents more

---

Key Diagnostic Features of Fibrillary Glomerulonephritis

- Typically membranoproliferative or mesangial proliferative by light microscopy
- Smudgy polyclonal positivity for IgG and C3
- Randomly arranged fibrils by electron microscopy, Congo red negative

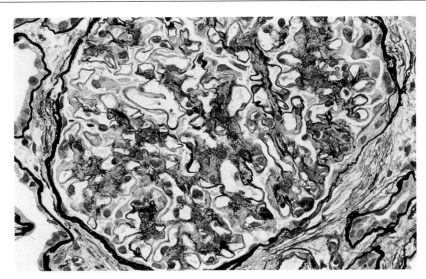

FIG. 1.120 Fibrillary glomerulonephritis. The light microscopic pattern varies from mesangial to membranoproliferative. This case shows moderate mesangial proliferation and occasional basement membrane double contours (Jones silver stain, ×400).

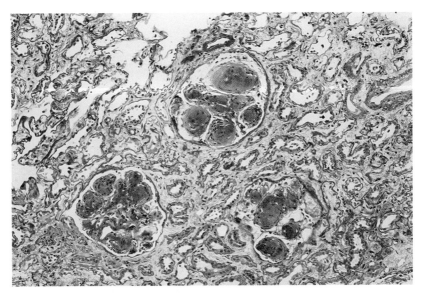

FIG. 1.121 Fibrillary glomerulonephritis. In some cases of fibrillary glomerulonephritis, there may be a lobular or nodular proliferative pattern, which may resemble diabetic nephropathy, as in this case (periodic acid Schiff, ×100).

commonly are associated with diffuse endocapillary proliferation and may be associated with worse outcome. Sclerosis is associated with more severe disease (Fig. 1.123). By definition, Congo red stains are negative. The interstitium shows interstitial fibrosis and tubular atrophy, proportional to glomerular changes. Rare cases had fibrillary deposits extending to the tubular basement membranes. Vessels do not show any specific lesions.

Immunofluorescence demonstrates prominent, smudgy IgG and lesser amounts of C3 in mesangial areas, and segmental, usually chunky, staining along GBMs, occasionally in a membranous pattern (Figs. 1.124, 1.125). Polyclonal IgG4 is the dominant or exclusive

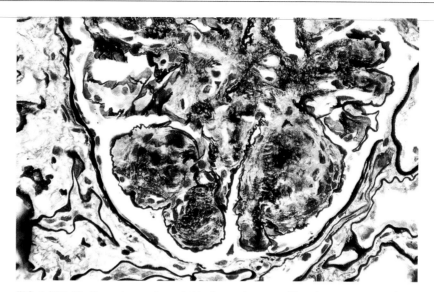

FIG. 1.122 Fibrillary glomerulonephritis. A membranoproliferative pattern is evident with mesangial and endocapillary proliferation and basement membrane reduplication and interposition (Jones silver stain, ×400).

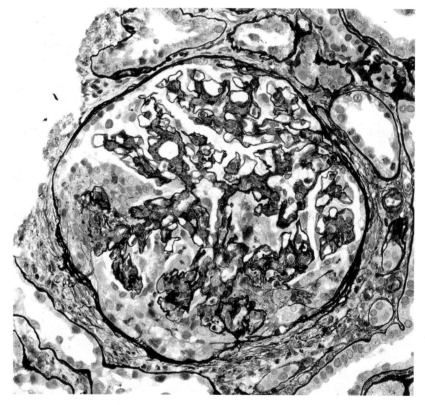

FIG. 1.123 Fibrillary glomerulonephritis. In our series, approximately one third of cases showed crescents. In this case, there is associated moderate mesangial proliferation, an important feature indicating by light microscopy that this crescentic lesion is likely not pauci-immune crescentic glomerulonephritis or anti-GBM antibody–mediated glomerulonephritis. Periglomerular fibrosis and early adhesions are also evident (Jones silver stain, ×400). *GBM,* glomerular basement membrane.

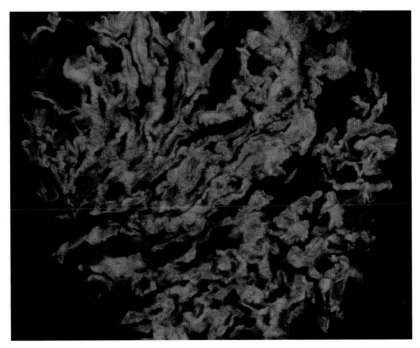

FIG. 1.124 Fibrillary glomerulonephritis. Immunofluorescence patterns in fibrillary glomerulonephritis mirror the light microscopic changes, ranging from mesangial to membranoproliferative or even membranous patterns. There is typically a smudgy positivity with particularly predominant mesangial staining. This case illustrates chunky mesangial staining and irregular, coarsely granular peripheral loop staining, corresponding to a light microscopic membranoproliferative pattern. Deposits typically stain for IgG and C3 and are polyclonal, but restricted to IgG4 subclass (anti-IgG, ×400).

subclass. In about half of cases, weaker IgA and IgM and C1q may also be detected. Rare cases of other patterns have been reported, with predominant IgA deposits, or distinct fibrillar deposits by electron microscopy but no immunoglobulin staining. Not infrequently, the deposits are so diffuse as to provide an apparent linear staining by immunofluorescence (Fig. 1.125). This may, especially in cases with crescents, lead to an initial erroneous impression of possible anti-GBM antibody–mediated glomerulonephritis. The smudgy, predominantly mesangial staining suggests the specific diagnosis, confirmed by electron microscopy and negative Congo red stain.

The electron microscopic findings are then confirmatory of the diagnosis of fibrillary glomerulonephritis, showing the presence of randomly aligned fibrils that resemble amyloid fibrils but are larger (Figs. 1.126-1.129). However, a precise distinction from amyloid cannot, in our experience, be made on fibril diameter alone. Fibril diameters in some series were 20-22 nm, with a range of 13-39 nm, contrasting amyloid cases with a mean of approximately 10 nm. However, in our series of fibrillary glomerulonephritis, there was some overlap, with average fibril diameter in fibrillary glomerulonephritis cases of 14 nm (range 10.4-18.4 nm). Therefore, it is critical to also use Congo red–negative staining and typical immunofluorescence staining, as described above, as diagnostic criteria. Electron microscopy may show fibrils in all glomerular compartments, including mesangium and basement membrane in intramembranous, subepithelial, and subendothelial locations. Additional dense deposits without distinct fibrillary composition have been observed in some cases (Fig. 1.128). Rare tubular basement membrane fibrillary deposits may occur (Fig. 1.130).

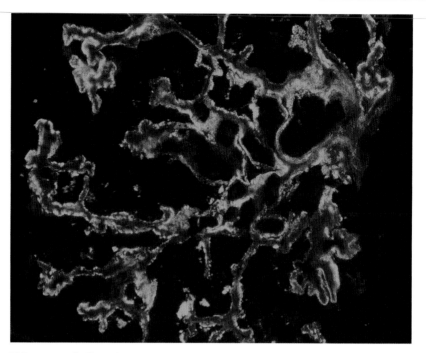

FIG. 1.125 Fibrillary glomerulonephritis may also show a membranous pattern of deposits in some cases, with corresponding coarsely granular peripheral loop deposits, along with coarse mesangial deposits as shown here (anti-IgG immunofluorescence, ×400).

Differential Diagnosis of Fibrils

- Fibrillary glomerulonephritis
  - LM: Proliferative, often crescents
  - IF: IgG polyclonal, smudgy
  - Congo red: Negative
  - EM: Fibrils random, 12-24 nm (mostly 18-20 nm)
- Immunotactoid glomerulopathy
  - LM: Proliferative
  - IF: IgG often clonal
  - Congo red: Negative
  - EM: Organized, parallel, microtubular (>30 nm)
- Amyloid
  - LM: Acellular, mesangial/lobular
  - IF: Monoclonal light chain for AL; no light chain for non-AL
  - Congo red: Positive
  - EM: fibrils random, 8-15 nm (mostly 10-12 nm)
- Cryoglobulinemic glomerulonephritis
  - LM: Proliferative, PAS-positive cryoplugs
  - IF: IgM, often clonal
  - Congo red: Negative
  - EM: Microtubular or vague, short fibrillary

EM, electron microscopy; *IF*, immunofluorescence; *LM*, light microscopy; *PAS*, periodic acid Schiff.

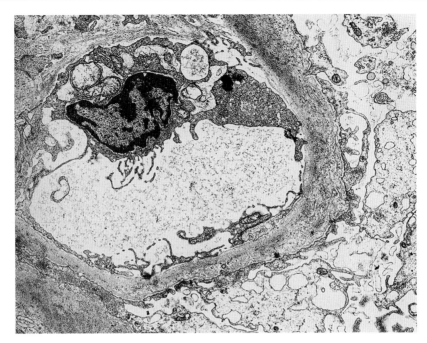

FIG. 1.126 Fibrillary glomerulonephritis. The deposits in fibrillary glomerulonephritis may be localized anywhere in the glomerulus. Randomly arranged fibrillar deposits, approximately 15 nm in diameter, permeate the thickened glomerular basement membrane, with overlying foot process effacement (transmission electron microscopy, ×4400).

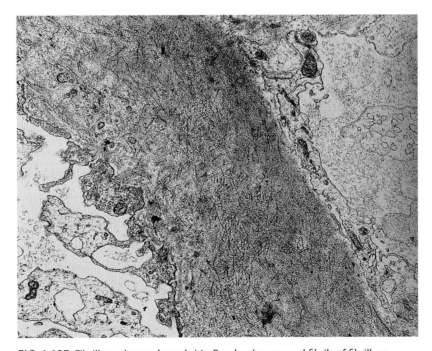

FIG. 1.127 Fibrillary glomerulonephritis. Randomly arranged fibrils of fibrillary glomerulonephritis permeate the glomerular basement membrane with blunting of overlying foot processes. The fibrils are slightly thicker than those seen in amyloid, but there may be overlap in fibril size in individual cases (transmission electron microscopy, ×7000).

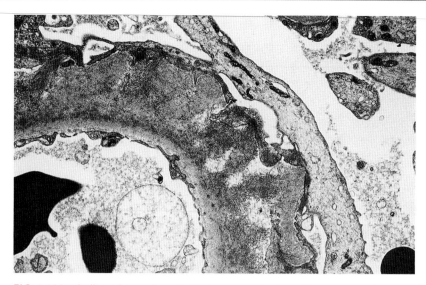

FIG. 1.128 Fibrillary glomerulonephritis. Large chunky deposits composed of randomly arranged fibrils are seen in this case of fibrillary glomerulonephritis, with interspersed more-amorphous deposits. The overlying foot processes are completely effaced (transmission electron microscopy, ×8000).

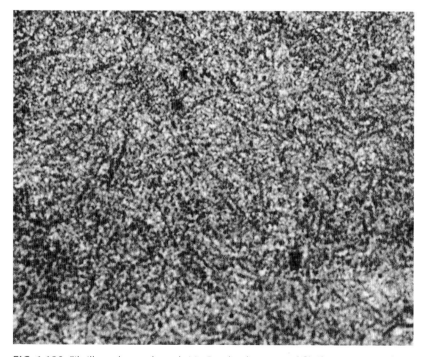

FIG. 1.129 Fibrillary glomerulonephritis. Randomly arranged fibrils, approximately 15 nm in diameter, in fibrillary glomerulonephritis, localized to the mesangium (transmission electron microscopy, ×15,000).

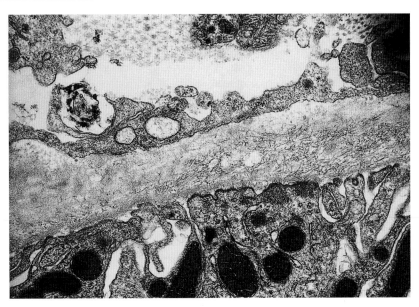

FIG. 1.130 Fibrillary glomerulonephritis. Rarely, there may be fibrillary deposits in tubular basement membranes in cases of fibrillary glomerulonephritis (transmission electron microscopy, ×7000). (Case shared by Dr Robert G. Horn.)

Etiology/Pathogenesis

The etiology of fibrillary glomerulonephritis is unknown. Amyloid P has been found to be bound to the fibrils. Cryoprecipitated mixed immunoglobulin–fibronectin complexes were detected in the serum of a patient with fibrillary glomerulonephritis who had no evidence of a systemic disease process. The immunoglobulin component was polyclonal and consisted of IgG, IgM, and heavy and light chains. These exciting findings indicate that serum precursors can lead to formation of fibrillary deposits. Occasional association with hepatitis C infection has been reported, but causality has not been proven. Importantly, fibrillary glomerulonephritis is not associated with excess incidence of lymphoproliferative disorders or monoclonality of deposits, in contrast to immunotactoid glomerulopathy.

Selected Reading

Alpers, C.E., 1992. Immunotactoid (microtubular) glomerulopathy: An entity distinct from fibrillary glomerulonephritis? American Journal of Kidney Disease 19, 185-191.

Alpers, C.E., Rennke, H.G., Hopper, J.J., et al., 1987. Fibrillary glomerulonephritis: An entity with unusual immunofluorescence features. Kidney International 31, 781-789.

Bridoux, F., Hugue, V., Coldefy, O., et al., 2002. Fibrillary glomerulonephritis and immunotactoid (microtubular) glomerulopathy are associated with distinct immunologic features. Kidney International 62, 1764-1775.

Churg, J., Venkataseshan, V.S., 1993. Fibrillary glomerulonephritis without immunoglobulin deposits in the kidney. Kidney International 44, 837-842.

Fogo, A., Quereshi, N., Horn, R.G., 1993. Morphologic and clinical features of fibrillary glomerulonephritis versus immunotactoid glomerulopathy. American Journal of Kidney Disease 22, 367-377.

Iskandar, S.S., Falk, R.J., Jennette, J.C., 1992. Clinical and pathological features of fibrillary glomerulonephritis. Kidney International 42, 1401-1407.

Korbet, S.M., Schwartz, M.M., Rosenberg, B.F., et al., 1985. Immunotactoid glomerulopathy. Medicine 64, 228-243.

Pronovost, P.H., Brady, H.R., Gunning, M.E., et al., 1996. Clinical features, predictors of disease progression and results of renal transplantation in fibrillary/immunotactoid glomerulopathy. Nephrology, Dialysis and Transplantation 11, 837-842.

Ray, S., Rouse, K., Appis, A., et al., 2008. Fibrillary glomerulonephritis with hepatitis C viral infection and hypocomplementemia. Renal Failure 30, 759-762.

Rosenmann, E., Eliakim, M., 1977. Nephrotic syndrome associated with amyloid-like glomerular deposits. Nephron 18, 301-308.

Rosenstock, J.L., Markowitz, G.S., Valeri, A.M., et al., 2003. Fibrillary and immunotactoid glomerulonephritis: Distinct entities with different clinical and pathologic features. Kidney International 63 (4), 1450-1461.

Schwartz, M.M., Lewis, E.J., 1980. The quarterly case: Nephrotic syndrome in a middle aged man. Ultrastructural Pathology 1, 575-582.

IMMUNOTACTOID GLOMERULOPATHY

The classification of lesions with organized non-amyloid fibrillar or microtubular deposits has been controversial. Some investigators have chosen to use the term *immunotactoid glomerulopathy* to refer to this entire group of disorders. We prefer to use the term *fibrillary glomerulonephritis* only for the amyloid-like, Congo red–negative form, as this may have implications for prognosis and pathogenesis. We will here discuss immunotactoid glomerulopathy, defined as large microtubular deposits typically >30 nm in diameter, often arranged in parallel arrays. This entity is very rare, less than 0.06% of adult native kidney biopsies. Patients are typically older than those with fibrillary glomerulonephritis, about 60-70 years versus about 50 years on average, and are mostly Caucasian. Patients present with nephrotic syndrome, hematuria, and some have hypocomplementemia. Importantly, there is associated monoclonal gammopathy and hematologic malignancy in about two thirds of patients, and deposits may stain in a monoclonal pattern. Patients do not generally have definable cryoglobulins, a disorder that may also give rise to organized deposits (see Cryoglobulinemic Glomerulonephritis). Renal survival appears better than in fibrillary glomerulonephritis, but published series have been too small and/or had too short follow-up for definitive analysis. In our six patients, renal function remained stable, whereas one patient in a series of patients reported by the Columbia group reached end stage in 2 months. Chemotherapy directed at the underlying lymphoproliferative disease led to remission of nephrotic syndrome in some patients with immunotactoid glomerulopathy. Recurrence in the transplant has been described for immunotactoid glomerulopathy, with a slower course of loss of GFR in the graft than in the native kidney.

Light microscopy shows a mesangioproliferative or membranoproliferative pattern (Figs. 1.131, 1.132). The GBM may show only double contours, or occasionally spikes. Tubules and interstitium show atrophy and fibrosis proportional to glomerular injury. Vessels do not show specific lesions. Crescents are rare. Congo red stains are by definition negative.

Immunofluorescence shows predominant IgG with lesser IgA and IgM in occasional cases (Fig. 1.133). C3 is also usually positive, with less frequent C1q. The staining is chunky, irregular along capillary loops and in the mesangium. It does not appear smudgy as does fibrillary glomerulonephritis deposits by immunofluorescence. The staining is usually stronger in capillary loops rather than in the mesangium, the converse of the pattern in fibrillary glomerulonephritis. Some cases may show monoclonal staining.

Immunotactoid Glomerulopathy Key Diagnostic Features

- Mesangial proliferative to membranoproliferative appearance by light microscopy
- Immunoglobulin and complement staining by immunofluorescence, may be clonal
- Deposits with microtubular or parallel array arrangement by electron microscopy

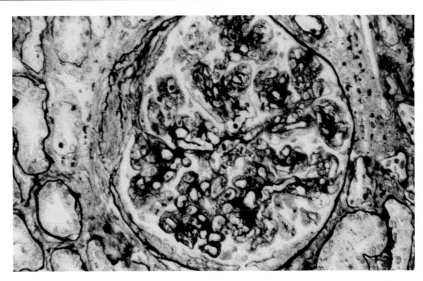

FIG. 1.131 Immunotactoid glomerulopathy. Light microscopic changes typically are those of a mesangial or membranoproliferative process, without crescents. Extensive glomerular basement membrane splitting and segmental adhesions are present in this case (Jones silver stain, ×200).

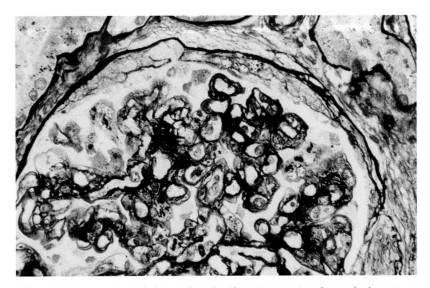

FIG. 1.132 Immunotactoid glomerulopathy. There is extensive glomerular basement membrane reduplication and interposition with mild mesangial and endocapillary proliferation (Jones silver stain, ×400).

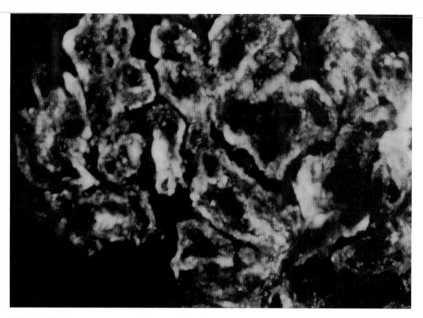

FIG. 1.133 Immunotactoid glomerulopathy. Immunofluorescence shows coarse positivity in a mesangial and membranoproliferative pattern, typically with IgG and C3. The subendothelial location of these deposits is evident by the smooth outer border of peripheral loop deposits. There are also chunky mesangial deposits (anti-IgG, immunofluorescence ×400).

Electron microscopy shows large microtubular deposits, usually >30 nm in diameter and sometimes >50 nm. The microtubules have a hollow core and are frequently arranged in parallel arrays, and may have a "stacked wood" arrangement (Figs. 1.134, 1.135). The distribution mirrors that seen by immunofluorescence, with predominant subendothelial and mesangial deposits. Some cases also have subepithelial or intramembranous deposits.

Etiology/Pathogenesis

Immunotactoid glomerulopathy, defined by microtubular deposits, often in organized arrays, is significantly more frequently associated with monoclonal protein and hematopoietic malignancy than is fibrillary glomerulonephritis. Further, these immunotactoid deposits stain monoclonally in about two thirds of cases. The clinical improvement of proteinuria when treatment was directed at the hematopoietic disorder, with parallel improvement of hematologic parameters, further supports a role for monoclonal proteins in some of these patients.

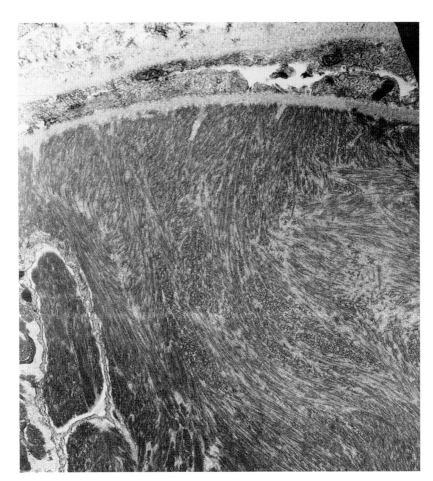

FIG. 1.134 Immunotactoid glomerulopathy. The specific diagnosis of immunotactoid glomerulopathy is made by electron microscopy. The deposits are microtubular and/or organized in parallel arrays, appearing like "kindling wood stacked up for the winter." The tubules are frequently 30-50 nm in diameter and are here seen both in longitudinal and cross section, revealing their tubular nature. A similar appearance may be seen in some cases of cryoglobulinemic glomerulonephritis (transmission electron microscopy, ×12,000).

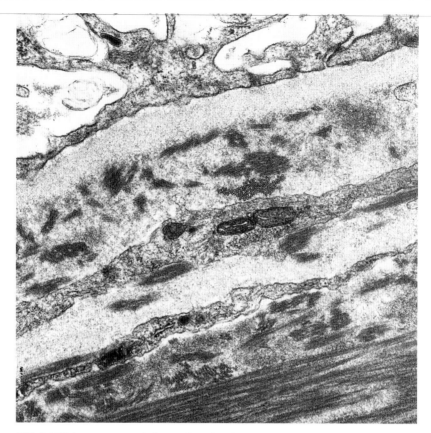

FIG. 1.135 Immunotactoid glomerulopathy. The microtubular nature of the deposits in immunotactoid glomerulopathy is illustrated, with microtubules cut in cross and longitudinal orientation. The deposits are intramembranous and subendothelial, with associated foot process effacement and interposition (transmission electron microscopy, ×26,000).

Selected Reading

Alpers, C.E., 1992. Immunotactoid (microtubular) glomerulopathy: An entity distinct from fibrillary glomerulonephritis? American Journal of Kidney Disease 19, 185-191.

Bridoux, F., Hugue, V., Coldefy, O., et al., 2002. Fibrillary glomerulonephritis and immunotactoid (microtubular) glomerulopathy are associated with distinct immunologic features. Kidney International 62, 1764-1775.

Fogo, A., Quereshi, N., Horn, R.G., 1993. Morphologic and clinical features of fibrillary glomerulonephritis versus immunotactoid glomerulopathy. American Journal of Kidney Disease 22, 367-377.

Korbet, S.M., Schwartz, M.M., Rosenberg, B.F., et al., 1985. Immunotactoid glomerulopathy. Medicine 64, 228-243.

Pronovost, P.H., Brady, H.R., Gunning, M.E., et al., 1996. Clinical features, predictors of disease progression and results of renal transplantation in fibrillary/immunotactoid glomerulopathy. Nephrology, Dialysis and Transplantation 11, 837-842.

Rosenstock, J.L., Markowitz, G.S., Valeri, A.M., et al., 2003. Fibrillary and immunotactoid glomerulonephritis: Distinct entities with different clinical and pathologic features. Kidney International 63, 1450-1461.

Glomerular Diseases That Cause Hematuria or Nephritic Syndrome: Immune Complex

ACUTE POSTINFECTIOUS GLOMERULONEPHRITIS

Postinfectious glomerulonephritis presents as acute nephritic syndrome. Classically, this condition follows streptococcal infection. Other bacterial, viral, mycotic, or even protozoan infections may give rise to the same type of glomerulonephritis. Staphylococcal infection can cause postinfectious glomerulonephritis with IgA-dominant staining pattern. In tropical climates, skin infection rather than throat infection may lead to acute glomerulonephritis. Acute poststreptococcal glomerulonephritis is more common in children and young adults, with boys affected more than girls. Patients with typical poststreptococcal glomerulonephritis following a pharyngitic infection usually have a rapid course with rapid resolution, and thus are not biopsied. Biopsies therefore may overrepresent more severe lesions. A small subset of patients has persistent renal dysfunction long-term after the acute nephritis subsides. Unrecognized subclinical disease related to postinfectious glomerulonephritis may also contribute to chronic renal disease. Children with this lesion have an excellent prognosis when the infection is transient. In a large series of postinfectious glomerulonephritis in predominantly adult patients, the majority of patients had glomerulosclerosis on rebiopsy 3-15 years from onset. When IgA-dominant poststaphylococcal glomerulonephritis occurred superimposed on diabetes nephropathy, prognosis was particularly ominous, with most patients reaching end-stage kidney disease.

The light microscopic characteristic features in the acute phase are diffuse, exudative proliferative glomerulonephritis, with prominent endocapillary proliferation (Fig. 1.136) and numerous neutrophils (Figs. 1.137-1.144). The proliferative lesions are diffuse and global.

Key Diagnostic Features of Acute Postinfectious Glomerulonephritis

- Exudative proliferative appearance, with numerous polymorphonuclear leukocytes, by light microscopy
- IgG and strong C3 by immunofluorescence, irregular, chunky mesangial and capillary wall pattern
- Hump-type subepithelial deposits by electron microscopy

Differential Diagnosis of Postinfectious Glomerulonephritis

- Endocapillary proliferation with PMNs may also be seen in cryoglobulinemic glomerulonephritis.
- Subacute postinfectious glomerulonephritis has a membranoproliferative or mesangial proliferative appearance.
- Differential diagnosis of deposits with prominent or dominant C3 includes:
  - Lupus nephritis or lupus-like conditions—usually full-house staining by IF, reticular aggregates by EM
  - Glomerulonephritis C3—lack of PMNs, usually no Ig staining, may also have rare hump-type deposits
  - Dense deposit disease—only C3 staining by IF, characteristic dense deposits by EM
  - IgA-dominant postinfectious glomerulonephritis—may differentiate from IgA nephropathy by PMNs, frequent hump-type deposits, dominant C3, and usually kappa>lambda by IF

EM, electron microscopy; *IF,* immunofluorescence; *PMN,* polymorphonuclear leukocyte.

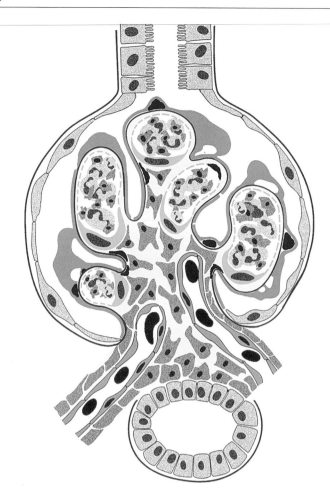

FIG. 1.136 Acute postinfectious glomerulonephritis. There is an exudative proliferation with numerous polymorphonuclear leukocytes and endocapillary proliferation, with scattered mesangial and large hump-shaped subepithelial deposits.

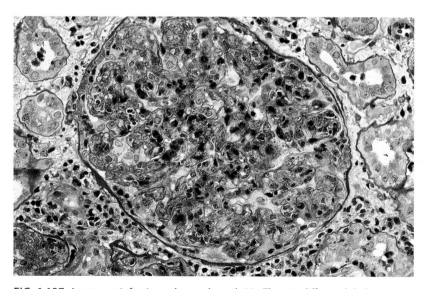

FIG. 1.137 Acute postinfectious glomerulonephritis. There is diffuse, global exudative proliferation with prominent endocapillary proliferation and numerous neutrophils. There is also surrounding inflammation in the tubulointerstitium (periodic acid Schiff, ×400).

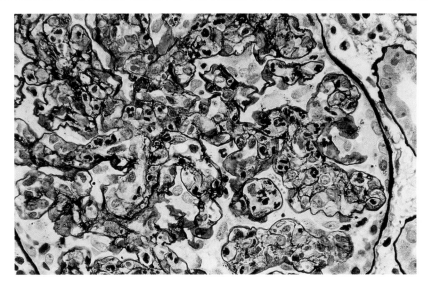

FIG. 1.138 Acute postinfectious glomerulonephritis. The numerous polymorphonuclear leukocytes filling capillary lumens are clearly demonstrated, along with endocapillary proliferation and segmental interposition (Jones silver stain, ×400).

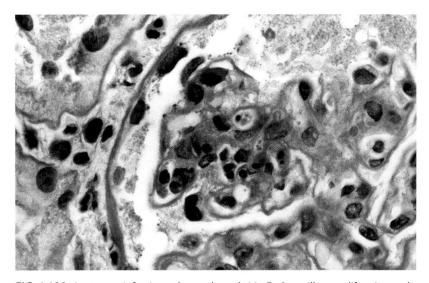

FIG. 1.139 Acute postinfectious glomerulonephritis. Endocapillary proliferation and numerous polymorphonuclear leukocytes both within capillary loops and within the mesangial area are present. Deposits are not visualized here, although they may occasionally be seen by light microscopy (see Fig. 1.144) (hematoxylin and eosin, ×1000).

Small hump-shaped deposits may occasionally be visualized even by light microscopy with silver, trichrome, or toluidine blue stains (Fig. 1.144). Crescents are present in severe cases and may portend worse prognosis (Fig. 1.140). When biopsy is performed later in the course, the neutrophilic infiltrate is less prominent with remaining diffuse mesangial hypercellularity (Figs 1.141-1.143).

By immunofluorescence, scattered fine or large chunky deposits are present along the GBM, along with scattered mesangial deposits. The deposits typically stain with IgG

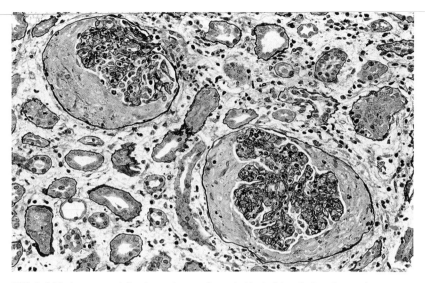

FIG. 1.140 Acute postinfectious glomerulonephritis. In biopsied patients, there may frequently be crescents as these patients typically have an unusual clinical course with more severe injury. The cellular crescents are associated with endocapillary proliferation and abundant polymorphonuclear leukocytes. There is also associated extensive edema and tubulointerstitial inflammation (Jones silver stain, ×100).

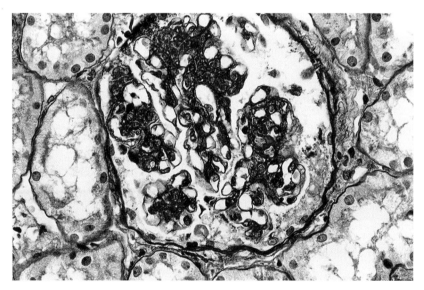

FIG. 1.141 Acute postinfectious glomerulonephritis. In the latter stages following onset of the disease, there may be less prominent neutrophilic infiltrate with focal segmental mesangial and/or endocapillary proliferation. Immunofluorescence and electron microscopy studies are then key in pointing to a postinfectious etiology (periodic acid Schiff, ×200).

with even more prominent C3 staining after the first few weeks. IgM and IgA staining is absent or minimal, except in cases caused by staphylococcal infection, where IgA may be dominant.

Three immunofluorescence patterns of typical poststreptococcal postinfectious glomerulonephritis have been described: starry sky, garland, and mesangial patterns (Figs. 1.145-1.148). The starry sky or garland patterns are seen early in the course of the disease, with garland-type

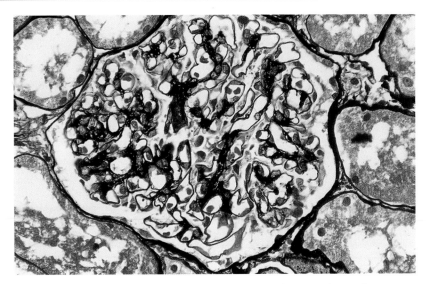

FIG. 1.142 Acute postinfectious glomerulonephritis. In this case of postinfectious glomerulonephritis, there is only segmental mesangial proliferation with very segmental endocapillary extension of the proliferation. No polymorphonuclear leukocytes remain at this late state where deposits are visualized in the mesangial area and at 9 o'clock, confirmed by immunofluorescence and electron microscopy studies (Jones silver stain, ×200).

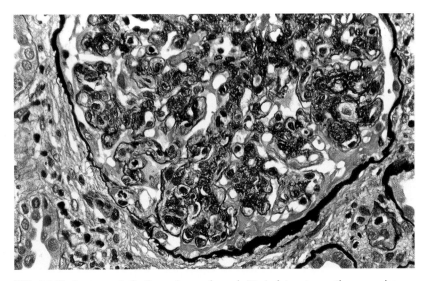

FIG. 1.143 Acute postinfectious glomerulonephritis. In later stages, there may be also diffuse, global endocapillary proliferation. In this case, there is extensive glomerular basement membrane reduplication, and polymorphonuclear leukocytes still remain. The postinfectious etiology was strongly suggested by immunofluorescence findings with predominant C3 and hump-shaped, rare deposits by electron microscopy (Jones silver stain, ×400).

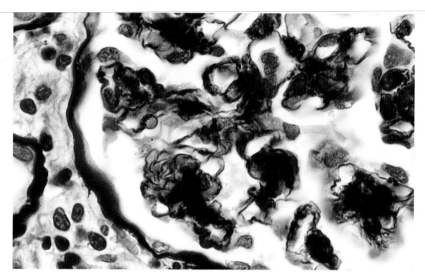

FIG. 1.144 Acute postinfectious glomerulonephritis. Large, hump-shaped deposits may occasionally be seen by light microscopy (Jones silver stain, ×1000).

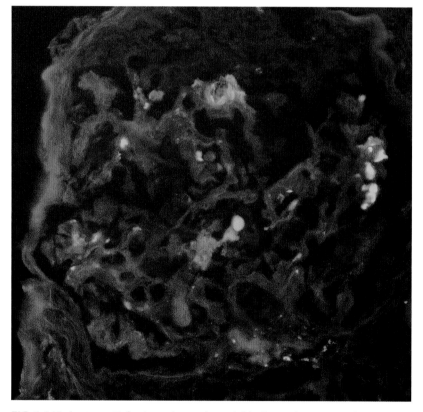

FIG. 1.145 Acute postinfectious glomerulonephritis. Starry sky pattern of immunofluorescence positivity is shown, with coarse, irregularly distributed fluorescence along the glomerular basement membrane, along with some mesangial staining (anti-IgG immunofluorescence, ×400).

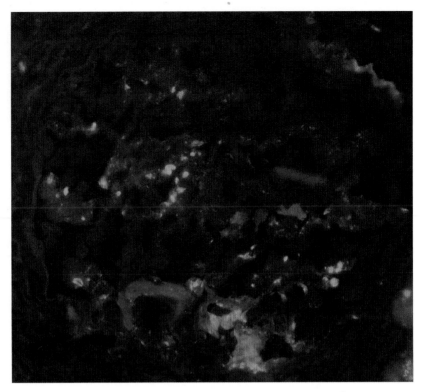

FIG. 1.146 Acute postinfectious glomerulonephritis. C3 positivity is often even stronger than IgG in postinfectious glomerulonephritis. This is the same case as in Figure 1.129, with predominant starry sky pattern, with occasional segments with thicker, more elongated deposits, so-called garland pattern (bottom) (anti-C3 immunofluorescence, ×400).

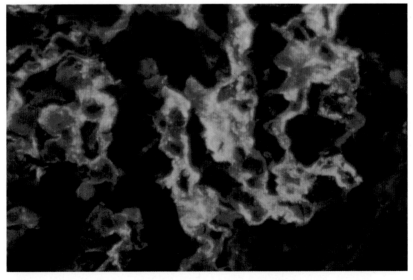

FIG. 1.147 Acute postinfectious glomerulonephritis. A more extensive garland pattern with elongated peripheral loop deposits is illustrated, along with occasional small mesangial deposits (anti-C3 immunofluorescence, ×400).

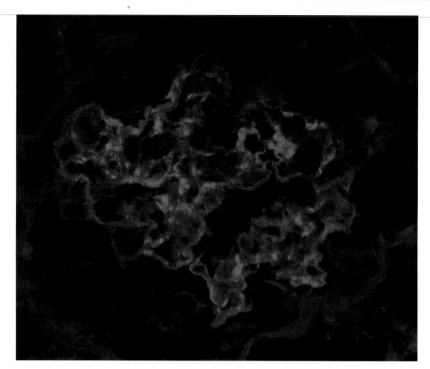

FIG. 1.148 Acute postinfectious glomerulonephritis. In the more chronic phase of the disease, mesangial deposits may be predominant, usually with less endocapillary proliferation and exudation, as illustrated here. There are very few, scattered subepithelial deposits, corresponding to rare hump-type deposits by electron microscopy (anti-C3 immunofluorescence, ×400).

deposits extending to the peripheral loops, associated with an exudative hypercellular glomerular lesion. Starry sky refers to the irregularly distributed coarse fluorescence positivity along the GBM. The garland pattern shows thicker, more elongated deposits along the capillary wall, is more commonly present in adults, and has been associated with worse prognosis (Fig. 1.147).

By electron microscopy, there are scattered subepithelial, hump-shaped deposits overlying the GBM without surrounding basement membrane reaction (Figs. 1.149-1.151). These hump deposits are particularly numerous in the acute phase and may be variegated. Occasional mesangial and subendothelial deposits are present. When biopsies are performed at a later stage, peripheral hump-type deposits are more rare. Hump-shaped deposits may then only be present in the subepithelial area overlying the mesangium (the "notch" or "waist" area) (Fig. 1.151). In the more chronic phase of the disease, mesangial deposits predominate, usually with less endocapillary proliferation and exudation. The finding of even rare hump-type subepithelial deposits strongly points to an infectious etiology of an immune complex glomerulonephritis, and it is quite helpful in suggesting etiology when biopsy is done in the more chronic phase where only mesangial proliferation or focal membranoproliferative changes are present by light microscopy. Note that patients with C3 glomerulonephritis may also have occasional hump-type deposits. Thus, clinical correlation is essential. Evidence of previous clinically silent postinfectious glomerulonephritis with healed "incidental" postinfectious lesions, deduced by presence of these hump-type subepithelial deposits by electron microscopy, was detected in about 10% of biopsies in one retrospective study. These deposits were associated with a variety of other renal lesions and may be additional contributors to progressive renal damage.

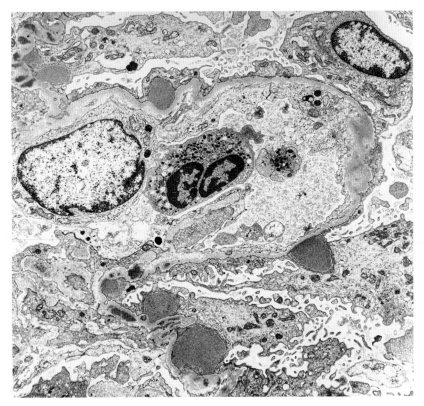

FIG. 1.149 Acute postinfectious glomerulonephritis. There is an intraluminal polymorphonuclear leukocyte, a platelet and endocapillary proliferation, with scattered intramembranous and large hump-shaped deposits without surrounding basement membrane reaction (transmission electron microscopy, ×3000).

Etiology/Pathogenesis

The immunopathogenesis of poststreptococcal glomerulonephritis has been studied extensively. Numerous streptococcal antigens have been proposed as the target antigen, including streptococcal exotoxin B (Spe B) and streptococcal GAPDH. Both of these antigens activate the alternative complement pathway, resulting in low serum complements, and have affinity for glomerular proteins and plasmin. Staphylococcal antigens may function as superantigens, and they can cause an IgA-dominant postinfectious glomerulonephritis. When these antigens are deposited in glomeruli, plasmin can then contribute to glomerular damage by activating proteolysis. Whether circulating immune complexes deposit in the glomeruli, or the antigens traverse the GBM and bind to sites within the glomerulus and stimulate antibody and subsequent complement activation, is not determined. Individual variability in susceptibility to glomerulonephritis after infection with presumed "nephritogenic" strains of bacteria is linked to HLA class II allelic variation, with resistance to disease in those patients with reduced immune responsiveness. The presence of humps in some patients with C3 glomerulonephritis could possibly represent increased susceptibility to infection-triggered initiation of injury in a patient with abnormal complement regulation. Such patients frequently have persistant and/or recurring disease flares, and even recurrence in transplants.

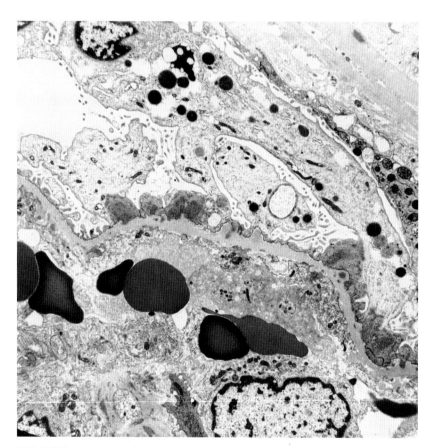

FIG. 1.150 Acute postinfectious glomerulonephritis. More continuous areas of hump-shaped subepithelial deposits are present, corresponding to the garland pattern by immunofluorescence. Rare small intramembranous and subendothelial deposits (bottom) are also present, along with endocapillary proliferation (transmission electron microscopy, ×3000).

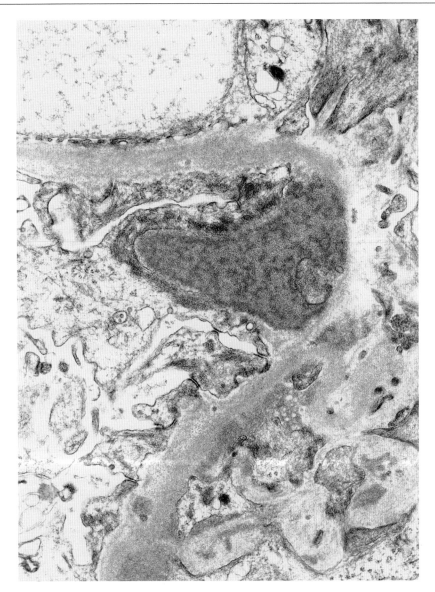

FIG. 1.151 Acute postinfectious glomerulonephritis. Small mesangial deposits and a large, variegated, hump-shaped deposit located subepithelially in the waist region are present. This area is the last place where hump-shaped deposits persist. The presence of even rare hump-shaped deposits is a useful, but not pathognomonic, indicator of an underlying infectious etiology for an immune complex glomerulonephritis (transmission electron microscopy, ×25,625).

Selected Reading

Baldwin, D.S., Gluck, M.C., Schacht, R.G., et al., 1974. The long-term course of poststreptococcal glomerulonephritis. Annals of Internal Medicine 80, 342-358.

Edelstein, C.L., Bates, W.D., 1992. Subtypes of acute postinfectious glomerulonephritis: A clinico-pathological correlation. Clinical Nephrology 38, 311-317.

Haas, M., 2003. Incidental healed postinfectious glomerulonephritis: a study of 1012. renal biopsy specimens examined by electron microscopy. Human Pathology 34, 3-10.

Haas, M., Racusen, L.C., Bagnasco, S.M., 2008. IgA-dominant postinfectious glomerulonephritis: a report of 13 cases with common ultrastructural features. Human Pathology 39, 1309-1316.

Kanjanabuch, T., Kittikowit, W., Eiam-Ong, S., 2009. An update on acute postinfectious glomerulonephritis worldwide. Nature Review Nephrology 5, 259-269.

Kotb, M., Norrby-Teglund, A., McGeer, A., et al., 2002. An immunogenetic and molecular basis for differences in outcomes of invasive group A streptococcal infections. Nature Medicine 8 (12), 1398-1404.

Lewy, J.E., Salinas-Madrigal, L., Herdson, P.B., et al., 1971. Clinico-pathologic correlations in acute poststreptococcal glomerulonephritis. A correlation between renal functions, morphologic damage and clinical course of 46 children with acute poststreptococcal glomerulonephritis. Medicine (Baltimore) 50, 453-501.

Nasr, S.H., Markowitz, G.S., Stokes, M.B., et al., 2008. Acute postinfectious glomerulonephritis in the modern era: experience with 86 adults and review of the literature. Medicine (Baltimore) 87, 21-32.

Sagel, I., Treser, G., Ty, A., et al., 1973. Occurrence and nature of glomerular lesions after group A streptococci infections in children. Annals of Internal Medicine 79 (4), 492-499.

Sorger, K., Balun, J., Hubner, F.K., et al., 1983. The garland type of acute postinfectious glomerulonephritis: morphological characteristics and follow-up studies. Clinical Nephrology 20, 17-26.

Sorger, K., Gessler, M., Hubner, F.K., et al., 1987. Follow-up studies of three subtypes of acute postinfectious glomerulonephritis ascertained by renal biopsy. Clinical Nephrology 27, 111-124.

Sorger, K., Gessler, U., Hubner, F.K., et al., 1982. Subtypes of acute postinfectious glomerulonephritis. Synopsis of clinical and pathological features. Clinical Nephrology 17, 114-128.

IgA NEPHROPATHY

IgA nephropathy (IgAN) is the most common glomerulonephritis in renal biopsies worldwide. Patients with IgAN present with hematuria, either microscopic or macroscopic, and varying proteinuria. Occasionally proteinuria may reach nephrotic range. The disease occurs in all age groups. The incidence of IgAN in African Americans and Africans is much lower than in other populations. The apparent higher incidence of IgA nephropathy in biopsy series from Japan likely reflects the practice of widespread screening urinalysis and frequent renal biopsy for isolated microscopic hematuria. The clinical presentation gives useful prognostic information in patients with IgA nephropathy, with worse prognosis in older male patients with hypertension, marked proteinuria, and increased creatinine at presentation and persistent microscopic hematuria. Prognosis is quite variable, with some patients showing rapid progression and approximately one third developing chronic renal failure over long-term, 30-year, follow-up. Recurrence of IgAN in the transplant occurs in up to 60% of patients, but morphologic recurrence does not equate to graft loss. When recurrence shows a proliferative or crescentic pattern, outcome may be worse.

The light microscopic appearance in IgA nephropathy varies from minimal mesangial expansion (Fig. 1.152) to diffuse proliferative lesions with crescents or widespread sclerosis.

Key Diagnostic Features of IgA Nephropathy

- IgA-dominant (or codominant) deposits by immunofluorescence
- Mesangial and occasionally subendothelial deposits by electron microscopy
- Variable light microscopic appearance; normal, mesangial proliferative, focal or diffuse proliferative, with or without crescents and/or sclerosis

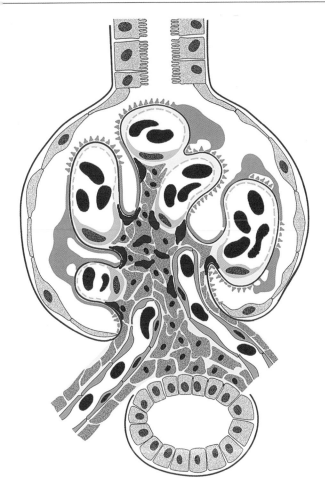

FIG. 1.152 IgA nephropathy. There is mesangial cell and matrix increase, with mesangial deposits.

There is often mesangial area increase due to increase in both mesangial cells, matrix, and deposits (Figs. 1.153-1.156). In some cases, deposits can be outlined on the silver stain as they are silver negative (Fig. 1.157). Endocapillary proliferation may be present, in either focal segmental or diffuse distribution, and is typically associated with extension of deposits to subendothelial areas of peripheral loops (Fig. 1.158). These deposits can result in mesangial interposition and GBM double contours. With severe injury, there may be segmental necrosis and crescents (Figs. 1.159, 1.160). In chronic cases, there is often segmental sclerosis, with proportional tubular atrophy and interstitial fibrosis (Figs. 1.161-1.163).

The relative frequency of proliferative lesions versus sclerosing lesions and minimal light microscopic findings likely reflects biopsy practices. In a large series, 13% of biopsies showed only minimal mesangial expansion, 6% showed diffuse mesangial hypercellularity, 80% showed focal segmental glomerulosclerosis and/or focal segmental proliferative lesions with crescents, and 1% showed an end-stage kidney. Classifications based on light microscopic appearance have been proposed, with parallels to the commonly used WHO classification for SLE nephritis (Tables 1.3, 1.4). The recent Oxford classification of IgAN (Table 1.5) is based on detailed examination of all lesions, selection of those reliably scoreable for further analysis, and then analysis with clinical correlation to arrive at a validated classification. The Oxford IgAN classification identified four morphologic features linked to worse prognosis, namely, any segmental glomerulosclerosis or adhesion, any endocapillary proliferation, even mild mesangial proliferation, and >25% tubulointerstitial fibrosis. Scoring mesangial proliferation was done by counting nuclei in each glomerulus in the most cellular mesangial area away from the vascular pole, with 3 nuclei/mesangial area defined as normal, and 4-5 nuclei given

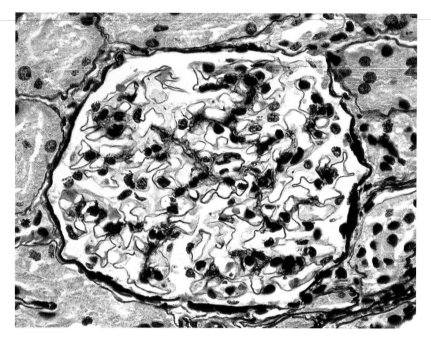

FIG. 1.153 IgA nephropathy. There may be inconspicuous changes by light microscopy with only minimal or no apparent increase in matrix. In these cases, the diagnosis rests on immunofluorescence and electron microscopy for a specific diagnosis of IgA nephropathy (Jones silver stain, ×200).

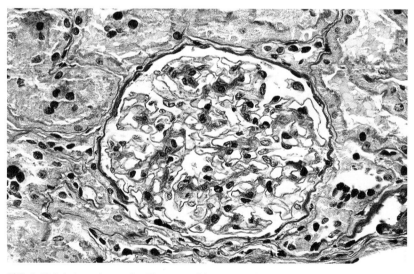

FIG. 1.154 IgA nephropathy. There is mild mesangial matrix expansion and a mild increase in mesangial cellularity, with three or more nuclei in most mesangial areas in this early case of IgA nephropathy (periodic acid Schiff, ×200).

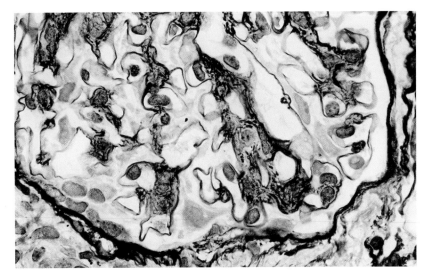

FIG. 1.155 IgA nephropathy. The expanded mesangial matrix is evident, with more lucent, weakly periodic acid Schiff–positive areas representing the immune deposits, verified by immunofluorescence and electron microscopy (Jones silver stain, ×1000).

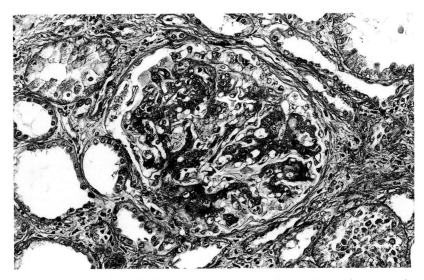

FIG. 1.156 IgA nephropathy. There is marked mesangial expansion, with segmental proliferation extending out to peripheral capillary loops, and early focal proliferative lesion (Masson trichrome stain, ×200).

a score of 1, 6-7 scored as 2, and ≥8 as 3. If even only half of glomeruli were hypercellular, that is, average score of ≥0.5, prognosis was worse. Of note, this classification was based on archival material, did not include patients with progression to end-stage kidney disease within a year or those with minimal proteinuria or with Henoch–Schönlein purpura. These limitations, and treatment variability, likely explain why crescents were not associated with worse outcome, as those patients with crescents were treated more aggressively. These morphologic predictors were confirmed to be valid in children in the Oxford series. Recent validation studies show similar results in other populations, including from North America, Europe, and China.

Henoch–Schönlein purpura may be thought of as the systemic counterpart of IgA nephropathy. The lesions in the kidney are indistinguishable, and differentiation is made based on

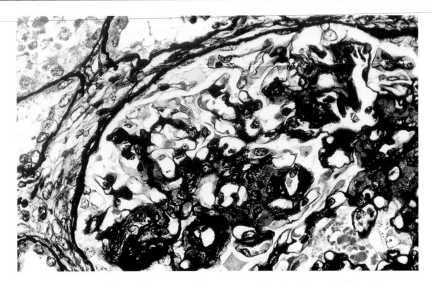

FIG. 1.157 IgA nephropathy. Massive deposits are visualized as periodic acid Schiff-positive areas within the mesangium in this case of advanced IgA nephropathy with mesangial proliferation and segmental sclerosis (top upper right) (Jones silver stain, ×400).

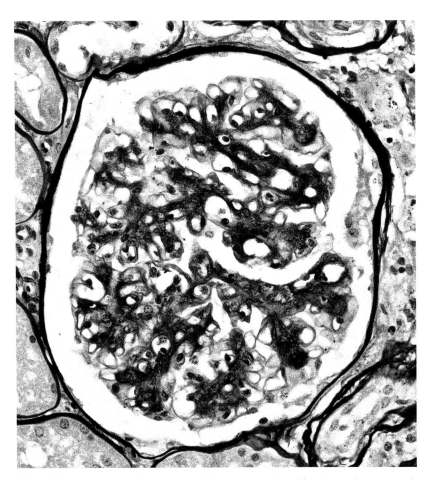

FIG. 1.158 IgA nephropathy. There is diffuse mesangial proliferation with segmental endocapillary proliferation and occasional peripheral basement membrane reduplication, evidence of deposits extending to peripheral loops (Jones silver stain, ×200).

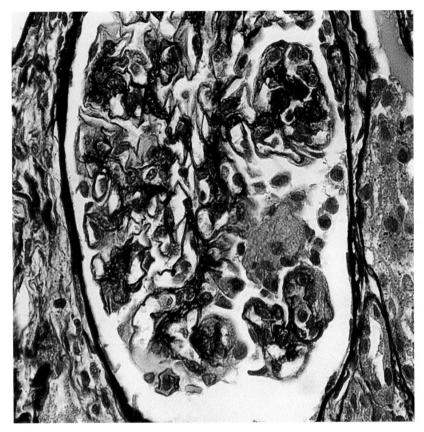

FIG. 1.159 IgA nephropathy. Mild mesangial proliferation is associated with segmental peripheral capillary loop double contours and endocapillary proliferation, and a small area of segmental fibrinoid necrosis (Jones silver stain, ×400).

Key Differential Diagnosis of IgA Nephropathy

- IgA nephropathy versus lupus nephritis: When IgA staining is equally strong as IgG, lupus nephritis may enter the differential. C1q positivity is rare in IgA nephropathy, and frequent in lupus nephritis. The presence of reticular aggregates also strongly favors lupus nephritis.
- IgA nephropathy versus IgA-dominant postinfectious glomerulonephritis: The presence of hump-type deposits, dominant C3, and an exudative appearance with polymorphonuclear leukocytes within the endocapillary proliferative lesions favor a postinfectious etiology. In IgA nephropathy, lambda is usually, but not invariably, stronger than kappa. Stronger kappa than lambda staining slightly favors postinfectious etiology.
- IgA nephropathy versus cryoglobulinemic glomerulonephritis: If IgA and IgM are codominant, cryoglobulinemic glomerulonephritis should be excluded. Cryoglobulinemic glomerulonephritis typically has clonal shift with kappa or lambda dominance and may have PAS-positive intracapillary cryoplugs and substructure of deposits by electron microscopy.

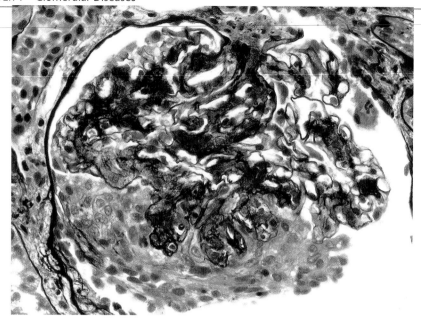

FIG. 1.160 IgA nephropathy. The underlying IgA nephropathy giving rise to the crescentic injury is evident by moderate mesangial proliferation with segmental peripheral capillary loop alteration (right). In addition, characteristic IgA positivity by immunofluorescent and electron microscopic demonstration of well-defined deposits were present (Jones silver stain, ×200).

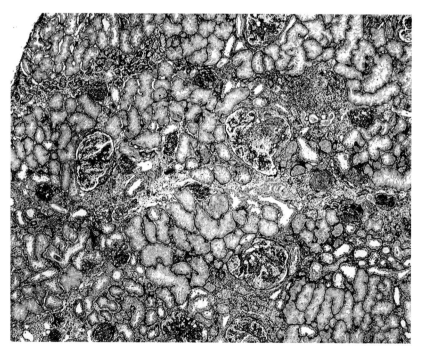

FIG. 1.161 IgA nephropathy. With ongoing injury, there may be extensive glomerulosclerosis, both segmental and global, often with associated more active lesions of endocapillary proliferation and cellular or fibrocellular crescents. Numerous adhesions with thickened areas of Bowman's capsule, indicative of past healed proliferative lesions, are present, in addition to the extensive global sclerosis and segmental sclerosis. There is associated tubulointerstitial atrophy and fibrosis (Jones silver stain, ×100).

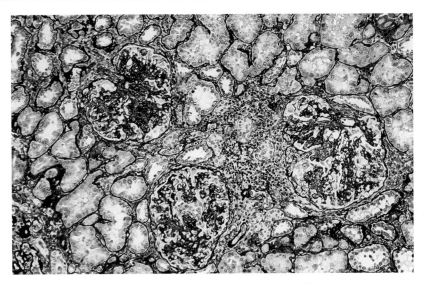

FIG. 1.162 IgA nephropathy. Mild to moderate mesangial proliferation, segmental endocapillary proliferation, early cellular crescent formation (left and top) with numerous adhesions, indicative of organization of past active lesions are present. There is early tubulointerstitial fibrosis, and active tubulointerstitial infiltrate surrounds the glomeruli with early crescentic injury and disruption of Bowman's capsule (Jones silver stain, ×200).

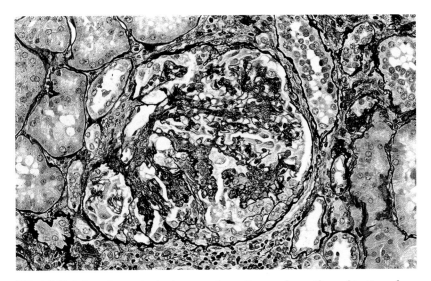

FIG. 1.163 IgA nephropathy. Lesions may be quite complex, with combination of adhesions, small cellular crescents, mesangial and endocapillary proliferation with peripheral basement membrane splitting. There is also early surrounding tubulointerstitial fibrosis and inflammation (Jones silver stain, ×200).

TABLE 1-3 Haas Classification of IgA Nephropathy

I	Minimal or no mesangial hypercellularity.
II	Focal and segmental glomerulosclerosis without cellular proliferation*
III	Focal proliferative glomerulonephritis*
IV	Diffuse proliferative glomerulonephritis
V	≥40% global glomerulosclerosis, and/or ≥40% cortical tubular atrophy

*Focal refers to <50% of glomeruli with the lesion.
FSGS, focal segmental glomerulosclerosis.

TABLE 1-4 WHO Classification of IgA Nephropathy

I	Minimal lesion
II	Minor changes with small segmental proliferation
III	Focal and segmental glomerulonephritis (<50% involved)
IV	Diffuse mesangial lesions with proliferation and sclerosis
V	Diffuse sclerosing glomerulonephritis affecting >80% of glomeruli

TABLE 1-5 Oxford Classification of IgA Nephropathy

Variable	Definition	Score
Mesangial hypercellularity	Scored from 0 to 3*	M0 0.5 M1>0.5
Segmental glomerulosclerosis	Sclerosis in segmental pattern, or the presence of an adhesion	S0 – absent S1 – present
Endocapillary hypercellularity	Hypercellularity due to increased number of cells within glomerular capillary lumina causing narrowing of the lumina	E0 – absent E1 – present
Tubular atrophy/interstitial fibrosis	Percentage of cortical area involved by tubular atrophy/interstitial fibrosis	T0 – 0-25% T1 – 26-50% T2 – >50%

*Mesangial score should be assessed in periodic acid Schiff–stained sections. Up to three mesangial cells in a mesangial area away from the vascular pole is scored as 0, four or five as 1, six or seven as 2, and eight or more as 3. Average score is calculated based on all glomeruli, excluding those with global sclerosis or global endocapillary proliferation. Mathematically, if more than half of glomeruli have mesangial hypercellularity, the score will be >0.5, and precise derivation of the mesangial score is then not necessary.

clinical pathologic features. The International Study of Kidney Disease in Children has used a classification for renal disease in patients with Henoch–Schönlein purpura (see "Henoch–Schönlein Purpura").

Immunofluorescence microscopy reveals the definitive characteristic of dominant or codominant deposits of IgA. These deposits may be confined to the mesangium (Fig. 1.164) or extend to subendothelial location of peripheral capillary loops, typically associated with proliferative lesions (Fig. 1.165). C3 is almost invariably present, but C1q is rarely positive. The immunofluorescence positivity for IgA is diffuse and global, although the light microscopic lesions may be focal and segmental. Of note, lambda staining is typically more predominant than kappa staining, in contrast to predominance of kappa in other polyclonal immune complex diseases. IgG and/or IgM may also be present, but by definition, are not present in greater intensity than IgA.

By electron microscopy, deposits are found in the mesangial areas, underlying the paramesangial GBM (Figs. 1.166, 1.167). There is increased mesangial matrix, and mesangial cellularity may also be increased. Subendothelial deposits are typically present in cases with

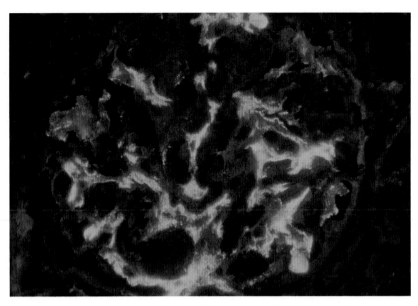

FIG. 1.164 IgA nephropathy. Definitive diagnosis is made by dominant or codominant staining with IgA in a predominantly mesangial pattern, as shown here. The mesangial location results in a "pruned shrub" appearance (anti-IgA immunofluorescence, ×400).

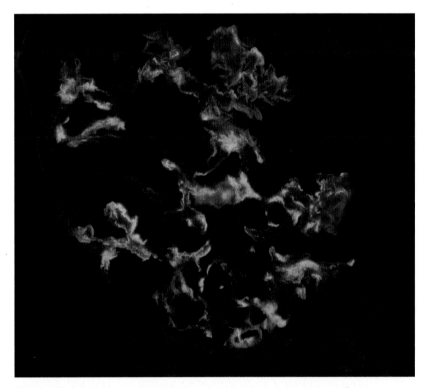

FIG. 1.165 IgA nephropathy. Definitive diagnosis is made by immunofluorescence, showing dominant or codominant IgA staining in the mesangium. In cases with more active lesions, there is frequent extension to peripheral capillary loops, as seen segmentally in this case (left) (anti-IgA immunofluorescence, ×400).

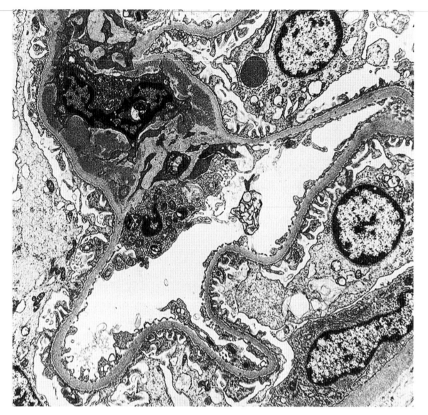

FIG. 1.166 IgA nephropathy. The deposits are in the mesangial area, underneath the paramesangial basement membrane. In this case, there is no extension of deposits to peripheral loops, and there was only mesangial proliferation by light microscopy (transmission electron microscopy, ×3000).

endocapillary proliferation, and extend out from the mesangial area (Fig. 1.168). Occasionally, there may be subepithelial or intramembranous deposits. Foot processes are effaced over areas with sclerosis. The distribution of deposits mirrors the immunofluorescence pattern (Fig. 1.169).

Etiology/Pathogenesis

The pathogenesis of progressive injury in IgAN is unknown. Morphologic features provide additional prognostic information over the clinical findings (see above).

Interestingly, IgAN recurs in the transplant, and conversely, IgAN regressed when transplantation of kidneys with mild IgAN into patients with end-stage renal disease from other causes was inadvertently performed. These observations strongly indicate that IgAN has a systemic basis. The etiology of IgA nephropathy remains unknown. Current research has focused on abnormal mucosal immune reactivity, production of IgA with an abnormal hinge region resistant to proteolysis, IgG antiglycan antibodies produced in response to this IgA, and genetic factors. Antiglycan IgG antibodies were identified in serum of patients with IgAN. The hinge region of IgA1 usually has bound oligosaccharides that are O-linked to serine or threonine residues. Abnormal oligosaccharides are postulated to be causal in resistance to

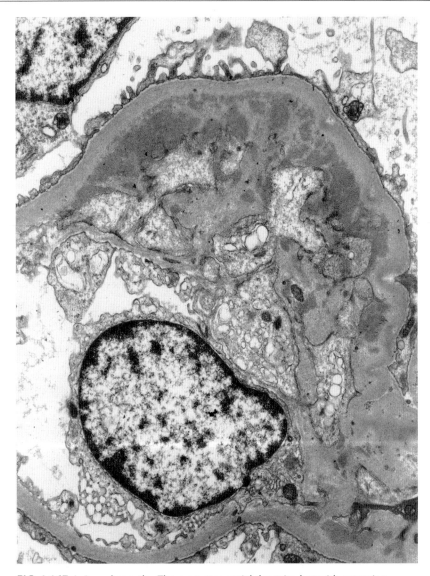

FIG. 1.167 IgA nephropathy. There are mesangial deposits, but with extension toward the peripheral loop basement membranes (transmission electron microscopy, ×17,125).

proteolysis of the IgA deposits. In support of this hypothesis, the deposits in IgAN are predominantly IgA1 subclass, which accounts for 90% of serum IgA, while IgA2 comprises 60% of IgA in secretions. African Americans commonly have a form of IgA1 with deletion of these hinge region amino acids, which could explain the rarity of IgAN in this population. Abnormal mucosal plasma cell production of J chain, required for transport of IgA into mucosal secretions, may also contribute to IgAN. Studies in familial IgA nephropathy have identified linkage to a region of chromosome 6. Whether this gene plays a role in sporadic IgAN is not known.

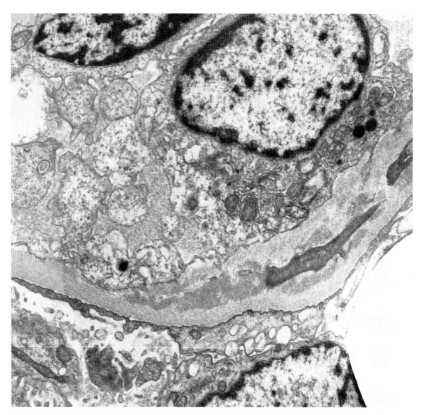

FIG. 1.168 IgA nephropathy. Extension of deposits to peripheral loop is often associated with mesangial interposition. Overlying foot processes show diffuse effacement, and there is associated endocapillary proliferation (transmission electron microscopy, ×17,125).

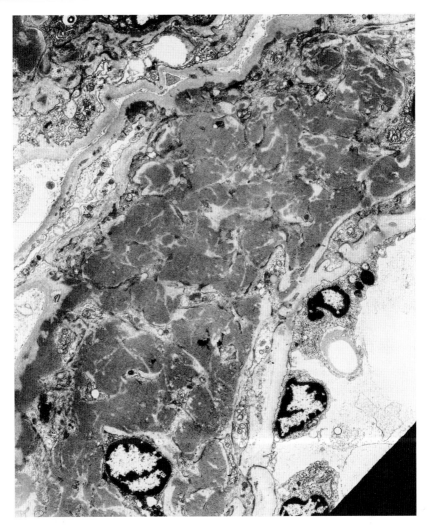

FIG. 1.169 IgA nephropathy. Deposits may be quite massive (same case as Fig. 1.157) (transmission electron microscopy, ×3000).

Selected Reading

Berger, J., 1969. IgA glomerular deposits in renal disease. Transplantation Proceedings 1, 939-944.

Berger, J., Hinglais, N., 1968. Les depots intercapillaires d'IgA-IgG. Journal of Urology 74, 694-695.

D'Amico, G., Imbasciati, E., Di Belgioso, G.B., et al., 1985. Idiopathic IgA mesangial nephropathy. Clinical and histological study of 374 patients. Medicine 64, 49-60.

D'Amico, G., Imbasciati, E., Barbiano Di Belgioso, G., et al., 1985. Idiopathic IgA mesangial nephropathy. Clinical and histological study of 374 patients. Medicine 64, 49-60.

Donadio, J.V., Grande, J.P., 1997. Predicting renal outcome in IgA nephropathy. Journal of the American Society of Nephrology 8, 1324-1332.

Emancipator, S.N., 1994. IgA nephropathy: morphologic expression and pathogenesis. American Journal of Kidney Disease 23, 451-462.

Floege, J., 2004. Recurrent IgA nephropathy after renal transplantation. Seminars in Nephrology 24, 287-291.

Frohnert, P.P., Donadio, J.V., Velosa, J.A., et al., 1997. The fate of renal transplants in patients with IgA nephropathy. Clinical Transplantation 11, 127-133.

Gharavi, A.G., Yan, Y., Scolari, F., et al., 2000. IgA nephropathy, the most common cause of glomerulonephritis, is linked to 6q22-23. Nature Genetics 26, 354-357.

Haas, M., 1997. Histologic subclassification of IgA nephropathy: A clinicopathologic study of 244 cases. American Journal of Kidney Disease 29, 829-842.

Herzenberg, A.M., Fogo, A.B., Reich, H.N., et al., 2011. Validation of the Oxford classification of IgA nephropathy. Kidney Interational (epub ahead of print).

Ibels, L.S., Gyory, A.Z., 1994. IgA nephropathy: analysis of the natural history, important factors in the progression of renal disease, and a review of the literature. Medicine (Baltimore) 73, 79-102.

Lee, S.M.K., Rao, V.M., Franklin, W.A., et al., 1982. IgA nephropathy: Morphologic predictors of progressive renal disease. Human Pathology 13, 314-322.

Radford Jr., M.G., Donadio Jr., J.V., Bergstralh, E.J., et al., 1997. Predicting renal outcome in IgA nephropathy. Journal of the American Society of Nephrology 8, 199-207.

Suzuki, H., Fan, R., Zhang, Z., et al., 2009. Aberrantly glycosylated IgA1 in IgA nephropathy patients is recognized by IgG antibodies with restricted heterogeneity. Journal of Clinical Investigation 119, 1668-1677.

Working Group of the International IgA Nephropathy Network and the Renal Pathology Society, Cattran, D.C., Coppo, R., Cook, H.T., et al., 2009. The Oxford classification of IgA nephropathy: rationale, clinicopathological correlations, and classification. Kidney International 76, 534-545.

Working Group of the International IgA Nephropathy Network and the Renal Pathology Society, Roberts, I.S., Cook, H.T., Troyanov, S, et al., 2009. The Oxford classification of IgA nephropathy: pathology definitions, correlations, and reproducibility. Kidney International 76, 546-556.

Working Group of the International IgA Nephropathy Network and the Renal Pathology Society, Coppo, R., Troyanov, S., Camilla, R, et al., 2010. The Oxford IgA nephropathy clinicopathological classification is valid for children as well as adults. Kidney International 77, 921-927.

Secondary Glomerular Diseases

Diseases Associated with Nephrotic Syndrome
MONOCLONAL IMMUNOGLOBULIN DEPOSITION DISEASE

Monoclonal immunoglobulin production may be seen as a consequence of multiple myeloma, Waldenström macroglobulinemia, or B-cell lymphoma or represent monoclonal gammopathy of undetermined significance (MGUS). Multiple myeloma is the most common underlying disease in monoclonal immunoglobulin deposition disease (MIDD) and accounts for 40-50% of pure MIDD. The incidence of overt multiple myeloma is even greater in patients with MIDD associated with light chain cast nephropathy (>90%). In patients with multiple myeloma, approximately 5% are found to have MIDD at autopsy. The diagnosis of MIDD by renal biopsy often precedes other clinical evidence of dysproteinemia (70%) and is commonly the presenting disease, which leads to the discovery of multiple myeloma. Some 15-30% of patients with MIDD on renal biopsy may not have a detectable urine or serum monoclonal protein. Conversely, not all patients with monoclonal protein have related renal disease. Of note, about 60% of our biopsied patients with monoclonal protein had unrelated renal disease. Most had MGUS detected by screening tests as part of the workup for their renal disease. The spectrum of diagnoses in these patients reflected that seen in our general adult renal biopsy population. Thus, diabetic nephropathy and FSGS were the most common diseases in these proteinuric MGUS patients.

The most common monoclonal immunoglobulin–mediated nephropathies include AL-amyloidosis light chain cast nephropathy, cryoglobulinemia (type I and II), light chain cast nephropathy, and the MIDDs. The MIDDs are characterized by non-Congophilic, non-fibrillar electron-dense deposits distributed in various tissues. MIDD predominantly affects the kidneys, but can also commonly involve the heart and liver. Non-amyloid glomerular MIDD is divided into three categories based on the type of immunoglobulin deposits: light chain deposition disease (LCDD), light and heavy chain deposition disease (LHCDD), and heavy chain deposition disease (HCDD). Among these three entities, LCDD is the most common and thus best understood with respect to its clinical and pathologic features and appears to have a slightly better prognosis than LHCDD or HCDD. LHCDD is less frequent, comprising less than 10% of MIDDs. HCDD has been reported in only 11 cases to date. MIDD may recur in the transplant. Rarely, monoclonal immunoglobulins may cause a proliferative glomerulonephritis with membranoproliferative appearance and IgG monoclonal deposits, often without a detectable serum or urine monoclonal protein (see below).

AMYLOIDOSIS

Amyloidosis is defined as the deposition of proteins that have the capacity to form beta-pleated sheets and are therefore resistant to degradation. Amyloid is a systemic disease, and different amyloids have somewhat differing propensities for tissue-specific involvement. The most common presentation of AA amyloidosis (due to active serum amyloid A protein) is that of renal disease, and AL amyloid (due to monoclonal light chain) also frequently involves the kidney. When amyloid involves the kidney, nearly half of patients have nephrotic range proteinuria, regardless of the peptide origin of the amyloid. Occasionally patients present with concentrating defects due to tubulointerstitial amyloid deposition. Additional extrarenal manifestations include carpal tunnel syndrome, peripheral neuropathy, liver dysfunction, and congestive heart failure due to cardiac amyloidosis. Cardiac involvement is rare in AA amyloidosis, contrasting the frequent heart abnormalities in AL and transthyretin (ATTR) amyloidosis. In a large U.S. series of mostly adult native kidney biopsies, amyloidosis was the diagnosis in 2% of renal biopsies, and AL amyloid was the most common type of amyloid. In contrast, in developing and Mediterranean countries, renal amyloid is more commonly AA amyloid. The age of the patients reflects the underlying conditions causing amyloid formation. Patients with amyloid due to light chain are typically older adults. In contrast, familial Mediterranean fever may result in amyloid even in early childhood.

The prognosis of patients with amyloidosis varies according to the type of amyloid and underlying associated condition. With AL amyloidosis, the median survival is only 1-2 years, contrasting up to 15-year survival with ATTR amyloidosis. For AL amyloidosis, treatment of the underlying plasma cell dyscrasia has been attempted with melphalan with remission in some patients. In some patients, there may be coexisting light chain cast nephropathy, with worse prognosis. Vigorous treatment and removal of the underlying inciting inflammation in AA amyloidosis may halt progression. Colchicine has been used in some cases of familial Mediterranean fever–associated AA amyloidosis, although the efficacy of this approach in other forms of amyloidosis has not been shown. Other forms of amyloid may be specifically diagnosed by immunostaining or mass spectroscopy.

By light microscopy, there may be only minimal mesangial expansion or segmental areas of amorphous, acellular pale eosinophilic material ("cotton candy" appearance) (Figs. 1.170, 1.171). The glomeruli may also have massive amyloid deposits and show a nodular appearance, typically without marked increase in cellularity (Figs. 1.172-1.174). The GBM may also have amyloid deposits, which typically are segmental, giving rise to irregular thickening with a feathery spike appearance on Jones silver stain (Figs. 1.175, 1.176). Amyloid deposits often also involve arterioles and arteries, with acellular chunky, pale material (Fig. 1.174). The interstitium and tubules may also show similar acellular, pale eosinophilic amyloid material (Fig. 1.177). Histologic pattern of renal involvement is not useful in differentiating various

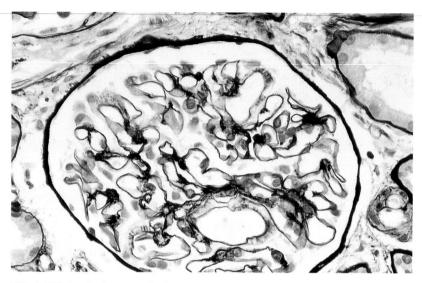

FIG. 1.170 Amyloidosis. Amyloid deposits may be small and inconspicuous by light microscopy. There is only minimal mesangial expansion, and occasional small feathery spikes along the peripheral basement membrane (5 o'clock). Amyloid deposition must be verified by Congo red positivity, and can also be verified by electron microscopy (Jones silver stain, ×400).

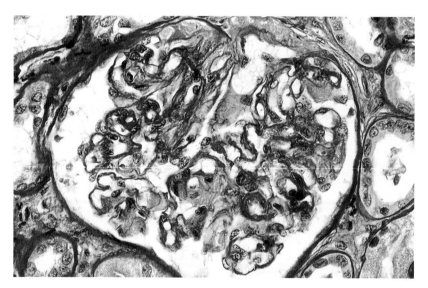

FIG. 1.171 Amyloidosis. There is very segmental amorphous, eosinophilic, fluffy "cotton candy" appearance material in the mesangium, and very segmentally along the capillary wall (Jones silver stain, ×400).

forms of amyloid, although amyloid derived from the fibrinogen alpha chain are localized to glomeruli, whereas apolipoprotein AI-derived amyloid preferentially involves the medulla. A recent classification describes extent of amyloid; whether minimal class I, mesangial class II, focal MPGN Class III, diffuse MPGN class IV, membranous class V, or advanced renal amyloidosis class VI.

Definitive diagnosis is made by Congo red stain detecting apple-green birefringence under polarized light (Figs. 1.178-1.180). This stain should be done on a section cut thicker than normal, 4-6 μm, to optimize detection of amyloid proteins. Preexposure of slides to potassium permanganate tends to abolish Congo red positivity of AA, but not AL amyloid, although

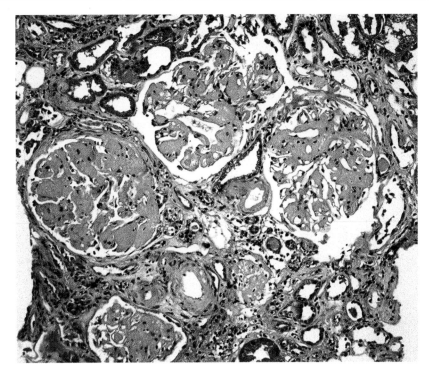

FIG. 1.172 Amyloidosis. Massive amyloid deposits are present in glomeruli and arterioles. There is a nodular appearance due to amorphous, acellular eosinophilic pale material, characteristic of amyloid (hematoxylin and eosin, ×100).

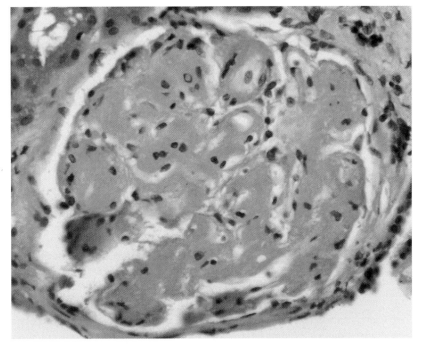

FIG. 1.173 Amyloidosis. The slightly chunky appearance of the amorphous, acellular amyloid deposits expanding the mesangial areas with focal extension to capillary loops is shown (hematoxylin and eosin, ×200).

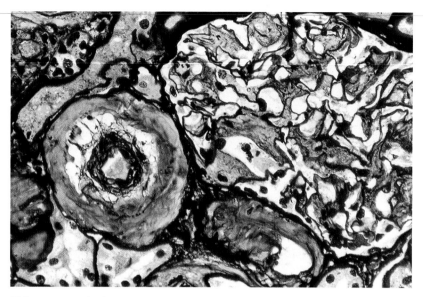

FIG. 1.174 Amyloidosis. There is massive amyloid deposition within the arteriole, and moderate expansion of the mesangium with amorphous, pale, "cotton candy appearance" material within the mesangium with occasional peripheral loop alteration (Jones silver stain, ×200).

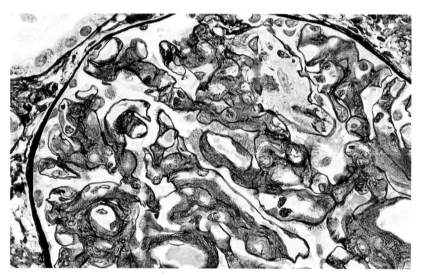

FIG. 1.175 Amyloidosis. Moderate mesangial expansion due to amyloid is shown, along with segmental feathery spikes. These are not as short and well defined as the spikes due to the glomerular basement membrane reaction in membranous glomerulonephritis, and appear rather like "the fringe on a rug." These feathery spikes may be seen with marked peripheral loop amyloid deposit due to the basement membrane reaction (Jones silver, ×400).

this technique is no longer in common use because of its insensitivity and the availability of antibodies to AA and light chain proteins, and other amyloids.

By immunofluorescence, AL amyloid may show positivity for the corresponding light chain in a smudgy pattern, mirroring the light microscopic distribution (Fig. 1.181). In non–light chain amyloid, immunofluorescence shows no specific staining (Fig. 1.182).

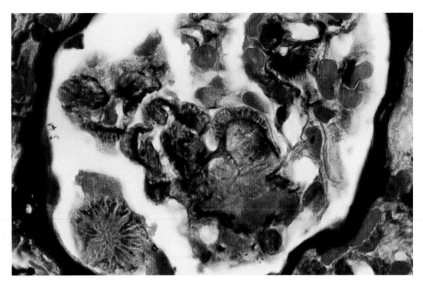

FIG. 1.176 Amyloidosis. Large feathery spike reaction due to amyloid infiltration of the peripheral capillary loop is shown, with a tangential section of such a spike reaction giving a corona appearance (bottom left) (Jones silver stain, ×400).

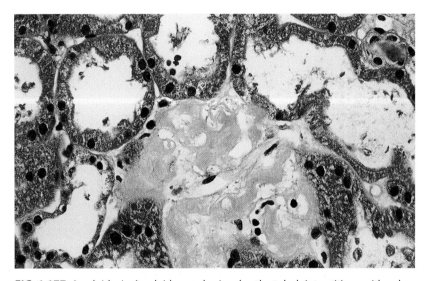

FIG. 1.177 Amyloidosis. Amyloid may also involve the tubulointerstitium, with pale, amorphous acellular areas, which should not be mistaken for areas of necrosis (hematoxylin and eosin, ×200).

Electron microscopy shows nonbranching 8-12-nm-diameter fibrils with random orientation (Figs. 1.183-1.185). Amyloid fibrils may be present in the mesangium, along the basement membrane, where they form the feathery spike appearance by light microscopy, in arterioles, and tubulointerstitium. Of note, the fibrils in fibrillary glomerulonephritis tend to be slightly thicker than amyloid fibrils, but there may be overlap in individual cases. Fibrillary glomerulonephritis also has distinct immunofluorescence findings, with prominent mesangial, and to lesser degree capillary wall staining with polyclonal IgG and complement, which also differentiates this entity from amyloid. Congo red staining should be used for ultimate, specific diagnosis of amyloid (see Differential Diagnosis of Fibrils under Fibrillary Glomerulonephritis). Although mass spectrometry may be useful to identify the specific type of amyloid, it may not detect minute deposits of amyloid seen by microscopy.

Text continued on page 141

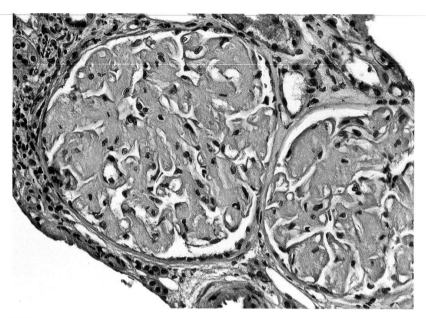

FIG. 1.178 Amyloidosis. Congo red positivity gives a specific diagnosis of amyloid. The specific positivity of the Congo red stain must be verified by viewing under polarized light (see Fig. 1.164) (Congo red, ×200).

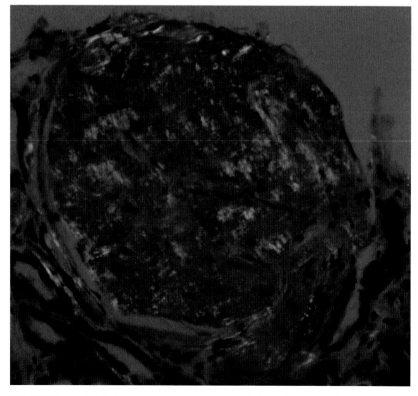

FIG. 1.179 Amyloidosis. Amyloid gives a characteristic apple-green birefringence when stained with Congo red and viewed under polarized light. There is amyloid deposition in the mesangial area, capillary loops, and weakly in the interstitium (Congo red under polarized light, ×200).

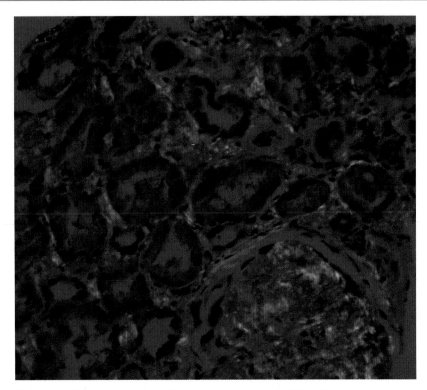

FIG. 1.180 Amyloidosis. Tubular involvement with amyloid is verified by apple-green birefringence under polarized light. By light microscopy, these deposits were not readily apparent (Congo red under polarized light, ×400).

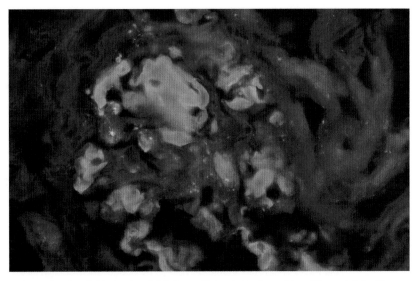

FIG. 1.181 Amyloidosis. Amyloid due to light chain deposition (AL amyloid) will often show preferential staining with the light chain. Lambda light chain more frequently is amyloidogenic than kappa light chain. The positivity is usually smudgy, and follows the distribution of amyloid seen by light microscopy (anti-lambda immunofluorescence, ×400).

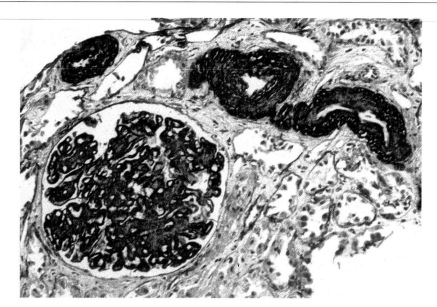

FIG. 1.182 Amyloidosis. Secondary amyloid due to the acute phase reactant protein may be diagnosed by specific immunostaining (AA amyloid). This patient had tuberculosis infection as the presumed underlying etiology of her extensive amyloid deposits (anti-AA immunohistochemistry, ×100).

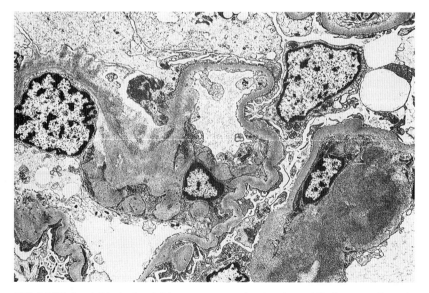

FIG. 1.183 Amyloidosis. Amyloid appears as randomly oriented fibrils, approximately 10 nm in diameter by electron microscopy. Fibrils can be found in the mesangium, the glomerular basement membrane, tubules, interstitium, and vessels. A specific diagnosis of amyloid should be verified by Congo red positivity, as there may be some overlap in fibril size with fibrillary glomerulonephritis. In this case, there is moderate expansion of the mesangium due to amyloid, with segmental capillary loop involvement (transmission electron microscopy, ×3000).

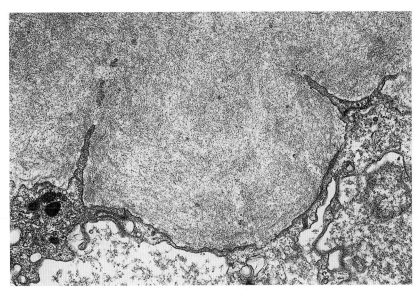

FIG. 1.184 Amyloidosis. Under higher magnification, the random, fibrillary arrangement of amyloid fibrils in the mesangium, underlying the endothelium, is apparent (transmission electron microscopy, ×20,000).

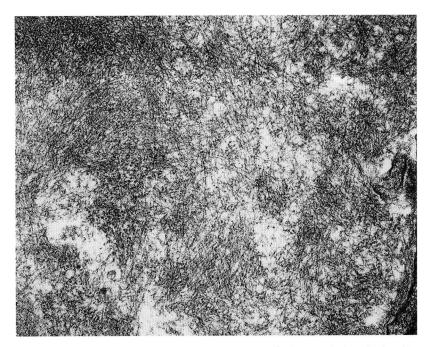

FIG. 1.185 Amyloidosis. Randomly oriented, 8-10 nm fibrils, typical of amyloid within the mesangium (transmission electron microscopy, ×25,000).

Etiology/Pathogenesis

Amyloid proteins are a group of proteins that share the common characteristic of the ability to form beta-pleated sheets, which are resistant to proteolysis. More than 20 different types of amyloid have been identified. Light chain (AL) amyloid is much more commonly lambda than kappa, likely reflecting the propensity of the molecules to form beta-pleated sheets. AA amyloid is due to the acute phase protein formed in response to chronic infection such as tuberculosis, osteomyelitis, or chronic inflammatory conditions such as rheumatoid arthritis. Other amyloids are associated with familial conditions (transthyretin), familial Mediterranean fever, or dialysis (β_2-microglobulin). Recent evidence has focused interest on amyloid P protein, which associates with the amyloid. Amyloid is resistant to proteolysis due at least in part to its binding to serum amyloid P component (SAP). Recent exciting results have been obtained with targeted pharmacologic or antibody-mediated depletion of SAP. A palindromic compound, abbreviated CPHPC, that acts as a competitive inhibitor of SAP binding to amyloid, or antibody to SAP resulted in crosslinking with amyloid, dimerization, and rapid clearance by the liver with decreased amyloid load in patients by whole body scintigraphy, or clearance of deposits in an experimental model, respectively. Inhibition of amyloid fibril formation by small molecules that appear to function by shifting the aggregation equilibrium away from the amyloid state has been successful in treating transthyretin amyloid.

Light Chain Deposition Disease

By light microscopy, glomeruli show varying degrees of mesangial proliferation (Figs. 1.186, 1.187). Early lesions consist of mild mesangial increase (Figs. 1.188-1.190). Over time, this typically progresses to nodular glomerular lesions. In many cases, lesions may by light microscopy be indistinguishable from nodular lesions of diabetic nephropathy (Figs. 1.190, 1.191).

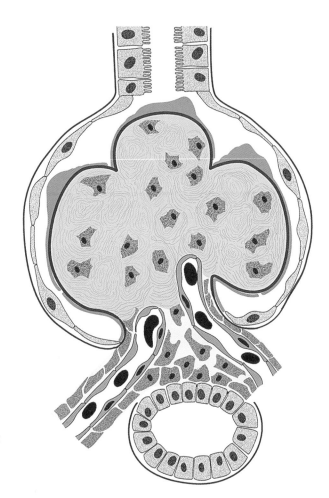

FIG. 1.186 LCDD. LCDD is characterized by nodular glomerulosclerosis, although GBMs are not as thick as in diabetic nephropathy. By electron microscopy and immunofluorescence, deposits of monoclonal light chain are visualized on the inner aspect of the GBM and outer aspect of the tubular basement membrane. *GBM*, glomerular basement membrane; *LCDD*, light chain deposition disease.

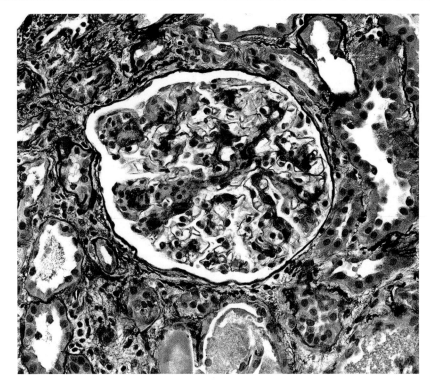

FIG. 1.187 LCDD. There may be only minimal mesangial expansion by light microscopy, with mild increase in mesangial cellularity and matrix. Specific diagnosis is made by immunofluorescence and confirmed by electron microscopy (Jones silver stain, ×200). *LCDD,* light chain deposition disease.

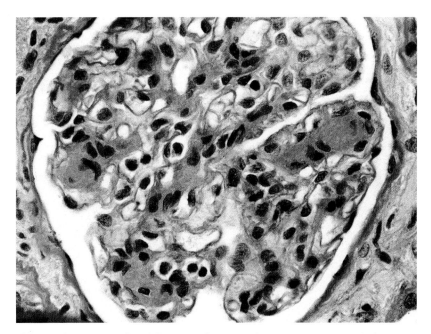

FIG. 1.188 LCDD. Small nodular areas of mesangial increase are present in this glomerulus (same case as Fig. 1.155) (hematoxylin and eosin, ×400). *LCDD,* light chain deposition disease.

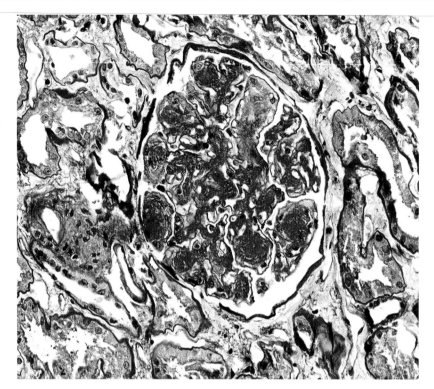

FIG. 1.189 LCDD. The characteristic nodular appearance of LCDD is illustrated. This may be difficult to distinguish from diabetes, although peripheral glomerular basement membranes are not quite as prominent as in diabetic nephropathy. Morphology of the nodules has been suggested to allow distinction between diabetic nephropathy and LCDD. However, in our experience, there is substantial overlap, and immunofluorescence and/or electron microscopy is necessary for diagnosis (periodic acid Schiff, ×200). *LCDD,* light chain deposition disease.

The nodules are PAS positive, lightly eosinophilic, PAS methenamine silver negative, and Congo red negative. Capillary microaneurysms may be present. Rarely, crescents are found. The nodular glomerular lesions of MIDD are similar by light microscopy to those found in other nodular glomerular diseases, including nodular diabetic glomerulosclerosis, amyloidosis, and membranoproliferative glomerulonephritis. There are several characteristics that have been proposed to distinguish MIDD from diabetic glomerulosclerosis. In MIDD, there tends to be multiple nodules within the glomerulus that generally stain PAS positive but methenamine silver PAS negative, and the efferent arterioles do not exhibit extensive hyalinosis. Conversely, diabetic glomerulosclerosis is characterized by solitary nodules within the glomerulus that stain PAS positive and methenamine silver PAS positive in the presence of extensive hyalinosis in the afferent and efferent arterioles. However, some patients with MIDD have silver positive nodules, and light microscopy alone does not allow definitive distinction from diabetic nephropathy in our experience (Figs. 1.190, 1.191). Other causes of nodular glomerulosclerosis may more readily be excluded by light microscopy: Amyloidosis is excluded from the differential diagnosis of MIDD by negative Congo red staining, and also the absence of fibrils on electron microscopy. Membranoproliferative glomerulonephritis is distinguished from MIDD by the presence of double contours of the GBM and dominant cellular proliferation. In addition, immunopathology and ultrastructural evaluation will differentiate the other glomerular diseases from MIDD.

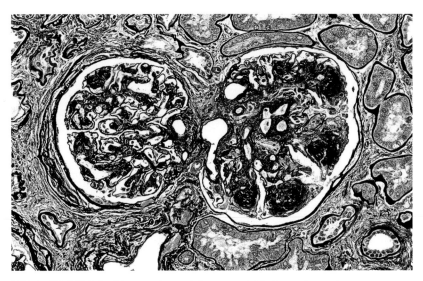

FIG. 1.190 LCDD. In this case, the nodules are variable from glomerulus to glomerulus and vary in number and in size, and stain with silver stain, all features postulated to allow distinction between diabetic nephropathy, which shows the aforementioned features, and light chain deposition disease, postulated to not show these features. There is even arteriolar hyalinization. However, immunofluorescence and electron microscopy studies confirmed the diagnosis of LCDD, corresponding to the patient's monoclonal protein (Jones silver stain, ×200). *LCDD,* light chain deposition disease.

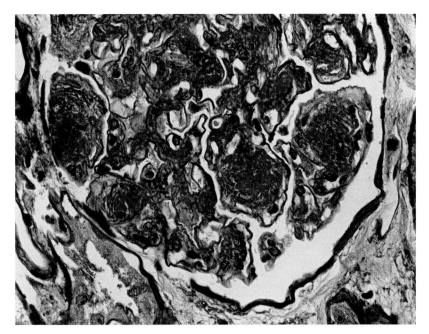

FIG. 1.191 LCDD. The expanded nodules of LCDD are shown. In this case, the glomerular basement membrane also appears slightly prominent by light microscopy, although immunofluorescence and electron microscopy studies confirmed the diagnosis of LCDD (periodic acid Schiff, ×400). *LCDD,* light chain deposition disease.

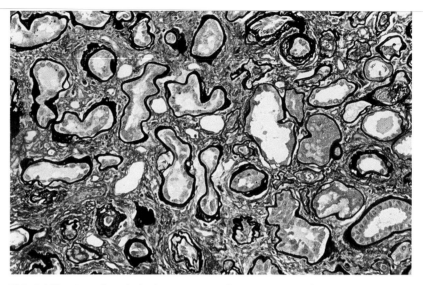

FIG. 1.192 LCDD. The tubular basement membranes are also affected by deposits in LCDD, and are commonly thick and refractile. However, this appearance overlaps with the thickening and fibrosis that occur with any tubulointerstitial fibrosis (Jones silver stain, ×200). *LCDD,* light chain deposition disease.

The renal tubular basement membranes in light chain deposition disease (LCDD) demonstrate "ribbon-like" thickening (Fig. 1.192). Tubular atrophy and interstitial fibrosis are typical findings with refractile, PAS-positive deposits found in both the tubular basement membranes and interstitium (occurring in 50% of cases of MIDD). PAS-positive deposits can also be found in the vascular basement membranes of arterioles and small interlobular arteries.

In some patients with MIDD, there is combined LCDD and light chain cast nephropathy, with attendant worse prognosis. Classic findings of light chain cast nephropathy with interstitial nephritis; severe tubular injury and interstitial fibrosis; and brittle, fractured casts with syncytial giant cell reaction are typically present. Of note, casts in light chain cast nephropathy may not stain monotypically in all cases, presumably due to nonselective proteinuria and/or abnormal monoclonal protein not recognized by standard commercial antibodies (see Light Chain Cast Nephropathy).

Definitive diagnosis of LCDD is by immunofluorescence (Figs. 1.193, 1.194). The pathognomonic finding of MIDD is the presence of monoclonal immunoglobulin deposits in the GBM and tubular basement membranes. Linear staining is present in the tubular basement membranes, GBM, often in the mesangium, and less often in interstitium and vascular basement membranes. The deposits in LCDD are most frequently kappa light chains, with a kappa to lambda case ratio of 9 : 1 in a large series. In contrast, AL amyloid most frequently is due to lambda light chain. Occasionally, deposits that appear typical for LCDD by electron microscopy in patients with known monoclonal protein fail to stain with either kappa or lambda antisera, perhaps reflecting altered antigenicity.

By electron microscopy, granular, amorphous deposits are present along the inner aspect of the GBM and the outer aspect of tubular basement membranes in LCDD (Figs. 1.195-1.198). Vascular basement membranes and mesangial nodules may also have deposits. The mesangial deposits are not sharply demarcated. Foot process effacement is variable. In general, there is no substructural organization within the deposits. Very rarely, there may be coexistent amyloid fibrils.

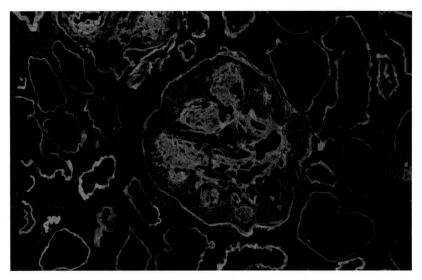

FIG. 1.193   LCDD. Specific diagnosis of LCDD is made by immunofluorescence, with monoclonal light chain, more commonly kappa, staining of glomeruli in tubular basement membranes (anti-kappa immunofluorescence, ×100). *LCDD,* light chain deposition disease.

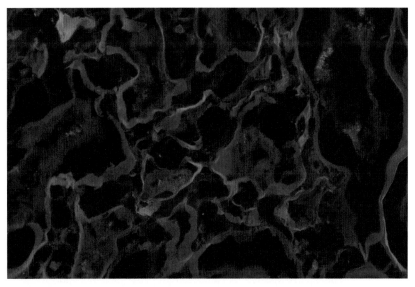

FIG. 1.194   LCDD. The tubular basement membrane staining in LCDD is illustrated (anti-kappa immunofluorescence, ×400). *LCDD,* light chain deposition disease.

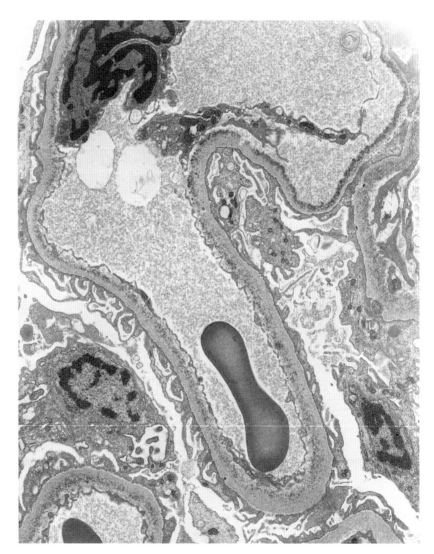

FIG. 1.195 LCDD. The deposits are finely granular and more amorphous than usual immune complexes, and generally are found along the internal aspect of the glomerular basement membrane, filling up the lamina rara interna, sometimes with extension to the lamina densa (transmission electron microscopy, ×11,250). *LCDD,* light chain deposition disease.

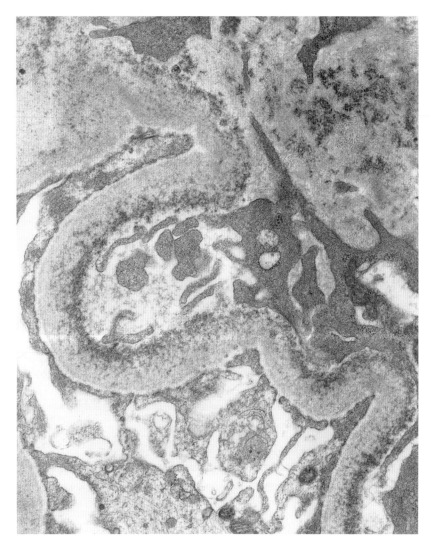

FIG. 1.196 LCDD. The granular, somewhat amorphous deposits of LCDD are shown. There is not a clear border between the deposits and the remaining GBM. Occasional granular deposits permeate into the lamina densa, but the deposits are mostly concentrated along the lamina rara interna (transmission electron microscopy, ×40,000). *GBM,* glomerular basement membrane; *LCDD,* light chain deposition disease.

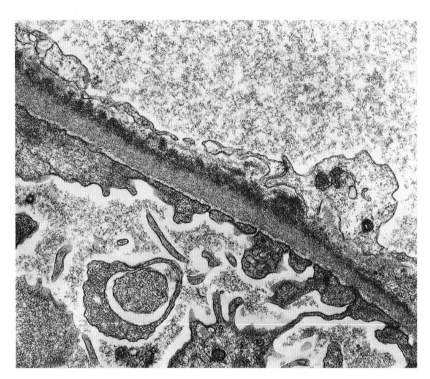

FIG. 1.197 LCDD. A thin granular line of deposits is shown in an early case of LCDD, with specific diagnosis confirmed by immunofluorescence (transmission electron microscopy, ×12,000). *LCDD,* light chain deposition disease.

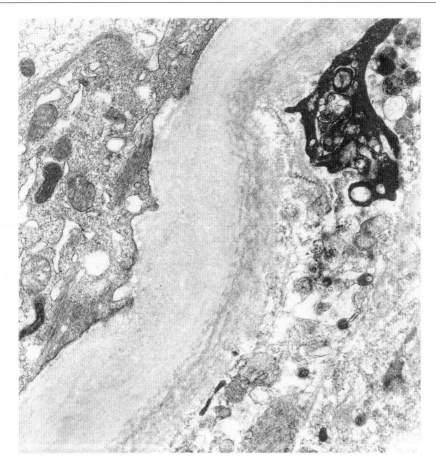

FIG. 1.198 LCDD. The deposits of the tubular basement membrane are granular, and typically along the outer aspects (transmission electron microscopy, ×4400). *LCDD, light chain deposition disease.*

Light and Heavy Chain Deposition Disease and Heavy Chain Deposition Disease

The clinical presentations of light and heavy chain deposition disease and heavy chain deposition disease (LHCDD and HCDD) are usually nephrotic syndrome with hypertension and hematuria. Some patients with HCDD may have hypocomplementemia. Interestingly, some HCDD and LHCDD patients have falsely positive hepatitis C antibody tests. Monoclonal protein in the blood may be present, but the truncated monoclonal heavy chain in HCDD may be difficult to detect in circulation.

Light microscopy in LHCDD and HCDD is indistinguishable from LCDD. There is mesangial proliferation or membranoproliferative or nodular lesions (Figs. 1.199-1.201). As in LCDD, crescents may occasionally be present. Definitive diagnosis and distinction of these MIDD diseases is made by immunofluorescence.

In LHCDD the immunofluorescence studies reveal both a monotypic heavy and light chain within the deposits, whereas in HCDD only a monotypic heavy chain is identified. The deposits are present along the GBM, mesangium, and tubular basement membranes (Figs. 1.202, 1.203). The predominant class of heavy chain in HCDD is gamma although rare cases of alpha have also been reported.

By electron microscopy, deposits in LHCDD have been divided into three differing types. These deposits may be punctate as in LCDD, confluent and homogenous as in immune

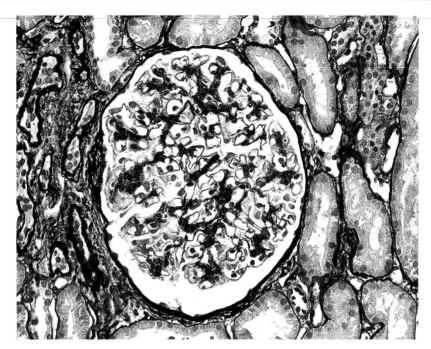

FIG. 1.199 LHCDD. The light microscopic appearance may range from minor mesangial expansion with increased mesangial matrix and cellularity to an overt nodular sclerosis. There is early surrounding tubulointerstitial fibrosis (Jones silver stain, ×100). *LHCDD,* light and heavy chain deposition disease.

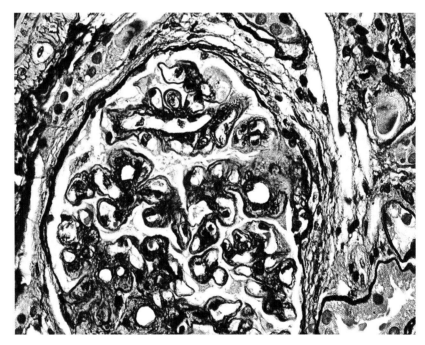

FIG. 1.200 LHCDD. A membranoproliferative pattern with increased mesangial cells and matrix is evident in this case of LHCDD, confirmed by immunofluorescence and electron microscopy. There is mesangial interposition, but no overt endocapillary proliferation (Jones silver stain, ×400). *LHCDD,* light and heavy chain deposition disease.

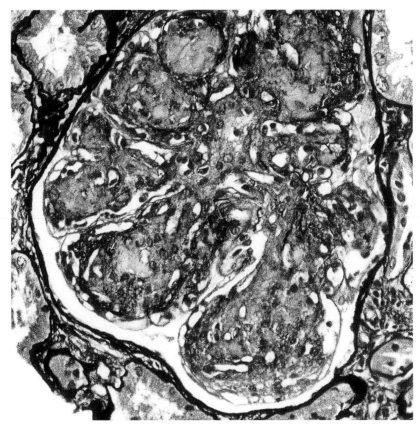

FIG. 1.201 LHCDD. This case demonstrated nodular glomerulosclerosis, indistinguishable by light microscopy from light chain deposition disease. Specific diagnosis was made by immunofluorescence and electron microscopy (Jones silver stain, ×200). *LHCDD,* light and heavy chain deposition disease.

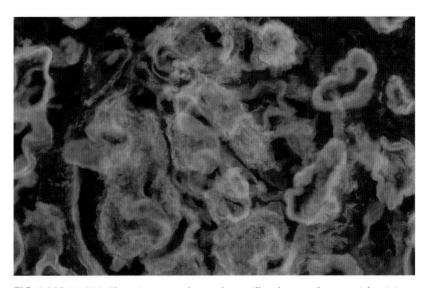

FIG. 1.202 LHCDD. There is strong glomerular capillary loop and mesangial staining in a smudgy, continuous pattern along the glomerular basement membrane. There is also tubular basement membrane staining (left) (anti-IgG immunofluorescence, ×400). *LHCDD,* light and heavy chain deposition disease.

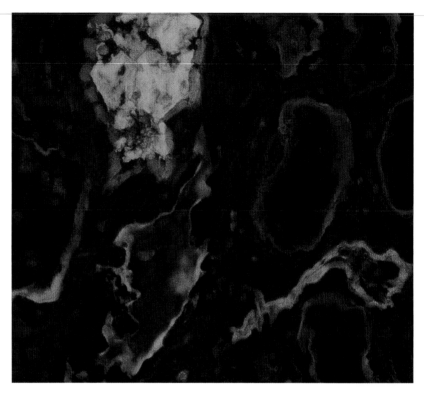

FIG. 1.203 LHCDD. The diagnosis of LHCDD was specifically confirmed by monoclonal staining with light chain, in addition to restricted heavy chain staining. Staining for lambda was negative (anti-kappa immunofluorescence, ×400). *LHCDD, light and heavy chain deposition disease.*

complex disease, or they may lack density and be invisible at the ultrastructural level (Figs 1.204-1.207). We have rarely observed combined subendothelial and subepithelial deposits in LHCDD (Fig. 1.205). In HCDD, the deposits appear finely granular, and ill defined, permeating the lamina densa of the GBM and the mesangial nodules. Finely granular deposits are also present within the tubular basement membranes and vascular basement membranes (Fig. 1.208).

Etiology/Pathogenesis of MIDD

The physicochemical properties of the monoclonal protein determine whether it results in light chain deposition disease (or LHCDD, or HCDD), amyloid, light chain cast nephropathy, or occasionally, combined lesions. Elegant experiments infusing monoclonal proteins from

---

Key Diagnostic Findings of Monoclonal Immunoglobulin Deposition Disease

- Monoclonal staining of glomeruli and tubules
- Variable light microscopic appearance – mesangial proliferative to nodular
- Amorphous deposits by electron microscopy

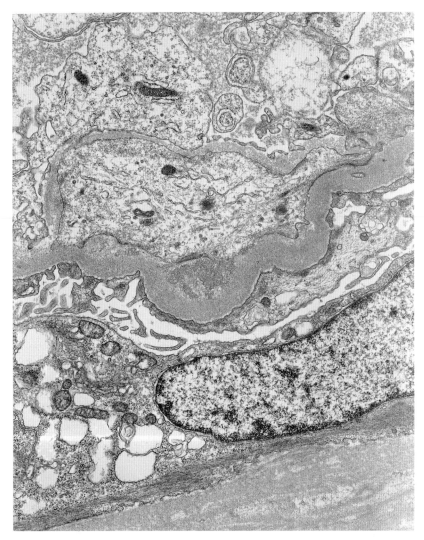

FIG. 1.204 LHCDD. Subendothelial deposits are present with a vague, coarsely fibrillar substructure. There is also mesangial interposition (transmission electron microscopy, ×20,250). *LHCDD,* light and heavy chain deposition disease.

patients into mice replicated the type of renal lesion caused by the monoclonal protein in patients in the mouse model. The predominance of kappa monoclonal light chain resulting in LCDD whereas lambda monoclonal protein more frequently manifests as amyloid is consistent with the dominant precursor proteins, Vkappa4 and Vlambda6, in LCDD and amyloidosis, respectively. Evidence supports that LHCDD and HCDD result from deletion of one of the heavy chain domains, resulting in truncated heavy chains both in the circulation and in the renal deposits. Gamma heavy chain is the most common Ig resulting in HCDD. The CH1 deletion of the heavy chain appears to play a key pathogenic role in these rare cases of HCDD, preventing binding to heavy chain binding protein in the endoplasmic reticulum and appropriate assembly with light chains.

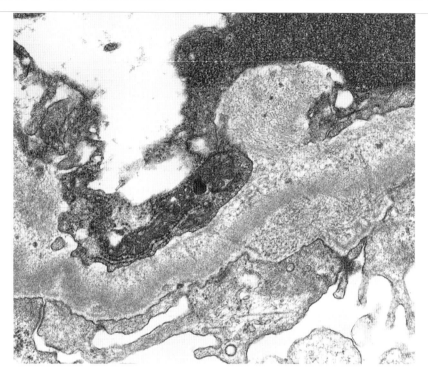

FIG. 1.205 LHCDD. Subendothelial and subepithelial deposits are present, with a coarsely fibrillar substructure. The specific diagnosis was verified by immunofluorescence (transmission electron microscopy, ×8000). *LHCDD,* light and heavy chain deposition disease.

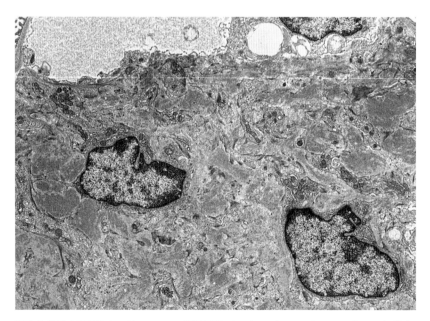

FIG. 1.206 LHCDD. In other cases of LHCDD, the deposits may be granular, as in light chain deposition disease, or appear as usual immune complex–type deposits, as in areas of this case. There are massive mesangial deposits, which extended into the subendothelial areas (transmission electron microscopy, ×8000). *LHCDD,* light and heavy chain deposition disease.

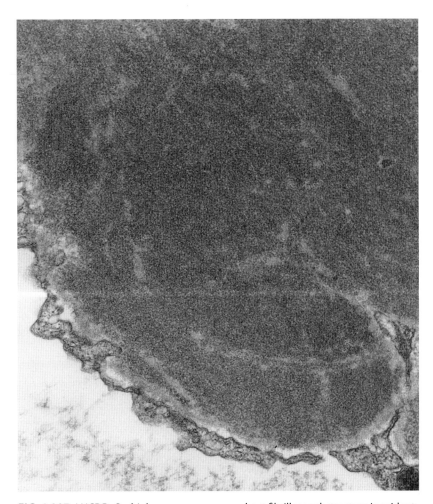

FIG. 1.207 LHCDD. On higher power, a vague, short fibrillary substructure is evident in this case of LHCDD (same case as in Fig 1.206) (transmission electron microscopy, ×40,000). *LHCDD,* light and heavy chain deposition disease.

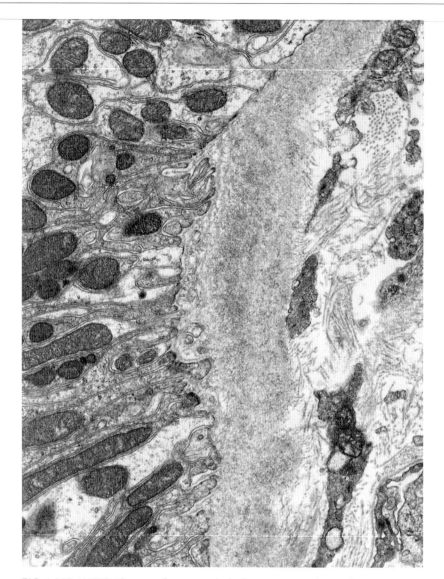

FIG. 1.208 LHCDD. There are frequent tubular basement membrane deposits in LHCDD. They are granular without discrete borders (transmission electron microscopy, ×25,625). *LHCDD,* light and heavy chain deposition disease.

Selected Reading

Amyloidosis

Bodin, K., Ellmerich, S., Kahan, M.C., et al., 2010. Antibodies to human serum amyloid P component eliminate visceral amyloid deposits. Nature 468, 93-97.

Dikman, S.H., Churg, J., Kahn, T., 1998. Morphologic and clinical correlates in renal amyloidosis. Human Pathology 12 (2), 160-169.

Faulk, R.H., Comenzo, R.L., Skinner, M., 1997. The systemic amyloidoses. New England Journal of Medicine 337, 898-909.

Glenner, G.G., 1980. Amyloid deposits and amyloidosis. The beta-fibrilloses. New England Journal of Medicine 302, 1283-1292.

Glenner, G.G., 1980. Amyloid deposits and amyloidosis: the beta-fibrilloses. New England Journal of Medicine 302, 1333-1343.

Hammarstrom, P., Wiseman, R.L., Powers, E.T., et al., 2003. Prevention of transthyretin amyloid disease by changing protein misfolding energetics. Science 31 299, 713-716.

Kyle, R.A., Gertz, M.A., 1995. Primary systemic amyloidosis: clinical and laboratory features in 474 cases. Seminars in Hematology 32, 45-59.

Looi, L.-M., Cheah, P.-L., 1997. Histomorphological patterns of renal amyloidosis: a correlation between histology and chemical type of amyloidosis. Human Pathology 28, 847-849.

Picken, M.M., 2007. New insights into systemic amyloidosis: the importance of diagnosis of specific type. Current Opinion Nephrology and Hypertension 16, 196-203.

Sen, S., Sarsik, B., 2010. A proposed histopathological classification, scoring and grading system for renal amyloidosis. Archives of Pathology and Laboratory Medicine 134, 532-544.

LCDD, LHCDD, and HCDD

Gallo, G., Picken, M., Buxbaum, J., et al., 1989. The spectrum of immunoglobulin deposition disease associated with immunocytic dyscrasias. Seminars in Hematology 26, 234-245.

Gallo, G.R., Feiner, H.D., Buxbaum, J.N., 1982. The kidney in lymphoplasmacytic disorders. Pathology Annual 17, 291-317.

Gallo, G.R., Lazowski, P., Kumar, A., et al., 1998. Renal and cardiac manifestations of B-cell dyscrasias with nonamyloidotic monoclonal light chain and light and heavy chain deposition diseases. Advances in Nephrology at Necker Hospital 28, 355-382.

Ganeval, D., Mignon, F., Preud'homme, J.L., et al., 1982. Visceral deposition of monoclonal light chains and immunoglobulins: a study of renal and immunopathologic abnormalities. Advances in Nephrology 11, 25-63.

Ganeval, D., Noel, L.H., Preud'homme, J.L., et al., 1984. Light-chain deposition disease: its relation with AL-type amyloidosis. Kidney International 26, 1-9.

Kambham, N., Markowitz, G.S., Appel, G.B., et al., 1999. Heavy chain deposition disease: The disease spectrum. American Journal of Kidney Disease 33, 954-962.

Lin, J., Markowitz, G.S., Valeri, A.M., et al., 2001. Renal monoclonal immunoglobulin deposition disease: the disease spectrum. Journal of the American Society of Nephrology 12, 1482-1492.

Paueksakon, P., Revelo, M.P., Horn, R.G, et al., 2003. Monoclonal gammopathy: significance and possible causality in renal disease. American Journal of Kidney Disease 42, 87-95.

Pirani, C.L., Silva, F., D'Agati, V., Chander, P., et al., 1987. Renal lesions in plasma cell dyscrasias: ultrastructural observations. American Journal of Kidney Disease 10, 208-221.

Preud'homme, J.L., Aucouturier, P., Touchard, G., et al., 1994. Monoclonal immunoglobulin deposition disease (Randall type). Relationship with structural abnormalities of immunoglobulin chains. Kidney International 46, 965-972.

Randall, R.E., Williamson Jr., W.C., Mullinax, F., et al., 1976. Manifestations of systemic light chain deposition. American Journal of Medicine 60, 293-299.

Sanders, P.W., Herrera, G.A., Kirk, K.A., et al., 1991. Spectrum of glomerular and tubulointerstitial renal lesions associated with monotypical immunoglobulin light chain deposition. Laboratory Investigation 64, 527-537.

Sanders, P.W., Herrera, G.A., 1993. Monoclonal immunoglobulin light chain-related renal diseases. Seminars in Nephrology 23, 324-341.

Solomon, A., Weiss, D.T., Kattine, A.A., 1991. Nephrotoxic potential of Bence Jones proteins. New England Journal of Medicine 324, 1845-1851.

PROLIFERATIVE GLOMERULONEPHRITIS WITH MONOCLONAL DEPOSITS

This unusual manifestation of monoclonal protein-related kidney disease differs from the MIDD group above in that there are no extraglomerular deposits. In a recent large series, half had nephrotic syndrome, about two thirds had renal insufficiency, and three fourths had

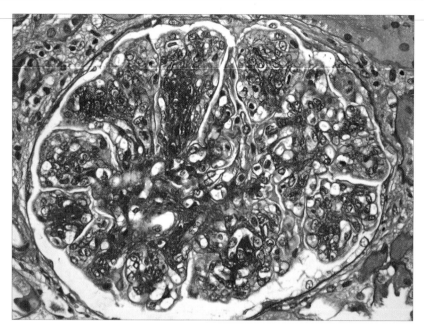

FIG. 1.209 PGNMID. There is diffuse and global endocapillary proliferation in PGNMID (periodic acid Schiff, ×400). (Case kindly shared by Samih H. Nasr, M.D., Consultant, Anatomic Pathology, Assistant Professor of Laboratory Medicine and Pathology, College of Medicine, Mayo Medical School and Vivette D'Agati, M.D., Professor of Pathology, New York- Presbyterian Hospital at the Columbia University Medical Center.) *PGNMID*, proliferative glomerulonephritis with monoclonal deposits.

Key Diagnostic Findings of Proliferative Glomerulonephritis with Monoclonal Deposits

- Monoclonal staining of glomeruli for IgG and light chain
- Membranoproliferative pattern by light microscopy (rarely membranous pattern, rarely crescents)
- Subendothelial and mesangial, rarely subepithelial, deposits by electron microscopy, indistinguishable by electron microscopy from usual-type immune complexes

---

hematuria. A serum monoclonal protein corresponding to the type identified in the glomeruli was identified in only a third of patients. Only one patient had myeloma, and development of myeloma was also rare during follow-up. About a third of the patients had complete or partial recovery, a third had persistent renal dysfunction, and about 20% progressed to end-stage renal disease. Poor prognosis was associated with higher initial serum creatinine, extent of glomerulosclerosis and interstitial fibrosis. Proliferative glomerulonephritis with monoclonal deposits (PGNMID) can recur in the transplant despite the absence of an M-spike. Lesions were variable, with proliferative or mesangial proliferative lesions, and responded to increased immunosuppression with cyclophosphamide or rituximab.

Light microscopy shows predominantly proliferative lesions, frequently with double contour GBMs and occasionally with membranous features. Crescents may occasionally be present (Figs. 1.209-1.211). Immunofluorescence showed mesangial and chunky capillary wall, or occasional membranous granular pattern staining for IgG, with monoclonal restriction, most commonly IgG3 and kappa (Fig. 1.212). Electron microscopy revealed granular, nonorganized mesangial and subendothelial with occasional segmental epimembranous or

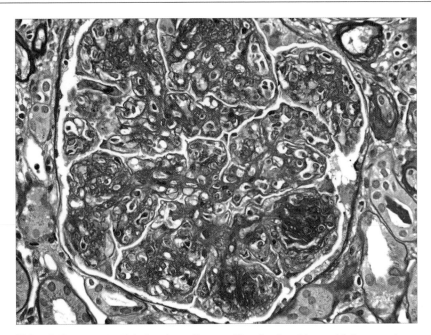

FIG. 1.210 PGNMID. Global endocapillary proliferation is evident, with frequent but segmental interposition (periodic acid Schiff, ×400). (Case kindly shared by Samih H. Nasr, M.D., Consultant, Anatomic Pathology, Assistant Professor of Laboratory Medicine and Pathology, College of Medicine, Mayo Medical School and Vivette D'Agati, M.D., Professor of Pathology, New York- Presbyterian Hospital at the Columbia University Medical Center.) *PGNMID,* proliferative glomerulonephritis with monoclonal deposits.

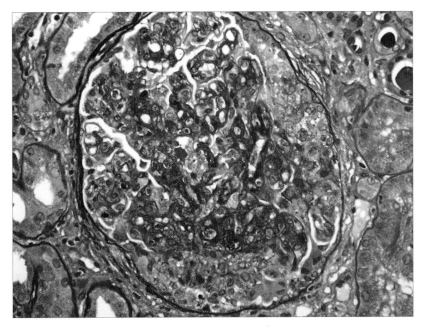

FIG. 1.211 PGNMID. There is endocapillary proliferation, and also small cellular crescent (periodic acid Schiff, ×400). (Case kindly shared by Samih H. Nasr, M.D., Consultant, Anatomic Pathology, Assistant Professor of Laboratory Medicine and Pathology, College of Medicine, Mayo Medical School and Vivette D'Agati, M.D., Professor of Pathology, New York- Presbyterian Hospital at the Columbia University Medical Center.) *PGNMID,* proliferative glomerulonephritis with monoclonal deposits.

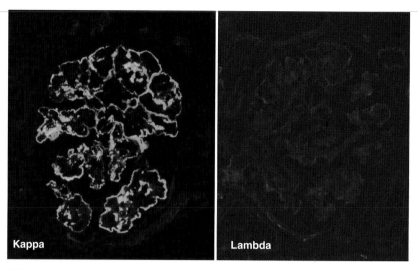

FIG. 1.212 PGNMID. Deposits stain with IgG, but show clonal restriction, staining most typically only with kappa, in a chunky irregular mesangial and capillary loop pattern. There are no deposits along tubular basement membranes (left panel anti-kappa, right panel anti-lambda immunofluorescence, ×400). (Case kindly shared by Samih H. Nasr, M.D., Consultant, Anatomic Pathology, Assistant Professor of Laboratory Medicine and Pathology, College of Medicine, Mayo Medical School and Vivette D'Agati, M.D., Professor of Pathology, New York- Presbyterian Hospital at the Columbia University Medical Center.) *PGNMID,* proliferative glomerulonephritis with monoclonal deposits.

Key Differential Diagnosis

- Membranoproliferative glomerulonephritis due to immune complexes (e.g., lupus nephritis, chronic infections) shows polyclonal staining of deposits (i.e., both kappa and lambda)
- Heavy chain deposition disease: differentiate by the presence of light and heavy chain monoclonal staining in PGNMID
- Light and heavy chain deposition disease: differentiate by the absence of tubular staining in PGNMID

PGNMID, proliferative glomerulonephritis with monoclonal deposits.

---

intramembranous deposits that are not distinguishable from usual immune complex–type deposits (Fig. 1.213). Tubular basement membranes show no deposits.

Etiology/Pathogenesis

IgG3 was found in about two thirds of PGNMID cases, although it is the rarest of the four IgG isotypes, and was associated with C3 deposition and in some cases hypocomplementemia. IgG3 is nephritogenic and avidly fixes complement, and its high molecular weight and anionic charge favor its localization to the glomerular capillary wall. In PGNMID, unlike heavy chain deposition disease (see above), no mutations of the constant regions of IgG were detected. Further elucidation of specific physicochemical features of IgG3 in PGNMID may shed light on its pathogenesis.

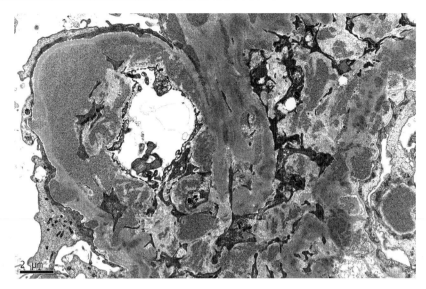

FIG. 1.213 PGNMID. By electron microscopy, deposits are widespread with numerous mesangial, subendothelial and occasional intramembranous or subepithelial deposits. Deposits appear as usual immune complexes with no distinct features by electron microscopy, and the specific diagnosis of PGNMID relies on immunofluorescence findings. Foot processes show extensive effacement and there is interposition (left) (transmission electron microscopy, ×8000). (Case kindly shared by Samih H. Nasr, M.D., Consultant, Anatomic Pathology, Assistant Professor of Laboratory Medicine and Pathology, College of Medicine, Mayo Medical School and Vivette D'Agati, M.D., Professor of Pathology, New York- Presbyterian Hospital at the Columbia University Medical Center.) *PGNMID,* proliferative glomerulonephritis with monoclonal deposits.

Selected Reading

Nasr, S.H., Sethi, S., Cornell, L.D., et al., 2010. Proliferative glomerulonephritis with monoclonal IgG deposits recurs in the allograft. Clinical Journal of the American Society of Nephrology 6, 122-132.

Nasr, S.H., Satoskar, A., Markowitz, G.S., et al., 2009. Proliferative glomerulonephritis with monoclonal IgG deposits. Journal of the American Society of Nephrology 20, 2055-2064.

HIV-ASSOCIATED NEPHROPATHY

Patients present with nephrotic-range proteinuria, often with rapid downhill course of GFR. Despite marked proteinuria, patients usually do not manifest edema or hypertension. Renal enlargement is common. HIVAN may precede other manifestations of HIV infection.

By light microscopy, there is a collapsing form of focal segmental glomerulosclerosis with collapse of the glomerular tuft and hyperplasia and hypertrophy of overlying visceral epithelial cells with prominent protein droplets (Figs. 1.214-1.219). This proliferation should not be mistaken for a crescent. The entire tuft or just segments of the glomerulus are collapsed with wrinkling of the GBM. Bowman's space may therefore appear dilated. With progressive disease, there may be solidification and segmental sclerosis and adhesions (Fig. 1.215). There are associated disproportionately severe tubulointerstitial lesions with cystic dilatation of tubules and tubular degeneration affecting all tubule segments (Fig. 1.216). Tubular epithelial cells often contain prominent protein droplets. The interstitium shows edema and a variable infiltrate with mainly lymphocytes and occasional monocytes and plasma cells (Fig. 1.216). With progression, there is interstitial fibrosis and tubular atrophy. Vessels do not show any specific changes.

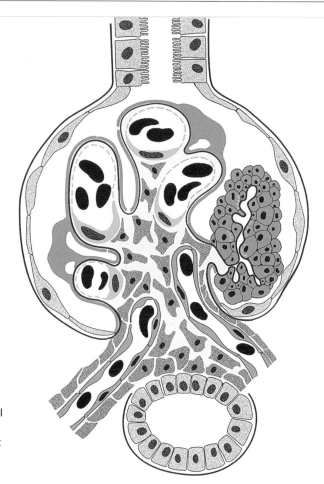

FIG. 1.214 HIVAN. There is segmental or global collapse of the capillary tuft with overlying visceral epithelial cell hyperplasia, without deposits. In addition, frequent reticular aggregates are present in the endothelial cell cytoplasm, seen by electron microscopy. *HIVAN*, HIV-associated nephropathy.

Key Diagnostic Features of HIV-Associated Nephropathy

- Segmental or global collapse of tuft with overlying visceral epithelial cell proliferation
- Microcystic tubular injury, often with interstitial inflammation
- Reticular aggregates

Differential Diagnosis of Collapsing Glomerular Lesions

- HIV-associated nephropathy (reticular aggregates by electron microscopy)
- Idiopathic variant of focal segmental glomerulosclerosis
- Associated with pamidronate or interferon treatment
- Severe ischemia (e.g., calcineurin inhibitor therapy or other causes of ischemia)
- Parvo virus
- Systemic lupus erythematosus (rare)

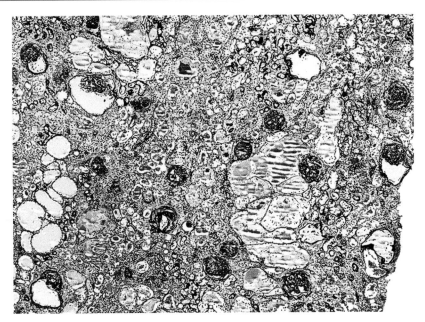

FIG. 1.215 HIVAN. There is disproportionately severe microcystic tubular injury with tubulointerstitial inflammation, and extensive glomerulosclerosis. Some of the glomeruli have retracted and collapsed, with apparent dilatation of Bowman's space (top left), in this autopsy specimen from a patient who died with HIVAN (Jones silver stain, ×100). *HIVAN,* HIV-associated nephropathy.

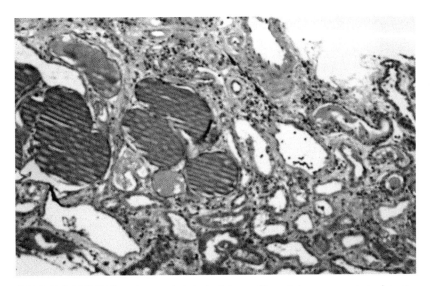

FIG. 1.216 HIVAN. The microcystic tubular injury with proteinaceous casts is shown, along with interstitial edema and early fibrosis, with a lymphoplasmacytic infiltrate (hematoxylin and eosin, ×200). *HIVAN,* HIV-associated nephropathy.

Immunofluorescence studies do not show immune complex deposits but may show nonspecific IgM and C3 in mesangial areas. The protein droplets in the podocytes may stain for any Ig, including IgG and IgA. The specific location and round, globular pattern of this staining allows distinction from immune complexes.

Electron microscopy demonstrates collapse of the tuft and proliferation of the podocytes with foot process effacement (Fig. 1.220). Reticular aggregates, also known as tubuloreticular

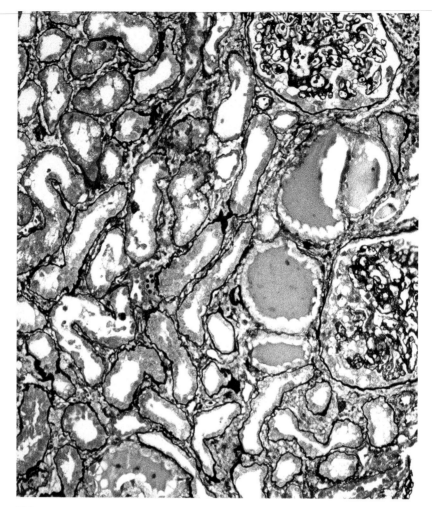

FIG. 1.217 HIVAN. There is microcystic tubular injury and collapse of the glomerular tuft with overlying visceral epithelial cell proliferation (Jones silver stain, ×200). *HIVAN*, HIV-associated nephropathy.

inclusions, are present in endothelial cell cytoplasm (Fig. 1.221) in HIV-infected patients, whether they have nephropathy or not. These ~25-nm-diameter structures are related to elevated levels of interferon-alpha and are present systemically in the endoplasmic reticulum, particularly in endothelial cells. Reticular aggregates are particularly numerous in patients with HIV infection or with SLE and are markers of the underlying systemic condition, not specifically of nephropathy. Reticular aggregates are less frequent in patients on highly active anti-retroviral treatment.

Etiology/Pathogenesis

The specific pathogenesis of HIVAN has not been determined. Some investigators have found HIV antigens in tubular epithelium, but this finding has not been widely confirmed. Whether HIV directly infects resident glomerular cells, and thereby causes the lesions, or whether injury is due to secondary cytokine effects, or both mechanisms contribute, has not been definitively proven. HIV transgenic mice and primates with simian AIDS have been extensively studied to elucidate the role of specific viral genes and systemic versus renal parenchymal factors in

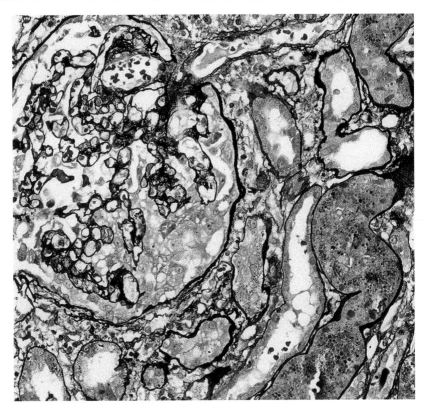

FIG. 1.218 HIVAN. The glomeruli show a collapsing form of injury, where the lobule is retracted and collapsed with overlying glomerular visceral epithelial cell hyperplasia, often with prominent protein droplets (Jones silver stain, ×200). *HIVAN,* HIV-associated nephropathy.

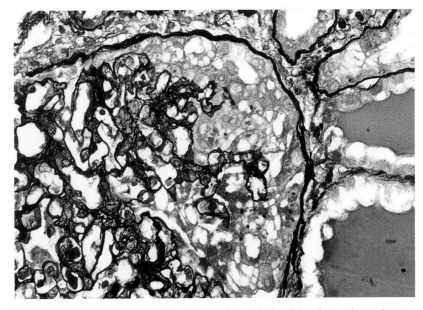

FIG. 1.219 HIVAN. The segmental collapse of the lobule of the glomerulus is shown with prominent overlying visceral epithelial cell proliferation, with protein droplets (Jones silver stain, ×400). *HIVAN,* HIV-associated nephropathy.

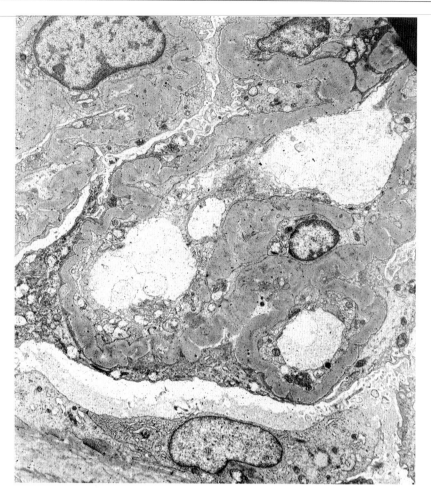

FIG. 1.220 HIVAN. There are no immune deposits, but affected glomeruli show extensive corrugation and collapse of the basement membrane, with overlying visceral epithelial cell hyperplasia and extensive foot process effacement. In distinction to idiopathic collapsing glomerulopathy, there frequently are numerous reticular aggregates in endothelial cell cytoplasm (transmission electron microscopy, ×8000). *HIVAN*, HIV-associated nephropathy.

injury. Direct infection with selected HIV genes of podocytes in mouse models caused a collapsing glomerulopathy.

The podocyte is a major target of injury in HIVAN. There is dedifferentiation of podocytes with loss of differentiation markers, such as the Wilms tumor antigen WT-1, and loss of cyclin-dependent kinase inhibitors, allowing proliferation of visceral epithelial cells, likely including parietal epithelial cells. HIVAN occurs much more commonly in African Americans with HIV infection than in Caucasians; 80-85% of HIVAN patients are African American. In contrast, Caucasian HIV-infected individuals with renal disease studied in Europe had various immune complex and nonimmune glomerular diseases rather than HIVAN. Lesions other than HIVAN, including usual FSGS, and immune complex lupus-like lesions, also occur in some black African patients with HIV. This increased susceptibility in African Americans has recently been linked to a mutation in apolipoprotein L1, ApoL1, which has protective effects against some trypanosomes. How this mutation could cause kidney disease is unknown.

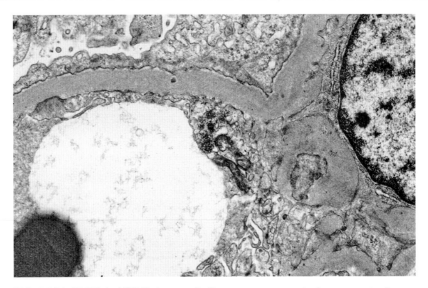

FIG. 1.221 HIVAN. In HIVAN, there typically are numerous reticular aggregates in endothelial cell cytoplasm throughout the body, a marker of HIV infection and high interferon levels (transmission electron microscopy, ×25,625). *HIVAN,* HIV-associated nephropathy.

Selected Reading

Alpers, C.E., Tsai, C.C., Hudkins, K.L., et al., 1997. Focal segmental glomerulosclerosis in primates infected with a simian immunodeficiency virus. AIDS Research in Human Retroviruses 13, 413-424.

Cohen, A.H., Nast, C.C., 1988. HIV-associated nephropathy. A unique combined glomerular, tubular, and interstitial lesion. Modern Pathology 1, 87-97.

Cohen, A.H., Sun, N.C., Shapshak, P., et al., 1989. Demonstration of human immunodeficiency virus in renal epithelium in HIV-associated nephropathy. Modern Pathology 2, 125-128.

D'Agati, V., Suh, J.I., Carbone, L., et al., 1988. Pathology of HIV-associated nephropathy: a detailed morphologic and comparative study. Kidney International 35, 1358-1370.

Fine, D.M., Fogo, A.B., Alpers, C.E., 2008. Thrombotic microangiopathy and other glomerular disorders in the HIV-infected patient. Seminars in Nephrology 28, 545-555.

Genovese, G., Friedman, D.J., Ross, M.D., et al., 2010. Association of trypanolytic ApoL1 variants with kidney disease in African Americans. Science 329, 841-845.

Kimmel, P.L., Phillips, T.M., Ferreira-Centeno, A., et al., 1993. HIV-associated immune-mediated renal disease. Kidney International 44, 1327-1340.

Nochy, D., Glotz, D., Dosquet, P., et al., 1993. Renal disease associated with HIV infection: a multicentric study of 60 patients from Paris hospitals. Nephrology, Dialysis and Transplantation 8, 11-19.

Rosenstiel, P., Gharavi, A., D'Agati, V., et al., 2009. Transgenic and infectious animal models of HIV-associated nephropathy. Journal of the American Society of Nephrology 20, 2296-2304.

Ross, M.J., Klotman, P.E., 2002. Recent progress in HIV-associated nephropathy. Journal of the American Society of Nephrology 13, 2997-3004.

Winston, J.A., Bruggeman, L.A., Ross, M.D., et al., 2001. Nephropathy and establishment of a renal reservoir of HIV type 1 during primary infection. New England Journal of Medicine 344, 1979-1984.

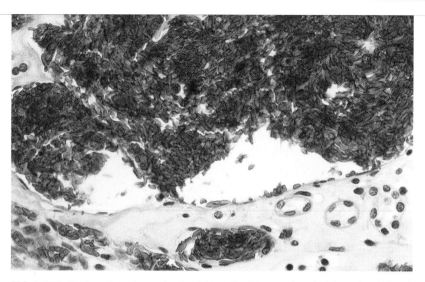

FIG. 1.222 Sickle cell nephropathy. In sickle cell crisis, massive sludging of red blood cells may occur in large vessels because of agglutination of the sickled red blood cells (hematoxylin and eosin, ×100).

SICKLE CELL NEPHROPATHY

Patients with sickle cell anemia are at risk for developing progressive renal disease, which initially manifests as microalbuminuria in childhood, progressing to overt proteinuria and progressive decrease in renal function after age 20 years. Some 5-8% of all sickle cell patients develop renal failure. Patients typically also have hematuria and urine-concentrating defects. The prognosis is poor when patients have nephrotic syndrome and sickle cell nephropathy, with two thirds developing renal failure and half dying within 2 years.

The most common renal diseases in sickle cell patients can be categorized as acute injury, including cortical infarcts, related to sickle cell crisis; acute or more insidious injury of the medulla resulting in papillary necrosis and/or fibrosis; and chronic glomerular injury manifesting as a secondary FSGS. Sickle cell crisis causes sludging of sickled red blood cells in vessels (Fig. 1.222). The medullary vasa recta are particularly vulnerable (Fig. 1.223). The occlusion of normal blood flow may cause cortical infarcts or occlude glomeruli with surrounding tubular injury (Fig. 1.224). Acute or more insidious injury due to subclinical sickling in the vasa recta can result in papillary necrosis, tubulointerstitial fibrosis, and urine-concentrating defects. In the more chronic glomerular injury of sickle cell nephropathy, there is remarkable glomerular enlargement by light microscopy (Fig. 1.225). The mesangium may be expanded, but there is no overt proliferation. Secondary lesions of focal segmental and global glomerulosclerosis can develop later in the course (Fig. 1.226). These lesions are predominantly hilar and have been associated with hyalinosis, lipid vacuoles, and foam cells. The GBM may be thickened and reduplicated, but without immune complex–type deposits (Figs. 1.226, 1.227). Hemosiderin may be present in the glomerulus, including podocytes, and in tubular epithelial cells (Figs. 1.228-1.230). There is proportional tubulointerstitial fibrosis in cases. Vessels show no specific lesions. In stable patients not undergoing sickle cell crisis, only rare sickled cells can be detected, even when overt sclerotic lesions are present.

Immunofluorescence microscopy typically shows only IgM, C3, and C1q in the sclerosed areas. Electron microscopy in sickle cell nephropathy with secondary focal segmental glomerulosclerosis shows subtotal foot process effacement overlying areas of sclerosis. Sickled cells may be detected (Fig. 1.231). In cases with GBM double contours by light microscopy, there typically is only mesangial interposition by electron microscopy without well-defined immune

Text continued on page 175

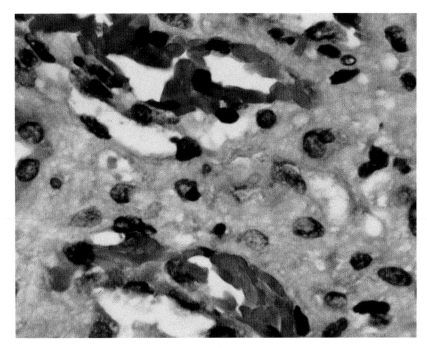

FIG. 1.223 Sickle cell nephropathy. Even without sickle cell crisis, there may be sickling of red blood cells in peritubular capillaries and in the vasa recta. There is surrounding edema and tubular injury in this patient who had sickle cell trait and died after extreme exertion and dehydration (hematoxylin and eosin, ×400).

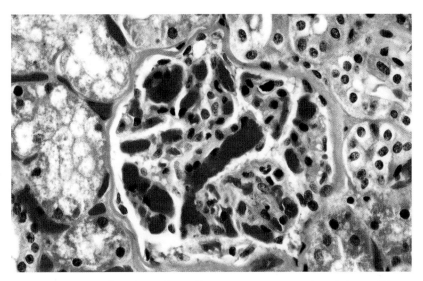

FIG. 1.224 Sickle cell nephropathy. Sickling may cause congestion of glomeruli in addition to peritubular capillaries. There is associated diffuse tubular injury and acute tubular necrosis in this patient who had acute sickle cell crisis (hematoxylin and eosin, ×200).

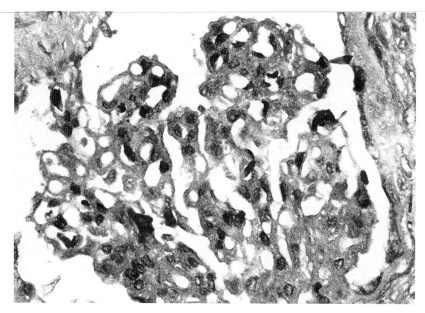

FIG. 1.225 Sickle cell nephropathy. Chronically, sickle cell patients may have glomerular lesions characterized by extreme glomerulomegaly, and a membranoproliferative and/or focal segmental sclerosis pattern of injury. Most often there are not immune complexes, and glomerular basement reduplication and mesangial proliferation are due to chronic endothelial injury. Rare sickled cells are present (right) (hematoxylin and eosin, ×200).

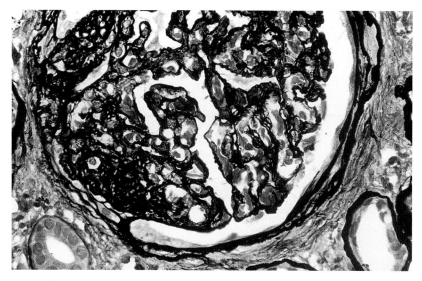

FIG. 1.226 Sickle cell nephropathy. The corrugated, double contour glomerular basement membrane in chronic sickle cell nephropathy is evident, along with mild congestion. There is segmental sclerosis (left), a secondary process presumed linked to the chronic endothelial injury (Jones silver stain, ×400).

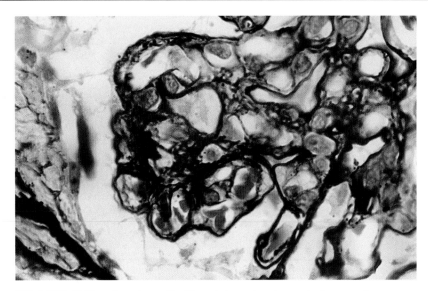

FIG. 1.227 Sickle cell nephropathy. There is irregular glomerular basement membrane double contour and corrugation, along with mild mesangial proliferation with rare sickled cells in peripheral loops. This patient had secondary focal segmental glomerulosclerosis and marked proteinuria and no immune deposits (Jones silver stain, ×1000).

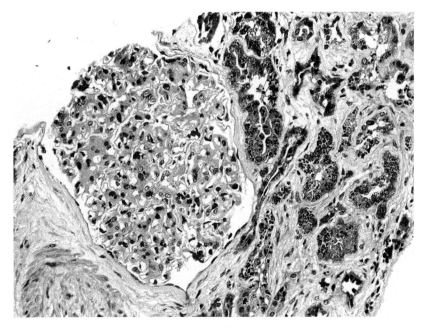

FIG. 1.228 Sickle cell nephropathy. As a result of chronic hemolysis, there may be hemosiderin present in tubules and even glomerular cells. The hemosiderin is seen as brown chunky pigment within tubules. There is associated mild tubular atrophy and interstitial fibrosis. The glomerulus is markedly enlarged with mild mesangial expansion (hematoxylin and eosin, ×200).

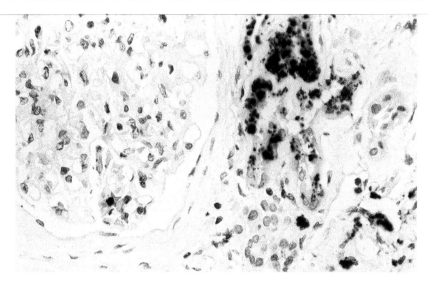

FIG. 1.229 Sickle cell nephropathy. Iron is readily and specifically demonstrated by a Prussian blue stain. There is iron within tubules, occasional interstitial macrophages and rare staining of glomerular resident cells (Prussian blue stain, ×200).

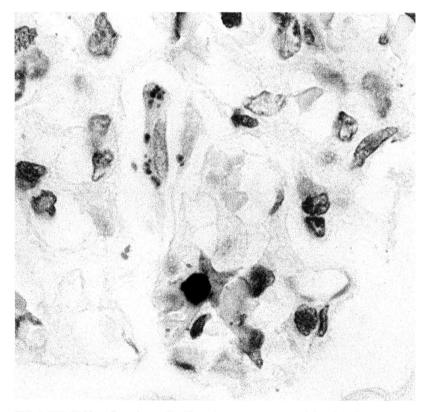

FIG. 1.230 Sickle cell nephropathy. There is apparent mesangial and podocyte localization of iron in this patient with chronic sickle cell nephropathy (Prussian blue stain, ×1000).

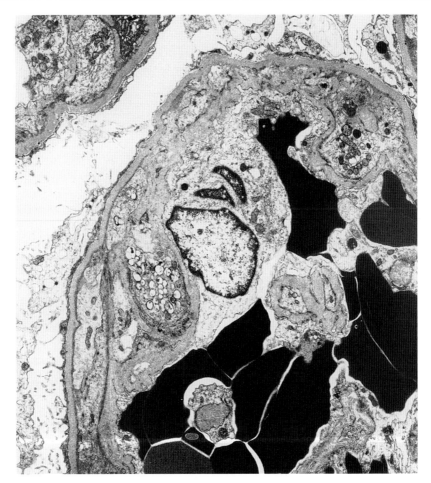

FIG. 1.231 Sickle cell nephropathy. The capillary loop is greatly distorted due to swollen endothelial cells and interposition without well-defined immune complexes. The capillary lumen is obliterated by sickled cells. The overlying foot processes are extensively effaced (transmission electron microscopy, ×19,000).

complex–type deposits (Fig. 1.231, 1.232). Sickle cell nephropathy can also recur in the transplant.

Etiology/Pathogenesis

Patients with either homozygous sickle cell disease or sickle cell thalassemia or hemoglobinopathy sickle cell may develop any renal disease related to sickling, including sickle cell nephropathy. Sickle cell trait may also result in significant sickling and even sickle cell crisis, but has only rarely been reported to cause sickle cell nephropathy. The pathogenesis of sickle cell crisis is related to decreased oxygen tension, particularly due to dehydration and exercise, triggering sickling. The vasa recta are particularly vulnerable because of relative hypoxia, low pH, and hypertonicity of the medulla, which all promote polymerization of the abnormal hemoglobin and sickling of RBCs. Papillary necrosis occurs secondary to the sickled RBCs occluding blood flow. In patients with gradual development of proteinuria and chronic renal insufficiency, the postulated pathogeneses relate to chronic hypoxia, endothelial injury related to iron/heme components and sickling of RBCs, imbalance in nitric oxide, and secondary mechanisms of marked glomerular hypertrophy/hypertension and hyperfiltration, all culminating in segmental sclerosis. Transgenic sickle cell mice are being studied to further elucidate

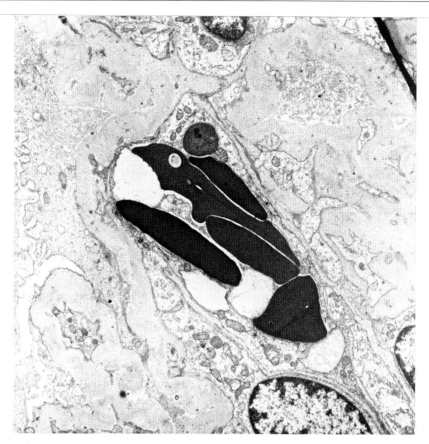

FIG. 1.232 Sickle cell nephropathy. There is marked mesangial matrix expansion and corrugation of the glomerular basement membrane. The capillary lumen is nearly occluded by sickled cells (transmission electron microscopy, ×21,000).

the pathogenesis of renal disease and efficacy of interventions. Clinical trials are ongoing to treat sickle cell patients with microalbuminuria, evidence of early renal injury, with angiotensin-converting enzyme inhibitors. Recently sickle cell trait has been postulated to modify risk for chronic kidney disease.

Selected Reading

Bernstein, J., Whitten, C.F., 1960. A histological appraisal of the kidney in sickle cell anemia. Archives in Pathology 70, 407-417.

Bhathena, D.B., Sondheimer, J.H., 1991. The glomerulopathy of homozygous sickle hemoglobin (SS) disease: morphology and pathogenesis. Journal of the American Society of Nephrology 1, 1241-1252.

Buckalew Jr., V.M., Someren, A., 1974. Renal manifestations of sickle cell disease. Archives of Internal Medicine 133, 660-669.

Elfenbein, I.B., Patchefsky, A., Schwartz, W., et al., 1974. Pathology of the glomerulus in sickle cell anemia with and without nephrotic syndrome. American Journal of Pathology 77, 357-374.

Falk, R.J., Scheinman, J., Phillips, G., et al., 1992. Prevalence and pathologic features of sickle cell nephropathy and response to inhibition of angiotensin-converting enzyme. New England Journal of Medicine 326, 910-915.

Pham, P.T., Pham, P.C., Wilkinson, A.H., et al., 2000. Renal abnormalities in sickle cell disease. Kidney International 57, 1-8.

Scheinman, J.I., 2003. Sickle cell disease and the kidney. Seminars in Nephrology 23, 66-76.

Shaw, C., Sharpe, C.C., 2010. Could sickle cell trait be a predisposing risk factor for CKD? Nephrology Dialysis Transplantation 25, 2403-2405.

FABRY DISEASE

Fabry disease is an X-linked deficiency of alpha-galactosidase A leading to accumulation of glycosphingolipids. Hemizygous males experience multisystem symptoms starting in infancy or childhood, with painful neuropathies and skin, cardiovascular, and renal disease. The early renal manifestations are a concentrating defect, with proteinuria appearing in adulthood, and renal failure developing by age 40-50 years. Patients also develop hemangiomas, conjunctival telangiectasias, corneal and lenticular opacities, and abnormal intestinal mobility. The typical skin lesion is the red nonblanching papular angiokeratoma corporis diffusum. Renal transplantation has obviated death from chronic renal failure, but does not provide sufficient normal enzyme to prevent systemic manifestations of disease. Patients with residual enzyme activity and heterozygous females often have milder course of the disease. However, heterozygous females may also be affected, depending on degree of lyonization of the mutated allele. Thus, some female carriers also develop significant disease, including end-stage kidney disease.

With standard processing, the accumulated galactosyl ceramide is extracted by xylene. Lectin histochemistry on Epon-embedded material to stain lysosomal sugar residues can be useful for specific diagnosis. By light microscopy, podocytes and tubular cells are prominently vacuolated (Figs. 1.233-1.235). With progressive disease, mesangial expansion and glomerulosclerosis develop, with proportional interstitial fibrosis and tubular atrophy. There may be segmental GBM double contours. Inclusions are also present early in Henle loop and especially the distal tubule, and occasionally in the proximal tubule (Figs. 1.236-1.238). Vascular sclerosis can be prominent even in early disease. Standard immunofluorescence may show IgM and C3 trapping in mesangial areas. By electron microscopy, inclusions in lysosomes are widespread and may be present in all renal cells. The inclusions vary in size and structure, and have been called myelin bodies, whorled or lamellated inclusions or zebra bodies (Figs. 1.239-1.241). The lamellated inclusions show alternating dark and light layers with a periodicity of 35-50Å. These inclusions are most prominently present in podocytes but also are variably present in endothelium, particularly of the peritubular capillary, tubules, and interstitial cells. Distal tubules also

---

Key Diagnostic Findings of Fabry Disease

- Vacuolization of cells, particularly podocytes, by LM
- Lysosomal inclusions in myelin bodies on toluidine blue EM scout sections
- Lysosomal inclusions by EM

EM, electron microscopy; *LM,* light microscopy.

Differential Diagnosis of Fabry Disease

- Hydrochloroquine or other drugs that inhibit lysosomes may result in similar inclusions.
- Vacuolization of podocytes may also be seen in other storage diseases such as Niemann-Pick, Gaucher.
- Extensive myelin bodies may also be seen in lecithin-cholesterol acyltransferase deficiency, but typically then are present throughout the glomerular basement membrane and not confined to the cells.

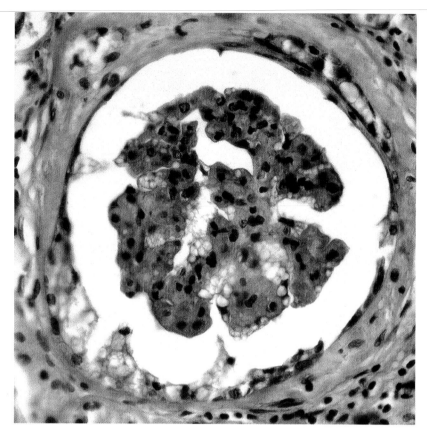

FIG. 1.233 Fabry disease. The podocytes and parietal epithelial cells show a vacuolated, honeycomb appearance resulting from accumulation of the abnormal glycosphingolipid in Fabry disease. Endothelial and mesangial cells are less prominently affected in this glomerulus (hematoxylin and eosin, ×200).

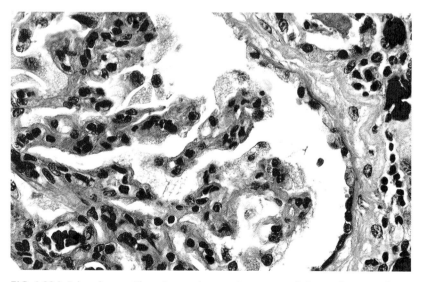

FIG. 1.234 Fabry disease. There is prominent enlargement of glomerular visceral epithelial cells with a vacuolated, honeycomb appearance. There is also associated mild mononuclear cell infiltrate. Lesser glycosphingolipid accumulation is present in the parietal epithelial cells (hematoxylin and eosin, ×200).

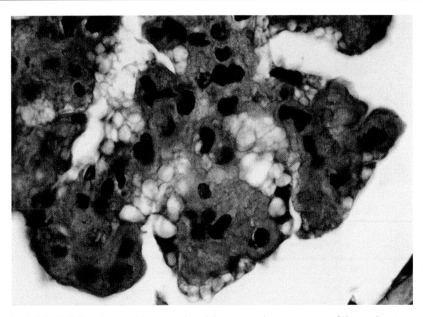

FIG. 1.235 Fabry disease. The vacuolated, honeycomb appearance of the podocytes is due to the accumulation of glycosphingolipid. Lesser accumulation in mesangial or endothelial cell is seen on the left, along with a mononuclear cell infiltrate (hematoxylin and eosin, ×400).

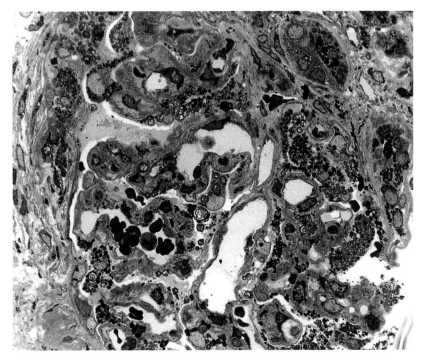

FIG. 1.236 Fabry disease. On the toluidine blue–stained plastic-embedded sections, the lysosomal inclusions and myelin bodies are numerous, especially in the podocytes. Surrounding tubular epithelium also shows this accumulated glycosphingolipid, with focal accumulation in parietal epithelial cells (toluidine blue, ×400).

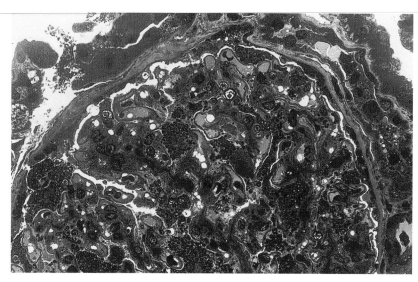

FIG. 1.237 Fabry disease. Massive accumulation of lysosomal inclusions and myelin bodies is present in podocytes with lesser accumulation in parietal epithelium and adjacent tubular epithelium (toluidine blue, ×400).

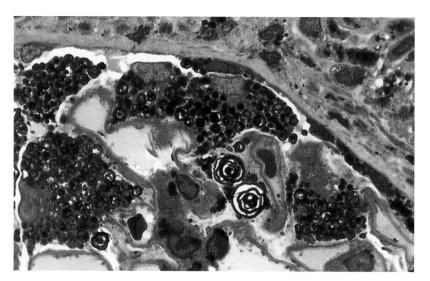

FIG. 1.238 Fabry disease. The myelin bodies and lysosomal inclusions, some of which are lamellated, are abundant in podocytes, with lesser accumulation in mesangial cells and adjacent proximal tubular cells and parietal epithelial cells (toluidine blue, ×1000).

show frequent inclusions. A recent large biopsy study of 59 adult patients, including 24 females, showed that chronic kidney disease stage correlated with severity of arterial and glomerular sclerosis. Significant changes, including segmental and global sclerosis, and interstitial fibrosis were seen even in patients with stage 1-2 chronic kidney disease with minimal proteinuria.

Etiology/Pathogenesis

Fabry disease is an X-linked recessive disease due to a deficiency of alpha-galactosidase. Disease occurs due to accumulation of intracellular glycosphingolipid globotriaosylceramide (Gb3). This enzyme is present in lysosomes throughout the body, and thus the disease manifestations

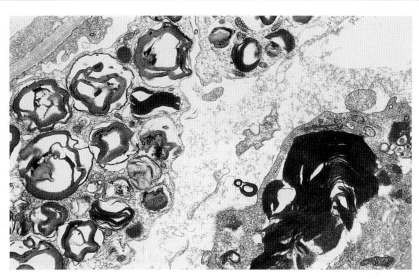

FIG. 1.239 Fabry disease. Lysosomal inclusions with lamellated structure are abundantly present in the podocyte. The glomerular basement membrane itself (upper left) is intact (transmission electron microscopy, ×12,000).

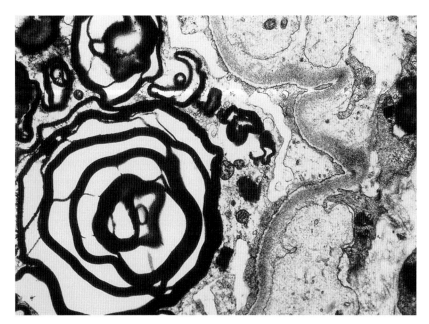

FIG. 1.240 Fabry disease. Lysosomal inclusion with so-called myelin body appearance in the podocyte (transmission electron microscopy, ×34,000).

are systemic. Its frequency is approximately 1:40,000 in the United States. Heterozygous females may also be affected, although typically with milder manifestations. Genetically engineered alpha-galactosidase A can now be used to treat patients with Fabry disease, resulting in decreased disease manifestations with decreased mesangial expansion and better preservation of GFR in some series. Renal disease has been postulated to be related to podocyte injury consequent to the marked accumulation of Gb3 in these cells. In other studies, decreased peritubular capillary inclusions correlated with improvement after replacement enzyme

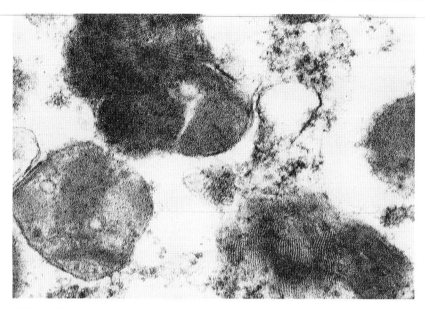

FIG. 1.241 Fabry disease. Dense lysosomal inclusions within tubular epithelium (transmission electron microscopy, ×34,000).

therapy. Early intervention in children has even resulted in cessation of proteinuria. Effect of intervention on other morphologic injury is unknown.

Selected Reading

Alroy, J., Sabnis, S., Kopp, J.B., 2002. Renal pathology in Fabry disease. Journal of the American Society of Nephrology 13 (Suppl 2):S134-S138.

Branton, M.H., Schiffmann, R., Sabnis, S.G., et al., 2002. Natural history of Fabry renal disease: influence of alpha-galactosidase A activity and genetic mutations on clinical course. Medicine (Baltimore) 81, 122-138.

Faraggiana, T., Churg, J., 1987. Renal lipidoses: a review. Human Pathology 18, 661-679.

Faraggiana, T., Churg, J., Grishman, E., et al., 1981. Light and electron microscopic histochemistry of Fabry's disease. American Journal of Pathology 103, 247-262.

Farge, D., Nadler, S., Wolfe, L.S., et al., 1985. Diagnostic value of kidney biopsy in heterozygous Fabry's disease. Archives of Pathological Laboratory Medicine 109, 85-88.

Fogo, A.B., Bostad, L., Svarstad, E., et al., all members of the International Study Group of Fabry Nephropathy (ISGFN) 2010. Scoring system for renal pathology in Fabry disease: report of the International Study Group of Fabry Nephropathy (ISGFN). Nephrology Dialysis Transplantation 25, 2168-2177.

Ojo, A., Meier-Kriesche, H.U., Friedman, G., et al., 2000. Excellent outcome of renal transplantation in patients with Fabry's disease. Transplantation 69, 2337-2339.

Schiffmann, R., Kopp, J.B., Austin 3rd, H.A., et al., 2001. Enzyme replacement therapy in Fabry disease: a randomized controlled trial. Journal of the American Medical Association 285, 2743-2749.

Sessa, A., Meroni, M., Battini, G., et al., 2001. Renal pathological changes in Fabry disease. Journal of Inherited Metabolic Disease 24 (Suppl 2), 66-70.

Thurberg, B.L., Rennke, H., Colvin, R.B., et al., 2002. Globotriaosylceramide accumulation in the Fabry kidney is cleared from multiple cell types after enzyme replacement therapy. Kidney International 62, 1933-1946.

Tøndel, C., Bostad, L., Hirth, A., et al., 2008. Renal biopsy findings in children and adolescents with Fabry disease and minimal albuminuria. American Journal of Kidney Disease 51, 767-776.

LIPOPROTEIN GLOMERULOPATHY

Lipoprotein glomerulopathy is a disorder with apparent autosomal recessive inheritance in some kindreds, with proteinuria and steroid-resistant nephrotic syndrome. Most described patients have been Japanese or Chinese, but the disease has also been rarely described in patients of other ethnicities. Males outnumber females. Patients are usually adult at presentation, although some patients were children. Patients typically have increased beta-lipoprotein and pre-beta-lipoprotein with elevated serum levels of apoE. Glomerular lesions identical to those observed in these patients also occur in patients with type III hyperlipoproteinemia. Approximately one third of patients show slowly progressive renal disease, and the lesions may recur in renal transplants.

The characteristic light microscopic lesion is one of intracapillary lipoprotein thrombi distending and enlarging glomeruli (Fig. 1.242). The mesangium may show mesangiolysis. In areas that do not show mesangiolysis, there is increased mesangial cellularity and matrix. The capillary wall can be thickened or split in response to this injury. The lipoprotein thrombi stain only lightly with PAS, and typically are vacuolated and laminated. The material stains positively for Oil red O and Sudan stain (Fig. 1.243). There may be associated segmental sclerosis, but in contrast to lecithin-cholesterol acyltransferase (LCAT) deficiency, there usually is no predominant foam cell change in the glomerulus, unless sclerosis has occurred. The tubulointerstitial changes are proportionate and follow glomerulosclerosis. There are no specific vascular lesions. By immunofluorescence, there may be IgM, C1q, and fibrinogen surrounding the lipoprotein thrombi, which contain beta-lipoprotein, apoB, and apoE. By electron microscopy, there are vacuolated or granular electron-dense or lucent deposits and thrombi, often with a concentric, laminated pattern with small lipid vacuoles (Fig. 1.244). The double contour of the capillary wall is determined by electron microscopy to be due to segmental lipid material between the endothelial cell and the GBM, with segmental mesangial interposition (Fig. 1.245).

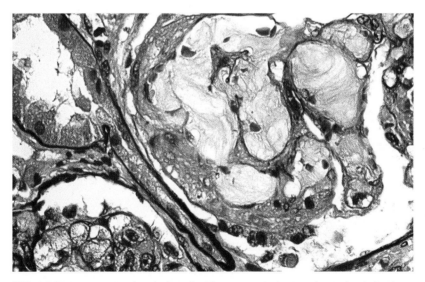

FIG. 1.242 Lipoprotein glomerulopathy. There are massive intraluminal pale lipid thrombi in the glomerular capillaries, distending the capillary lumens, with segmental GBM splitting (Jones silver stain, ×200). (Case 1.242-1.245 kindly provided by Dr. Barry Stokes). *GBM,* glomerular basement membrane.

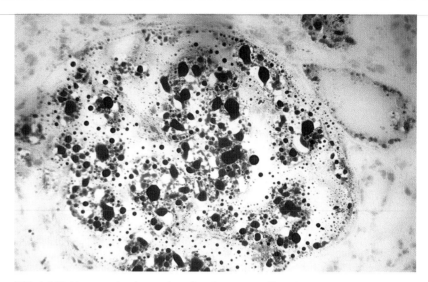

FIG. 1.243 Lipoprotein glomerulopathy. The intracapillary thrombi stain brightly positive for lipid (oil Red O stain, ×200).

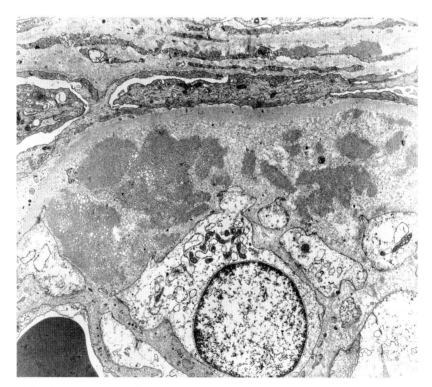

FIG. 1.244 Lipoprotein glomerulopathy. The intracapillary thrombi have a concentric, laminated pattern with small lipid vacuoles (transmission electron microscopy, ×8000).

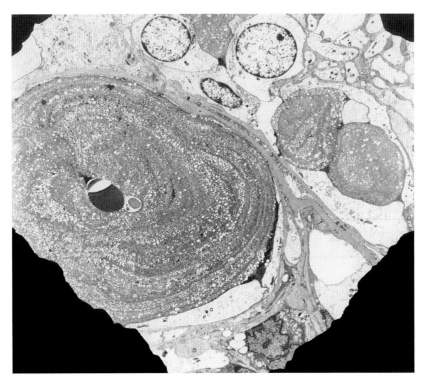

FIG. 1.245 Lipoprotein glomerulopathy. Occasional subendothelial/intramembranous deposits, with lipid vacuoles are present (transmission electron microscopy, ×18,000).

Selected Reading

Boumendjel, R., Papari, M., Gonzalez, M., 2010. A rare case of lipoprotein glomerulopathy in a white man: an emerging entity in Asia, rare in the white population. Archives of Pathology & Laboratory Medicine 134, 279-282.

Faraggiana, T., Churg, J., 1987. Renal lipidosis: A review. Human Pathology 18, 661-679.

Saito, T., Sato, H., Kudo, K., et al., 1989. Lipoprotein glomerulopathy: Glomerular lipoprotein thrombi in a patient with hyperlipoproteinemia. American Journal of Kidney Disease 132, 148-153.

Watanabe, Y., Ozaki, I., Yoshida, F., et al., 1989. A case of nephrotic syndrome with glomerular lipoprotein deposition with capillary ballooning and mesangiolysis. Nephron 521, 265-270.

LECITHIN-CHOLESTEROL ACYLTRANSFERASE DEFICIENCY

This systemic disorder is due to deficiency of LCAT, due to a mutation of the gene, which is on the long arm of chromosome 16. The disease was originally described in Scandinavian patients, but occurs worldwide, and is inherited as an autosomal recessive trait with varying plasma levels of lecithin-cholesterol acyltransferase in different kindreds. Patients have proteinuria, anemia, hyperlipidemia, corneal opacities, and accelerated atherosclerosis. Early kidney disease manifests as proteinuria, increasing in severity by the fourth and fifth decades, frequently progressing to nephrotic syndrome and end-stage renal disease. Genetic testing may be useful in diagnosis.

Light microscopy shows thickened capillary walls with irregular bubble appearance of the basement membranes (Figs. 1.246-1.249). The mesangium is expanded, often with a bubble

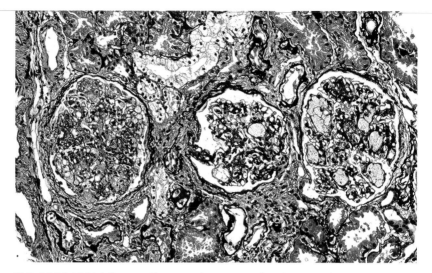

FIG. 1.246 LCAT deficiency. There may be nonspecific sclerosis and tubulointerstitial fibrosis. The glomerular basement membrane is irregular and thickened. The mesangium is expanded, and there is variable foam cell infiltrate within capillary lumens and in mesangial areas, as seen on the left (Jones silver stain, ×100). *LCAT,* lecithin-cholesterol acyltransferase.

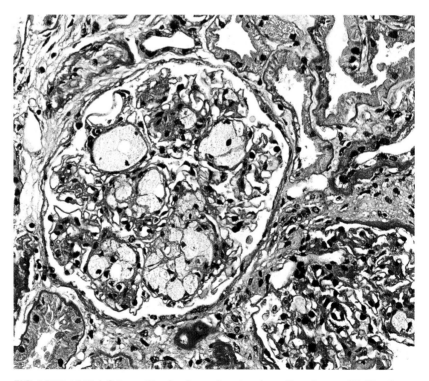

FIG. 1.247 LCAT deficiency. The focal prominent endocapillary foam cell infiltration is evident, with only minimal foam cells in the glomerulus on the left (periodic acid Schiff, ×200). *LCAT,* lecithin-cholesterol acyltransferase.

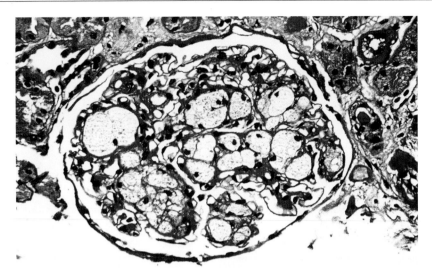

FIG. 1.248 LCAT deficiency. Segmental irregular peripheral capillary basement membranes are present, with prominent intracapillary and mesangial foam cells (hematoxylin and eosin, ×400). *LCAT,* lecithin-cholesterol acyltransferase.

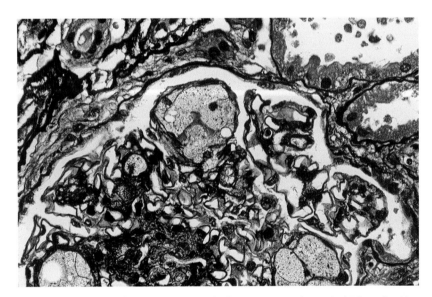

FIG. 1.249 LCAT deficiency. The glomerular basement membrane is thickened, with occasional double contours (bottom left). There are prominent intracapillary foam cells, with rare lipid vacuoles, and increased mesangial matrix (Jones silver stain, ×400). *LCAT,* lecithin-cholesterol acyltransferase.

appearance, with a variable foam cell infiltrate in capillaries and mesangial areas (Figs. 1.247-1.249). Foam cells may also be present in vessels and interstitium. In advanced cases, segmental sclerosis and hyalinosis are present. There are no immune complexes by immunofluorescence. Variable results have been reported with lipid stains. Electron microscopy reveals lacunae in basement membranes and mesangium-containing dense structures that appear solid or lamellar, or contain dense particles (striated membranous structures) (see Differential Diagnosis for Fabry Disease). Cells contain lipid inclusions (Fig. 1.250). The foot processes are effaced.

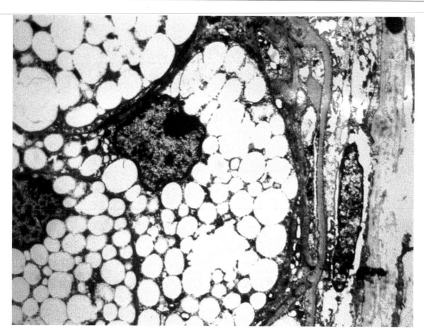

FIG. 1.250 LCAT deficiency. In the basement membrane, there may be lacuna, or solid or lamellar dense structures (not shown). Numerous lipid inclusions are seen within the intracapillary foam cells by electron microscopy (transmission electron microscopy, ×8000). *LCAT,* lecithin-cholesterol acyltransferase.

Etiology/Pathogenesis

LCAT is a catalyst for esterification of free cholesterol bound to low-density lipoprotein. LCAT deficiency is due to mutation of the gene. The different mutations result in varying enzyme levels, ranging from absolute absence in some kindreds, to 10-20% in some homozygotes. Heterozygotes may also have diminished LCAT activity. The gene frequency is about 2% in Scandinavia. Decreased LCAT activity results in abnormal lipid metabolism and accumulation of unesterified cholesterol, triglycerides, and phosphatidylcholine throughout the body. Lipid accumulations have been documented in aorta, other arteries, liver, spleen, and cornea. No effective therapy has been identified. Recently, knockout mice have been generated, creating a method for testing new gene therapy approaches. Renal transplantation does not restore normal lipid metabolism. Deposition of these lipid-related materials with foam cells in glomeruli recurs as early as 6 months after transplantation although renal function is usually maintained.

Selected Reading

Faraggiana, T., Churg, J., 1987. Renal lipidosis: A review. Human Pathology 18, 661-679.

Gjøne, E., 1981. Familial lecithin:cholesterol acyltransferase deficiency: a new metabolic disease with renal involvement. Advances in Nephrology 10, 167-185.

Hovig, T., Gjøne, E., 1974. Familial lecithin:cholesterol acyltransferase deficiency. Scandinavian Journal of Clinical Laboratory Investigation 33, 135-146.

Imbasciati, E., Paties, C., Scarpioni, L., et al., 1986. Renal lesions in familial lecithin-cholesterol acyltransferase deficiency: ultrastructural heterogeneity of glomerular changes. American Journal of Nephrology 6, 66-70.

Joosten, H., Strunk, A.L., Meijer, S., et al., 2010. An aid to the diagnosis of genetic disorders underlying adult-onset renal failure: a literature review. Clinical Nephrology 73, 454-472.

Lager, D.J., Rosenberg, B.F., Shapiro, H., et al., 1991. Lecithin cholesterol acyltransferase deficiency: ultrastructural examination of sequential renal biopsies. Modern Pathology 4, 331-335.

Lambert, G., Sakai, N., Vaisman, B.L., et al., 2001. Analysis of glomerulosclerosis and atherosclerosis in lecithin cholesterol acyltransferase-deficient mice. Journal of Biological Chemistry 276, 15090-15098.

HEREDITARY FOCAL SEGMENTAL GLOMERULOSCLEROSIS

Studies of the molecular biology of the podocyte and identification of genes mutated in rare familial forms of nephrotic syndrome or FSGS, such as nephrin, α-actinin-4 and podocin, have given important new insights into mechanisms of progressive glomerulosclerosis. Although there are no reliable morphologic clues as to the genetic nature of these diseases, an overview of the genetic mechanisms is provided.

CD2AP: Mutations of CD2AP, a key element interacting with nephrin in the slit diaphragm, have been detected in a few adult patients with proteinuria and FSGS without a family history of the disease.

ACTN4: Additional important genes interacting with the nephrin–CD2AP complex have been identified in rare cases of familial FSGS. Autosomal dominant FSGS is caused by mutation in α-actinin 4 (ACTN4), localized to chromosome 19q13. This is hypothesized to cause altered actin cytoskeleton interaction, causing FSGS through a gain-of-function mechanism, contrasting the loss-of-function mechanism implicated for disease caused by the nephrin mutation. Patients with ACTN-4 mutation progress to end stage by age 30 years, with rare recurrence in the transplant. Unusual cytoplasmic electron-dense aggregates in podocytes, perhaps representing accumulated abnormal fragments of α-actinin-4, have been observed.

Podocin: Podocin, another podocyte-specific gene (NPHS2), is mutated in autosomal recessive FSGS with an early onset in childhood with rapid progression to end stage. Podocin is an integral stomatin protein family member and interacts with the nephrin–CD2AP complex, indicating that podocin could serve in the structural organization of the slit diaphragm. In some series of steroid-resistant pediatric patients with nonfamilial forms of FSGS, a surprisingly high proportion, up to 25%, had podocin mutations. However, mutations of NPHS2 or WT-1 were not present in a recent study of African American children with FSGS and/or steroid-resistant nephrotic syndrome. Podocin mutations have been only very rarely detected in adult-onset steroid-resistant FSGS. Importantly, patients with podocin mutations are generally resistant to steroid therapy.

TRPC6: Familial FSGS has also been caused by mutations in the TRPC6 (transient receptor potential cation channel-6) ion channel gene located on chromosome 11q. The disease is autosomal dominant, with the mutation causing enhanced cell surface expression of the channel. TRPC6 is normally expressed on the podocyte. The mechanism for development of FSGS is not determined, but postulated to involve perturbed glomerular homeostasis and/or apoptosis related to exaggerated calcium responses to, for example, angiotensin.

PLCE1: Diffuse mesangial sclerosis or FSGS in a large kindred was recently linked to a truncating mutation of phospholipase C epsilon (PLCE1), and two of these patients responded to steroid therapy. PLCE1 is expressed in the glomerulus where it is postulated to play a key role in development, perhaps by interacting with other proteins that are crucial for the development and function of the slit diaphragm.

Mitochondrial tRNA[Leu(UUR)]: Mitochondrial cytopathy is due to a mutation of mitochondrial DNA in tRNA[Leu(UUR)]. Patients have myopathy, stroke, encephalopathy, and occasionally diabetes mellitus, hearing problems, cardiomyopathy, and FSGS with unusual hyaline lesions in arterioles. Some patients with FSGS without full-blown features of mitochondrial cytopathy have also been reported to have this mitochondrial mutation. Several developed diabetes or hearing loss after onset of proteinuria in adolescence, with biopsy showing multinucleated podocytes and dysmorphic mitochondria. However, there may not be any discernible morphologic findings.

INF2: Recently, mutation in INF2, which encodes a member of the formin family of actin-regulating proteins, was linked to autosomal dominant familial FSGS. Patients had variable, occasional nephrotic-range proteinuria but not full-blown nephrotic syndrome, adult onset, and frequently progressed to end-stage renal disease. The dysregulation of actin within podocytes is postulated to cause the disease. Morphologically, the FSGS was of usual type, with subtotal foot process effacement and prominent actin bundles in foot processes by electron microscopy.

Selected Reading

Bertelli, R., Ginevri, F., Caridi, G., et al., 2003. Recurrence of focal segmental glomerulosclerosis after renal transplantation in patients with mutations of podocin. American Journal of Kidney Diseases 41, 1314-1321.

Boute, N., Gribouval, O., Roselli, S., et al., 2000. NPHS2, encoding the glomerular protein podocin, is mutated in autosomal recessive steroid-resistant nephrotic syndrome. Nature Genetics 24, 349-354.

Brown, E.J., Schlöndorff, J.S., Becker, D.J., et al., 2010. Mutations in the formin gene INF2 cause focal segmental glomerulosclerosis. Nature Genetics 42, 72-76.

Chernin, G., Heeringa, S.F., Gbadegesin, R., et al., 2008. Low prevalence of NPHS2 mutations in African American children with steroid-resistant nephrotic syndrome. Pediatric Nephrology 23, 1455-1460.

Hildebrandt, F., Heeringa, S.F., 2009 Apr. Specific podocin mutations determine age of onset of nephrotic syndrome all the way into adult life. Kidney International 75, 669-671.

Hinkes, B., Wiggins, R.C., Gbadegesin, R., et al., 2006. Positional cloning uncovers mutations in PLCE1 responsible for a nephrotic syndrome variant that may be reversible. Nature Genetics 38, 1397-1405.

Hotta, O., Inoue, C.N., Miyabayashi, S., et al., 2001. Clinical and pathologic features of focal segmental glomerulosclerosis with mitochondrial tRNALeu(UUR) gene mutation. Kidney International 59, 1236-1243.

Kaplan, J.M., Kim, S.H., North, K.N., et al., 2000. Mutations in ACTN4, encoding alpha-actinin-4, cause familial focal segmental glomerulosclerosis. Nature Genetics 24, 251-256.

Kim, J.M., Wu, H., Green, G., et al., 2003. CD2-associated protein haploinsufficiency is linked to glomerular disease susceptibility. Science 300, 1298-1300.

Ruf, R.G., Lichtenberger, A., Karle, S.M., et al., 2004. Arbeitsgemeinschaft Fur Padiatrische Nephrologie Study Group: Patients with mutations in NPHS2 (podocin) do not respond to standard steroid treatment of nephrotic syndrome. Journal of the American Society of Nephrology 15, 722-732.

Winn, M.P., Conlon, P.J., Lynn, K.L., et al., 2005. A mutation in the TRPC6 cation channel causes familial focal segmental glomerulosclerosis. Science 308, 1801-1804.

Woroniecki, R.P., Kopp, J.B., 2007. Genetics of focal segmental glomerulosclerosis. Pediatric Nephrology 22, 638-644.

Diseases Associated with Nephritic Syndrome or RPGN: Immune Mediated

LUPUS NEPHRITIS

Both autopsy and biopsy studies of patients with the clinical diagnosis of SLE have documented that renal involvement is a frequent and serious complication of the disease, making renal biopsy an important part of the clinical management of these patients. The nature of

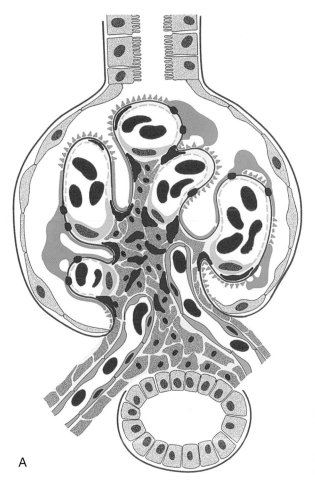

A

FIG. 1.251 (a) Lupus nephritis manifests in various forms. Mesangial lupus nephritis (WHO Type II) is characterized by predominantly mesangial proliferation and is due to mesangial deposits, with rare possible deposits in other compartments.

the lesion on renal biopsy gives direct information relating to the severity of the autoimmune response within the kidney and aids in the selection of appropriate therapies and the prediction of both short- and long-term outcome in individual patients. The various patterns of lupus nephritis (Fig 1.251) must be considered in the context of the potential pathogenetic mechanisms that are involved in their evolution. Analysis in this way not only gives a basis to correlate with clinical outcome but also offers a rationale for therapeutic manipulation. For these reasons, many clinicians advocate renal biopsy as a routine part of the evaluation for all patients with SLE.

The classification scheme for lupus nephritis (LN) was initially developed by the World Health Organization (WHO) as a basis for clinical application (Table 1.6). It combines all morphologic modalities of biopsy interpretation, including immunofluorescence and light and electron microscopic findings, and it thus represents a major improvement over previous classifications. A modification of this classification system, along with an assessment of severity and chronicity, is now in general use and has been accepted by clinical nephrologists and renal pathologists alike. A more detailed subclassification has been suggested by the pathology advisory group of the International Study of Kidney Diseases in Children (ISKDC), but this seems to be of greater value for investigative purposes than for general clinical use. The most recent modification of the previous WHO classification proposed by a joint committee of the International Society of Nephrology and the Renal Pathology Society (ISN/RPS) is more comprehensive (Table 1.7). It eliminates a class for biopsies with no significant findings and

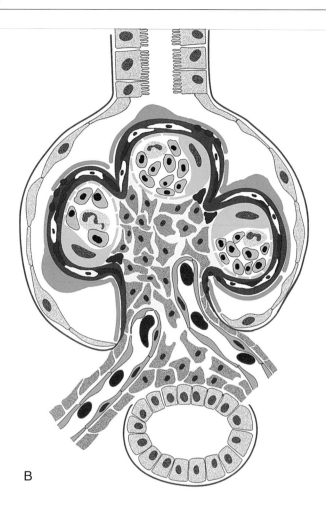

FIG. 1.251 Cont'd   (b) Lupus nephritis may also present as a proliferative lesion when there are subendothelial deposits, with endocapillary proliferation and GBM double contours. In lupus nephritis of the proliferative type, there will frequently be small, scattered subepithelial deposits as well.

B

emphasizes the role of light microscopy and immunofluorescence without requiring electron microscopy. These classifications do have the limitation of focusing on the glomerular lesions while attributing much less significance to tubular, interstitial, and vascular lesions. A recent assessment of the ISN/RPS classification has been published that demonstrates its utility in clinicopathologic studies. Studies addressing the relationship between lupus nephritis IV-S (with segmental lesions) and lupus nephritis IV-G (with global lesions) have failed to consistently identify a significantly worse outcome in IV-S than IV-G but its use has increased the percentage of lupus nephritis biopsies meeting criteria for class IV. A subset of class IV-S lupus nephritis patients show lesions with dominant segmental necrotizing/crescentic lesions with sparse immune complexes. These lesions have been suggested to perhaps be related to antineutrophil cytoplasmic antibodies (ANCAs) (see below). In addition, the issue of how to quantify largely sclerosed glomeruli in differentiating class II focal versus class IV diffuse lupus nephritis is complex. An ongoing review and reassessment of these and other issues of lupus classification will address these and other challenges. Other studies have shown that the new classification provides beneficial pathologic information relevant to the long-term renal outcome and the optimal therapy preventing end-stage renal disease and/or death. Most importantly, the ISN/RPS classification has improved interobserver reproducibility and provides a standardized approach to renal biopsy interpretation needed to compare outcome data across centers and studies.

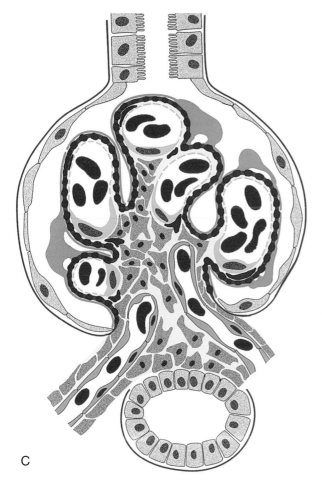

C

FIG. 1.251 Cont'd   (c) In the membranous form of lupus nephritis, there are global subepithelial deposits, as in idiopathic membranous glomerulonephritis, with additional mesangial deposits. GBM, glomerular basement membrane.

TABLE 1-6 1995 Modified Original Classification of Lupus Glomerulonephritis

I. Normal Nil

II. Pure mesangiopathy
   A. Normal by light microscopy but deposits present
   B. Moderate mesangial hypercellularity

III. Segmental and focal proliferative glomerulonephritis
   A. Active necrotizing
   B. Active and sclerosing
   C. Sclerosing

IV. Diffuse proliferative glomerulonephritis
   A. Without segmental necrotizing lesions
   B. With segmental necrotizing lesions
   C. With segmental active and sclerotic lesions
   D. Inactive, sclerotic

V. Diffuse membranous glomerulonephritis
   A. Pure membranous
   B. Associated with lesions in group IIA or IIB

VI. Advanced sclerosing glomerulonephritis

TABLE 1-7 2002 ISN/RPS Classification of Lupus Glomerulonephritis

Class I	Minimal mesangial LGN
	Normal glomeruli by LM, but mesangial immune deposits by IF and/or EM
Class II	Mesangial proliferative LGN
	Purely mesangial hypercellularity of any degree and/or mesangial matrix expansion by LM with immune deposits, predominantly mesangial with none or few, isolated subepithelial and/or subendothelial deposits by IF and/or EM, not visible by LM
Class III	Focal LGN (involving <50% of the total number of glomeruli)
	Active or inactive focal, segmental, and/or global endo- and/or extracapillary GN, typically with focal, subendothelial immune deposits, with or without focal or diffuse mesangial alterations
	Class III(A) Purely active lesions: active focal proliferative LGN
	Class III(A/C) Active and chronic lesions: active and sclerotic focal proliferative LGN
	Class III(C) Chronic inactive with glomerular scars: inactive sclerotic focal LGN
	• Indicate proportion of glomeruli with active and with sclerotic lesions
	• Indicate the proportion of glomeruli with fibrinoid necrosis and/or cellular crescents
Class IV	Diffuse segmental (IV-S) or global (IV-G) LGN (involving ≥50% of the total number of glomeruli either segmentally or globally)
	Active or inactive diffuse, segmental, or global endo- and/or extracapillary GN with diffuse subendothelial immune deposits, with or without mesangial alterations. This class is divided into diffuse segmental (IV-S) when >50% of the involved glomeruli have segmental lesions, and diffuse global (IV-G) when >50% of the involved glomeruli have global lesions.
	Class IV(A) Active lesions: diffuse segmental or global proliferative LGN
	Class IV(A/C) Active and chronic lesions: diffuse segmental or global proliferative and sclerotic LGN
	Class IV(C) Inactive with glomerular scars: diffuse segmental or global sclerotic LGN
	• Indicate the proportion of glomeruli with active and with sclerotic lesions
	• Indicate the proportion of glomeruli with fibrinoid necrosis and/or cellular crescents
Class V	Membranous LGN
	Numerous global or segmental subepithelial immune deposits or their morphologic sequelae by LM and/or IF and/or EM with or without mesangial alterations
	• May occur in combination with III or IV, in which case both will be diagnosed
Class VI	Advanced sclerotic LGN
	90% of glomeruli globally sclerosed without residual activity

Recommend that all renal biopsy include description and semiquantification of active and sclerosing glomerular lesions, grading of tubular atrophy, interstitial inflammation and fibrosis, severity of arteriosclerosis or other vascular lesions.
EM, electron microscopy; *GN,* glomerulonephritis; *IF,* immunofluorescence; *LGN,* lupus glomerulonephritis; *LM,* light microscopy.

Histopathology

In this presentation, the histopathologic findings of the most recent version of the classification will be described as outlined in Table 1.7.

Class I Minimal Mesangial Lupus Nephritis

Class I LN contains lesions with minimal or no significant changes by light microscopy. Immunofluorescence, however, may present evidence of immune deposits that are confined to the mesangium, and electron microscopy reveals corresponding electron-dense deposits in this location (Figs. 1.252, 1.253).

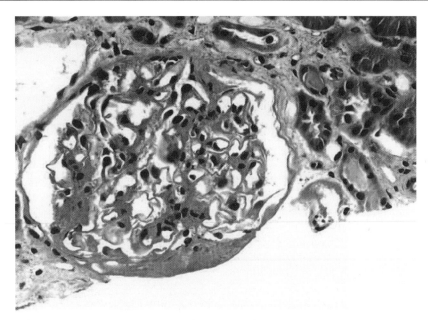

FIG. 1.252 Class I or minimal lupus glomerulonephritis. There is only minimal mild segmental mesangial widening. Peripheral capillary loops are entirely normal (hematoxylin and eosin, ×400).

Class II Mesangial Proliferative Lupus Nephritis

In Class II LN, light microscopy shows definite glomerular mesangial hypercellularity that is confined to the centrilobular areas away from the vascular pole (Fig. 1.254). There is no involvement of the peripheral glomerular capillary walls, and no segmental scars or crescents or necrosis. Immunofluorescence reveals mesangial immunoglobulin deposition (Fig. 1.255), and electron microscopy discloses dense deposits that are dominantly confined to the mesangial regions (Fig. 1.256). In some cases, deposits occasionally are seen in the paramesangial subendothelial areas, or scattered subepithelial deposits are present. Tubular, interstitial, and vascular changes are usually insignificant.

Patients with class II lesions generally have minimal clinical evidence of renal involvement, with mild to moderate proteinuria and/or hematuria and little or no evidence of renal insufficiency.

Class III Focal Lupus Nephritis

Class III is characterized by light microscopic findings of a focal glomerulonephritis. Less than 50% of the glomeruli are involved with either active or chronic lesions. These changes can be segmental or global and be proliferative, necrotizing, crescentic, sclerosing, or a combination of these alterations (Fig. 1.257). Endocapillary and extracapillary (i.e., crescent) cell proliferations with obliteration of the capillary lumina are often found in addition to generalized mesangial widening. Necrotic lesions may be either segmental or rarely global and are usually associated with crescent formations that progress to segmental scars with focal capsular adhesions. These lesions usually are superimposed on variable mesangial hypercellularity (Fig. 1.258). Immunofluorescence reveals peripheral chunky, irregular granular as well as mesangial deposits of immunoglobulins (Fig. 1.259), and electron microscopy demonstrates subendothelial deposits in addition to the presence of mesangial deposits (Fig. 1.260). The similarity of the immunofluorescence and electron microscopic findings of class III lesions with those

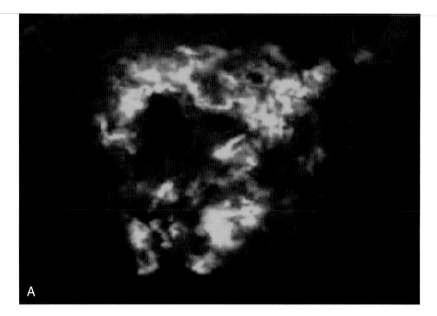

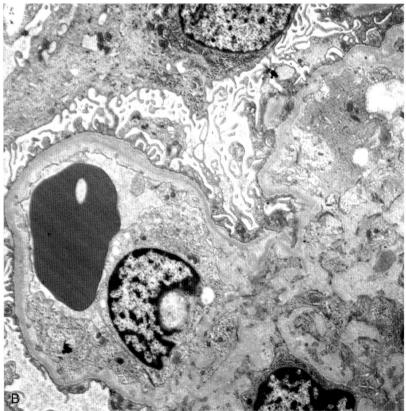

FIG. 1.253 Class I, minimal lupus glomerulonephritis. (a) Immunofluorescence of Class I shows immunoglobulin deposits in the mesangium. Most often this is IgG and may be accompanied by a similar pattern of deposition of C3 (anti-IgG immunofluorescence, ×400). (b) Electron microscopy in Class I reveals open peripheral capillary loops with well-preserved foot processes and endothelial cells. The mesangium contains an increase in mesangial matrix and small mesangial electron-dense deposits (transmission electron microscopy, ×4000).

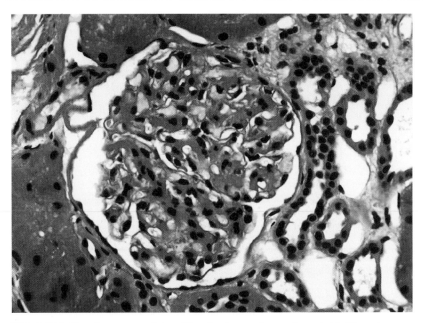

FIG. 1.254 Class II or mesangial proliferative lupus glomerulonephritis. There is more prominent mesangial widening than in Class I and there is a definite increase in mesangial cellularity. The peripheral capillary loops are normal. The adjacent tubules in interstitium are often uninvolved (hematoxylin and eosin, ×400).

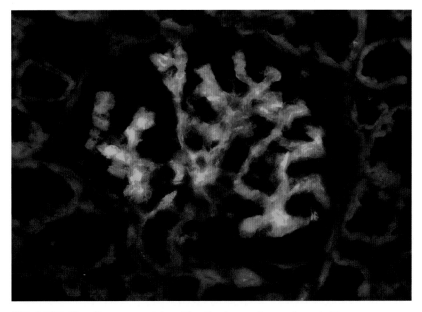

FIG. 1.255 Class II or mesangial proliferative lupus glomerulonephritis. Immunofluorescence of Class II reveals mesangial immunoglobulin deposition. The immunoglobulins deposited in lupus almost always include IgG but a full house of immunoglobulin deposition involving multiple immunoglobulins and complement is characteristic of lupus nephritis (anti-IgG immunofluorescence, ×400).

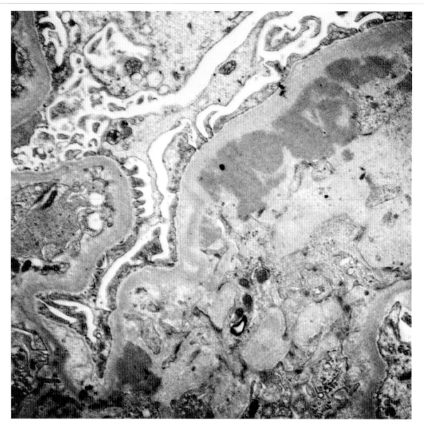

FIG. 1.256 Class II or mesangial proliferative lupus glomerulonephritis. Electron microscopy of Class II shows definite mesangial changes with abundant mesangial electron-dense deposits accompanying the increase in mesangial matrix. The electron-dense deposits correspond to the deposition of immunoglobulins and complement seen by immunofluorescence (transmission electron microscopy, ×5000).

of class IV suggests that these two classes actually may be variations of the same immunopathologic lesion, and that the focal nature of class III represents a quantitative rather than a qualitative difference.

Class III has been broken down into three subclasses: (1) active necrotizing lesions, (2) necrotizing and sclerosing lesions, and (3) purely sclerosing lesions. The clinical significance of this subclassification is not clear, however. The natural history of patients with class III lesions is similar to that of patients with class IV lesions, again suggesting that these two classes are a continuum of the same lesion.

Class IV Diffuse Lupus Nephritis

Class IV is the most common form of active lupus nephritis, and it is characterized by a diffuse global or segmental proliferative glomerulonephritis. Most, or all, of the glomeruli are involved. Glomeruli with active lesions show either mostly global (IV-G) or segmental (IV-S) endocapillary proliferation, often in a lobular pattern, and may also have necrosis and/or crescents (Figs. 1.261, 1.262). A controversial element in the ISN/RPS 2003 classification is the division of lupus nephritis class IV into subcategories based on predominance of segmental (IV-S) or global (IV-G) lesions. Some studies have suggested that despite similar treatment, lupus nephritis class IV-S had a worse prognosis than IV-G. It has also been suggested that the

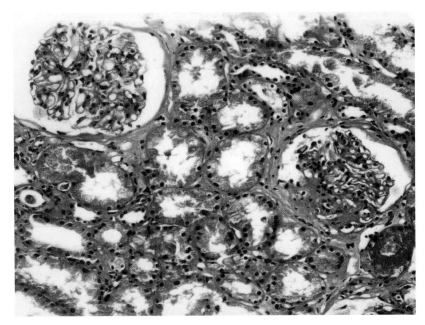

FIG. 1.257 Class III or focal and segmental lupus glomerulonephritis is characterized by focal involvement of glomeruli in which there are segmental lesions as demonstrated here with one entirely normal appearing glomerulus (left) adjacent to glomerulus with a segmental area of adhesion and necrosis (right) (hematoxylin and eosin, ×200).

pathogenesis of lupus nephritis class IV-S may be less dependent on glomerular immune deposits and is similar to that of ANCA-associated nephritis. As with Class III focal lesions, segmental areas of necrosis occasionally associated with focal areas of crescent formation can occur. Nuclear debris represented by hematoxyphil bodies also can be seen. Some segments of peripheral capillary loops can be dramatically thickened because of plaque-like massive subendothelial deposits to form the so-called wire loop lesion. Occasionally extensive deposits of immune complexes bulge into the capillary lumen, the so-called hyaline thrombi (which although smooth and glassy, i.e., "hyaline" in appearance, are not true thrombi and do not contain fibrin). Segmental areas of sclerosis with broad-based adhesions are an indicator either of sequelae of previous segmental necrosis and/or crescents.

The variety of lesions that can be encountered in this class ranges from diffuse mesangial hypercellularity without necrosis to a severe necrotizing and crescentic glomerulonephritis. Segmental and global areas of sclerosis may be present. The new subclassification is useful in separating these different patterns into active class IV lesion, IV (A), proliferative lesions that may also show necrosis and/or crescents; active and chronic class IV, IV (A/C), proliferative or necrotizing or crescentic active lesions combined with sclerosis and/or fibrous/fibrocellular crescents; and chronic class IV, IV(C), lesions of sclerosis and/or fibrous crescents (Fig. 1.263). About one quarter of cases exhibit lobular accentuation because of endocapillary proliferation with mesangial extension and cellular interposition around the peripheral loops, forming a pattern similar to that of other forms of membranoproliferative glomerulonephritis.

Immunofluorescence microscopy reveals a coarsely granular pattern of immunoglobulin deposition both in the mesangium and in the peripheral capillary walls (Fig. 1.264). Multiple immunoglobulins frequently are encountered and generally are accompanied by evidence of the activation of inflammatory mediators, such as a deposition of both classic and alternate complement components, fibrinogen, and properdin. This pattern has been termed a full-house pattern of immunoglobulin deposition.

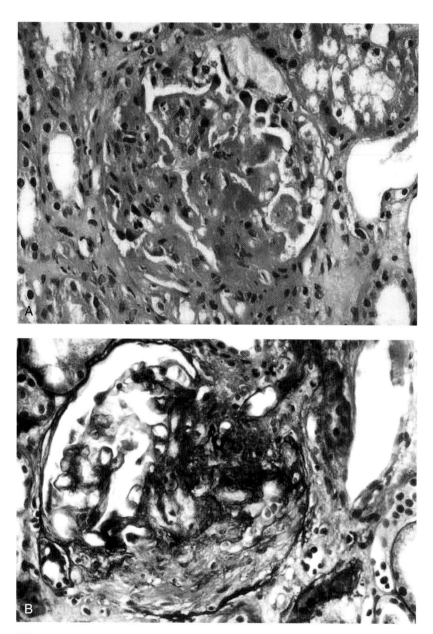

FIG. 1.258 Lupus nephritis. (a) Segmental changes can be merely proliferative or as demonstrated here necrotizing with adhesion to Bowman's capsule loss of the normal architecture. (b) In some instances, this progresses to the presence of epithelial crescents associated with collapse of the normal glomerular architecture (a, hematoxylin and eosin, ×400; b, Masson trichrome, ×400).

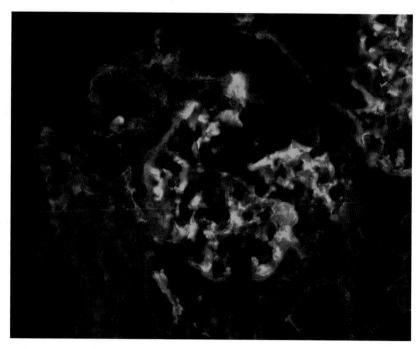

FIG. 1.259 Class III focal lupus nephritis. The mesangial and peripheral capillary deposition of immunoglobulins appears more prominent than in Class II (anti-IgG immunofluorescence, ×400).

Electron microscopic examination is similar to that seen with class III lesions (Fig. 1.265a-d). Abundant subendothelial deposits are accompanied by large mesangial deposits. These deposits generally are larger and more abundant than in other classes of lupus nephritis. Scattered epimembranous deposits often are present. Mesangial hypercellularity with circumferential cellular interposition is associated with the light microscopic pattern of a membranoproliferative glomerulonephritis. Occasionally, the electron-dense deposits show an organized (Fig. 1.265e) or crystalline pattern, which has been termed a fingerprint pattern. This organized appearance most frequently is seen in the presence of abundant endothelial deposits, but it can be present in all classes of lupus nephritis. The crystalline structure is thought by some to represent the presence of cryoglobulins, because similar structures are seen in patients with idiopathic mixed cryoglobulinemia. They also might represent a pattern of crystalline DNA. Endothelial cell swelling and proliferation are prominent, and occasional mitotic figures of glomerular cellular components suggest active proliferation and regeneration secondary to activation of inflammatory cytokines in growth factors. Intraendothelial tubular reticular inclusions (TRIs), also called reticular aggregates (Fig. 1.266) have been identified in a majority of patients with lupus nephritis. The significance of these structures is unclear, but some evidence suggests that they are induced by the cytokine γ-interferon. Class III and IV, focal and diffuse lesions respectively, represent the most severe form of glomerular involvement in patients with SLE, postulated to reflect that the subendothelial immune complexes have access to the humoral and cellular mediators of inflammation that are present in the circulation. Patients with class III or IV pathologic lesions usually have evidence of significant clinical renal disease, including proteinuria (frequently in the nephrotic range), renal insufficiency, and an active urinary sediment, and thus may show combined nephritic and nephrotic syndrome features. In some individual cases these lesions constitute the initial presentation of SLE, and in rare instances, these lesions are silent. The nature of the immunopathogenesis underlying the renal lesion in patients with class III or IV lesions suggests an unfavorable

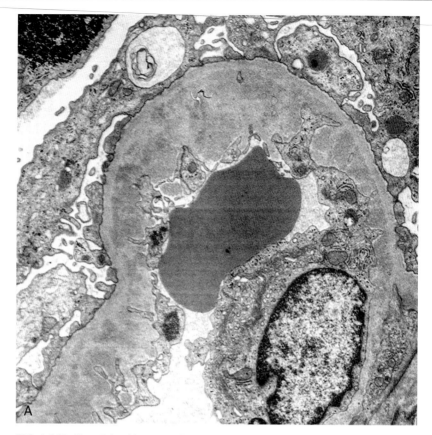

FIG. 1.260 Class III focal lupus nephritis. Electron microscopy in Class III is similar to the findings in Class IV diffuse lupus nephritis. (a) Subendothelial deposits are present in addition to mesangial deposits as seen in Classes I and II, minimal mesangial and mesangioproliferative lupus nephritis, respectively. (transmission electron microscopy, ×4000).

prognosis, with a high percentage of such patients eventually progressing to renal failure despite aggressive treatment. A major consequence of severe glomerular inflammation with necrosis is the development of both glomerular scarring and sclerosis, which results in decreasing glomerular filtration surface and contributes to progressive renal scarring and loss of function.

Class V Membranous Lupus Nephritis

The class V membranous LN lesion is a diffuse, membranous nephropathy. Light microscopy reveals a generalized diffuse thickening of the peripheral capillary walls, which on silver methenamine–Masson stains exhibits a so-called spike and dome pattern (Fig. 1.267). The spikes are outward projections of membrane-like material between domes that correspond to the subepithelial and intramembranous deposits that are seen on immunofluorescence and electron microscopy. Occasional subepithelial deposits may be present in any patient. To meet ISN/RPS criteria for diagnosis of class V membranous LN, more than half the glomeruli should show evidence of subepithelial deposits (e.g., spikes or holes by light microscopy, and/or granular capillary loop deposits by immunofluorescence) in more than half the loops. A variable degree of mesangial widening may be present, involving both an increase of mesangial cells and mesangial matrix and mesangial deposits.

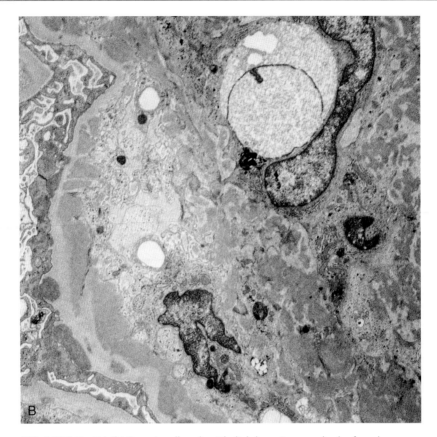

FIG. 1.260 Cont'd (b) Occasionally subepithelial deposits may also be found (transmission electron microscopy, ×4000).

Immunofluorescence demonstrates a classic confluent peripheral granular deposition of immunoglobulins and, occasionally, mesangial granular deposits (Fig. 1.268). Electron microscopy reveals a typical epimembranous nephropathy, with subepithelial and intramembranous deposits of varying electron density (Fig. 1.269). The pattern is essentially identical to that seen in idiopathic membranous nephropathy, except that mesangial deposits usually are present, along with tubuloreticular inclusions.

The modified WHO system used a subclassification to separate biopsies with prominent subepithelial deposits into Va, pure membranous nephritis; Vb, associated with lesions of Class II; Vc, associated with lesions of Class III; and Vd, associated with lesions of Class IV. While this classification is of interest from a historic and morphological view, it is not helpful from a clinical standpoint as patients with Vc and Vd should be treated as aggressively as patients with pure Class III or Class IV. Mixed lesions in the ISN/RPS are therefore designated as focal and membranous LN, Class III with Class V, and diffuse and membranous LN, Class IV with Class V, respectively, emphasizing the more aggressive lesions.

Class VI Advanced Sclerosing Lupus Nephritis

This class is essentially end-stage renal disease. Light microscopy reveals advanced glomerulosclerosis and interstitial fibrosis. Often it cannot be distinguished from chronic sclerosing lesions from other etiologies. The presence of immune deposits by immunofluorescence and electron microscopy, or a previous renal biopsy with lupus nephritis, are the only ways of ascertaining the diagnosis of this class of LN.

Text continued on page 212

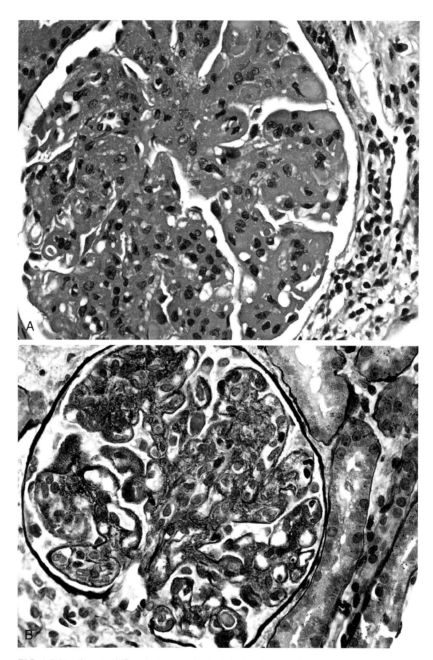

FIG. 1.261 Class IV diffuse lupus nephritis. (a) Class IV or diffuse lupus glomerulonephritis by light microscopy involves most or all of the glomeruli. In general, there is a marked increase in mesangial cellularity with lobular accentuation and double contours of the peripheral capillary loops (hematoxylin and eosin, ×400). (b) Silver methenamine (Jones) stains demonstrate the double contours and demonstrate the presence of subendothelial deposits lining along the capillary loops (×400).

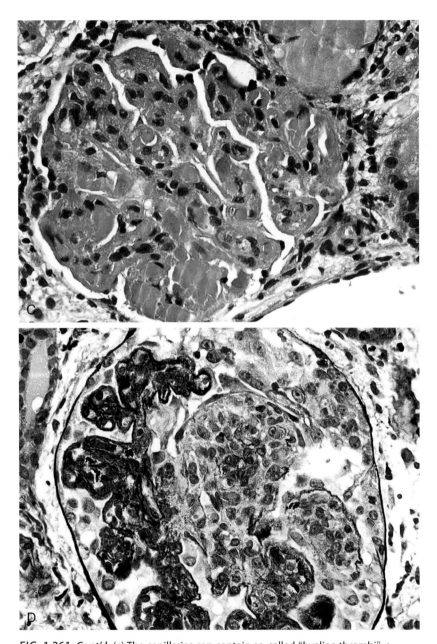

FIG. 1.261 Cont'd (c) The capillaries can contain so-called "hyaline thrombi", a lesion caused by massive subendothelial deposits bulging into the capillary lumen, hyaline thrombi and may be thickened to the point to be considered "wire loop" lesions, due to extensive subendothelial deposits (hematoxylin and eosin, ×400). (d) Segmental areas of necrosis are often associated with the presence of crescents (Masson trichrome, ×400).

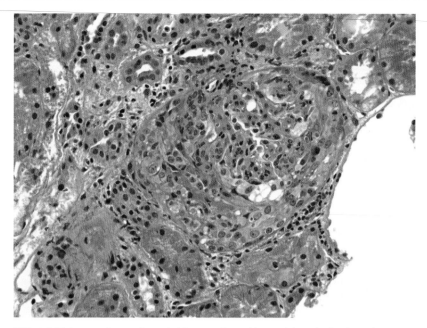

FIG. 1.262 Lupus glomerulonephritis complicated by antiphospholipid syndrome. There is thrombosis and necrosis (hematoxylin and eosin ×400).

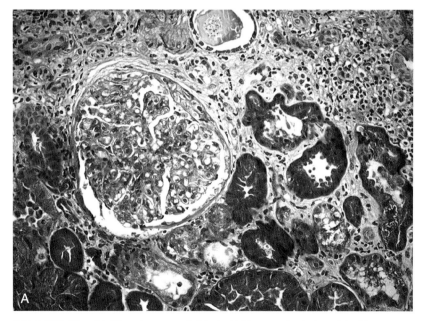

FIG. 1.263 Class IV diffuse lupus nephritis. (a, b) These active lesions (a) will eventually become sclerotic and are subclassified as IVc, namely, proliferative lesions with sclerosis (b) (Masson trichrome, a, ×200; b, ×400).

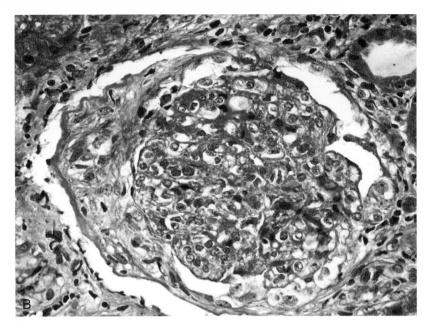

FIG. 1.263 Cont'd

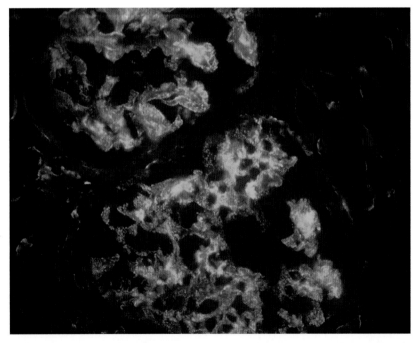

FIG. 1.264 Class IV diffuse lupus nephritis. Immunofluorescence reveals coarsely granular deposition of immunoglobulin in both the mesangium and in the peripheral capillary walls, the latter corresponding to subendothelial deposits (anti-IgG immunofluorescence, ×200).

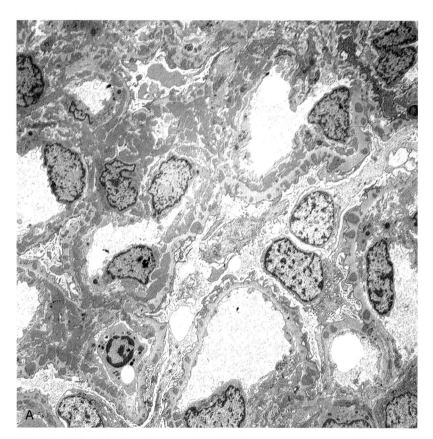

FIG. 1.265 Class IV diffuse lupus nephritis. (a) Electron microscopy reveals the presence of abundant subendothelial deposits lining all capillary loops. These are occasionally accompanied by subepithelial deposits in varying degrees. There are also numerous mesangial deposits (transmission electron microscopy, ×1500).

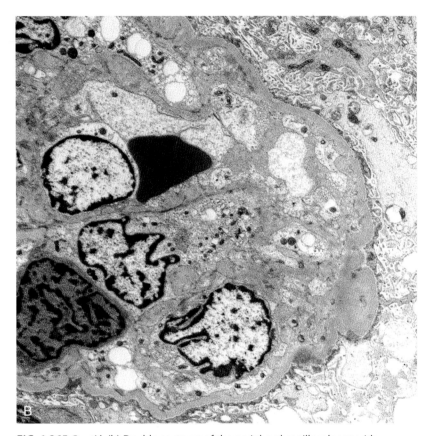

FIG. 1.265 Cont'd (b) Double contours of the peripheral capillary loops with mesangial/mononuclear cell interposition and capillary lumen leukocytic infiltration are also demonstrated (transmission electron microscopy, ×5000).

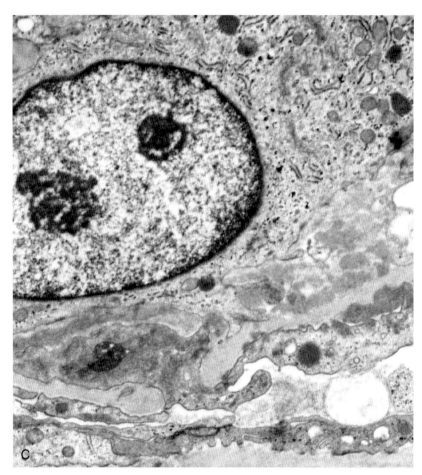

FIG. 1.265 Cont'd (c) Foci of necrosis can be seen with disruption of the glomerular basement membrane and extrusion of the endothelial cells through the gap (transmission electron microscopy, ×10,000).

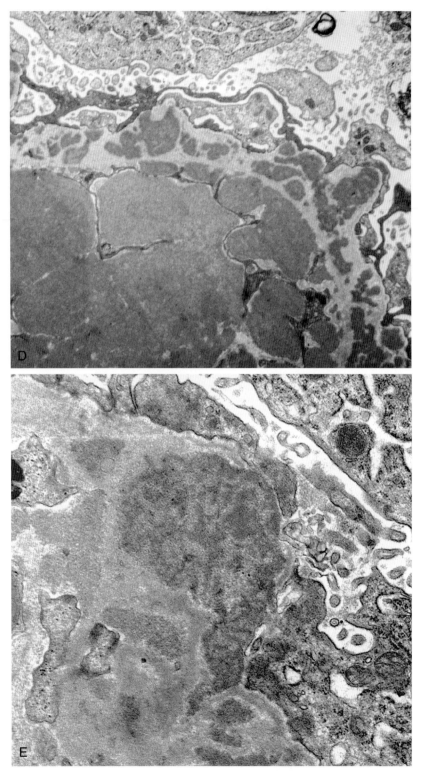

FIG. 1.265 Cont'd (d) The capillary lumen can contain large deposits that correspond to the "hyaline thrombus" seen on light microscopy. (e) The electron-dense deposits seen on electron microscopy often have an organized appearance, sometimes taking a fingerprint pattern (transmission electron microscopy, ×6000, ×10,000).

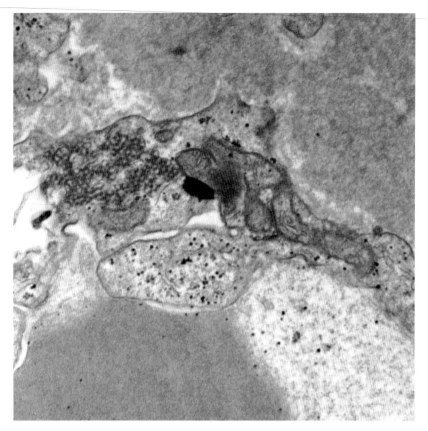

FIG. 1.266 Lupus nephritis. In the majority of patients with lupus, the endothelial cells contain reticular aggregates. The significance of these structures is still unclear, but they are associated with high levels of the cytokine alpha-interferon (transmission electron microscopy, ×15,000).

ATYPICAL PRESENTATIONS OF RENAL INVOLVEMENT IN SLE

Lupus Podocytopathy/Minimal Change Disease

Renal biopsies from patients with SLE who present with nephritic or nephrotic syndrome rarely show changes that are pathogenetically and morphologically unrelated to SLE. Although nephrotic syndrome is commonly associated with diffuse (ISN/RPS class IV) or membranous (ISN/RPS class V) lupus nephritis, several reports have described nephrotic syndrome in adult patients with minimal mesangial lupus nephritis (ISN/RPS class I) or mesangial proliferative lupus nephritis (ISN/RPS class II), sometimes with mesangial deposits of immunoglobulins (IgM or IgG) or complement (C1q or C3) and extensive foot process effacement by electron microscopy consistent with the podocytopathy of minimal change disease (Fig. 1.270). The pathogenesis of nephrotic syndrome with mesangial lupus nephritis is not clearly understood and several mechanisms have been postulated, including lupus nephritis itself, nonsteroidal anti-inflammatory drug (NSAID)–induced minimal change nephrotic syndrome and coincidental occurrence of idiopathic minimal change disease or focal segmental glomerulosclerosis. The prompt response of some such patients to corticosteroids with remission of proteinuria supports possible minimal change disease–like injury. The possibility that the spectrum of autoimmunity that is associated with SLE may include damage related to T cell–mediated immunity resulting in podocyte pathology and proteinuria is interesting but remains speculative.

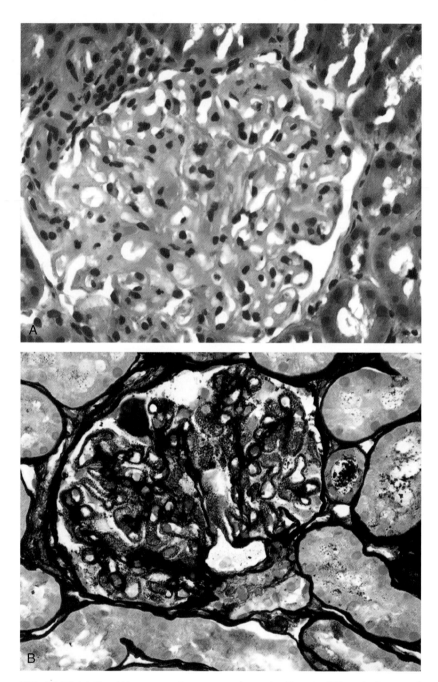

FIG. 1.267 (a) Class V lupus membranous nephropathy. There is diffuse thickening of the peripheral, capillary walls associated with an increase in mesangial matrix. Lobular accentuation is sometimes seen but is not associated with an increase in cellularity (hematoxylin and eosin, ×400). (b) Silver methenamine (Jones) stains reveal a spike and dome pattern to be present along the peripheral capillary loops. Where the wall of the capillaries is cut tangentially; there is a moth-eaten appearance of the capillary wall due to the deposits not staining with silver (Jones, ×400).

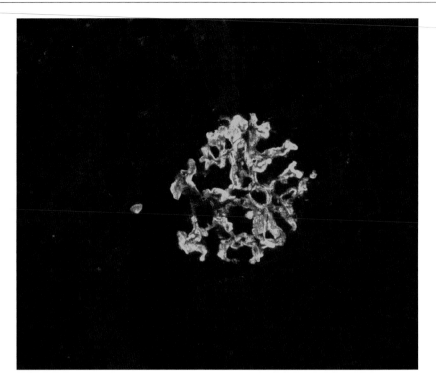

FIG. 1.268 Class V membranous lupus nephritis. Immunofluorescence reveals a peripheral granular deposition of immunoglobulin (anti-IgG immunofluorescence, ×400).

ANCA-Associated Nephritis

In patients with lupus nephritis with biopsy findings of prominent necrosis and crescent formation in the absence of significant endocapillary proliferation or subendothelial deposits, a role for ANCAs should be considered (Fig. 1.271). So-called pauci-immune necrotizing and crescentic glomerular nephritis differs from classical lupus nephritis in that glomerular necrosis and crescent formation are present in the absence of significant glomerular immune complex deposits. ANCAs have been implicated in the pathogenesis of ANCA-associated glomerulo-nephritis and are thought to directly target cytokine-primed neutrophils that express myelo-peroxidase (MPO) or proteinase 3 (PR3) at the cell surface. Recently, a novel ANCA has been shown to be directed against human lysosomal-associated membrane protein 2 (hLAMP2). After activation by an ANCA, neutrophils release cytokines, toxic oxygen metabolites, and lytic proteinases, leading to endothelial damage with subsequent GBM rupture, necrosis, and crescent formation. It is not clear if the ANCAs are part of the autoimmunity of lupus or an independent process superimposed on lupus. Some patients with classical LN with immune complex deposition may also have positive ANCA serology. In both instances, treatment options may include plasmapheresis in addition to immunosuppressive therapy.

Mixed Patterns and Transformation

Given the variability in the clinical and immunologic expression of disease that occurs in SLE, these classes and subclasses likely are not absolutely distinct clinicopathologic entities but rather represent different points in a continuum of disease. This is particularly evident in that transformation of renal lesions from one class to another can occur both spontaneously and as a result of treatment. The exact incidence of spontaneous transformation is difficult to determine, however, as relatively few serial biopsy studies have been performed in untreated

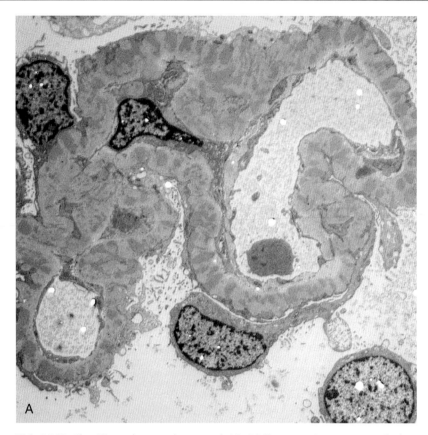

FIG. 1.269 Class V membranous lupus nephritis. (a) Electron microscopy reveals that there are numerous subepithelial deposits scattered throughout the peripheral capillary loops. There are no subendothelial deposits present. Mesangial deposits can be seen (transmission electron microscopy, ×4000).

patients. Further, recurrent lupus nephritis in renal transplants may be of same, or different, class as that seen in the native kidney. A number of studies do suggest that transformation occurs commonly and is particularly noted after various treatment protocols. Transformation from class III to class IV disease has been reported so frequently that most nephropathologists consider these classes to be morphologic variants of a single class of lesion with common immunofluorescence and electron microscopic patterns. Transformation of diffuse proliferative glomerulonephritis to a predominantly membranous nephropathy or a mesangial pattern has been observed in patients undergoing remission during the course of treatment.

Immunofluorescence Microscopic Features

One factor that has not been given enough consideration in the histopathologic evaluation of the glomerular lesion of patients with lupus nephritis is the role of immunoglobulin isotype and subclass. Most studies of the immunofluorescence microscopic findings in lupus nephritis have emphasized the deposition rather than the classes of immunoglobulins found.

In our own series of patients with lupus nephritis, IgG was most frequently present, followed by IgM and IgA. Less often, IgE is detected and usually is confined to the peripheral capillary wall. In LN class III and IV (focal and diffuse, respectively), peripheral granular and mesangial deposits appear concurrently. With equal frequency, IgM and IgG are detected in class II mesangioproliferative LN, and V, membranous LN, disease. IgE is identified most

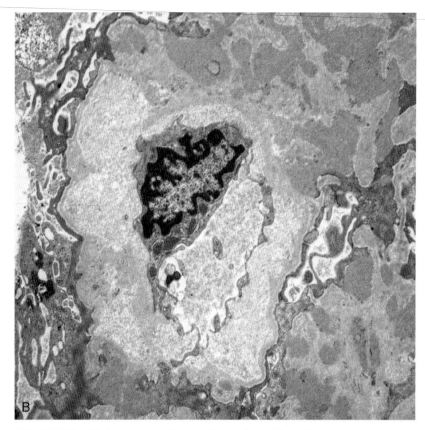

FIG. 1.269 Cont'd (b) In more advanced forms of class V membranous lupus nephritis, some of the deposits may be totally intramembranous and show evidence of resorption (transmission electron microscopy, ×8000).

frequently in class IV diffuse lupus nephritis and appears to be associated with necrosis in some class IV patients. These findings are similar to those of other studies.

IgG and IgM are the classes of immunoglobulin that most commonly are deposited, and although IgA is found frequently, it is not as common, nor is its distribution as extensive, as that of the other two immunoglobulins. In one study, IgG2 was found more frequently than other subclasses. Because subclasses IgG2 and IgG4 do not readily activate complement, a mild lesion would be expected to occur with these subclasses rather than with IgG1 or IgG3. This analysis, however, showed a poor correlation between IgG subclass and the severity of the morphologic lesion. Deposition of IgE usually has not been identified specifically. When reported, however, it has been found infrequently and been thought to reflect part of the general autoimmune response associated with this clinical syndrome of SLE. Some recent reports have suggested that IgE deposits in lupus nephritis are associated with a poor prognosis.

The so-called full-house pattern of multiple immunoglobulin deposition is characteristic of SLE and does not indicate any difference in severity of the lesion from a pattern of one immunoglobulin alone. Complement components, including the membrane attack complex, fibrinogen, and properdin, usually are associated with the presence of immunoglobulins, particularly in the more severe classes of disease. Less frequently, C4 is found in Class II mesangioproliferative LN, and class IV diffuse LN disease, which correlates with a lower activity index. The pattern of deposition usually is coarsely granular and corresponds to the dense deposits that are seen on electron microscopy. Occasionally, a purely linear pattern similar to that seen with anti-GBM antibody is found, but no pathologic or clinical implications for this type of deposition have been identified.

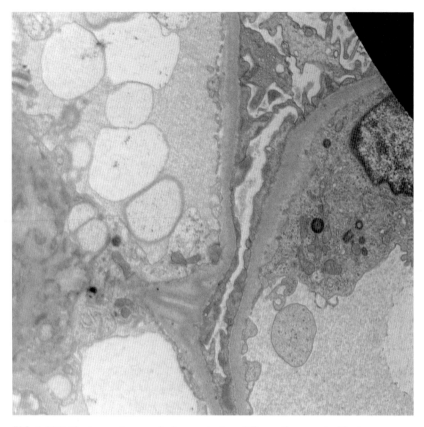

FIG. 1.270 Electron micrograph demonstrating diffuse effacement of foot processes in a patient with lupus and nephrotic syndrome. No electron-dense deposits are present (transmission electron microscopy, ×2000).

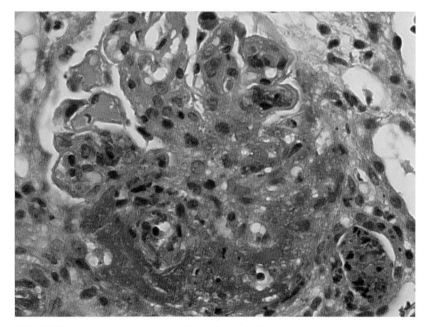

FIG. 1.271 Crescentic necrotizing glomerulonephritis and minimal mesangial proliferation and deposits in a patient with active lupus and significant titers of antineutrophil cytoplasmic antibody (hematoxylin and eosin, ×400).

Additional Pathologic Features

Although the ISN/RPS classification is based primarily on the glomerular changes, it should be recognized that tubular, interstitial and vascular lesions are an important part of the renal involvement and can contribute to the clinical picture. These additional pathologic features include vascular thrombosis and proliferative and sclerotic vascular lesions, including inflammatory vasculitis and tubular interstitial lesions. These complicating lesions occasionally are the predominant ones leading to clinical evidence of renal involvement. In addition, these lesions may become active or progress independently of the primary glomerular lesion. Thus, they should be evaluated independently as additional comorbid factors that may relate to specific additional therapeutic maneuvers or that have different prognostic significance.

Vascular Lesions

Vascular lesions were not considered in the establishment of the WHO or ISN/RPS classifications or in the currently used activity and chronicity indices. Vascular lesions are common and may include intravascular thrombosis, arterial and arteriolosclerosis, and necrotizing vasculitis. Of particular importance is the occurrence of glomerular capillary thrombosis signifying intravascular coagulation (Fig. 1.272). A pattern similar to that seen in adult hemolytic uremic syndrome, with multiple capillary and arteriolar thrombi containing fibrinogen, has been associated with the clinical course of rapidly progressive renal failure and is best diagnosed as thrombotic microangiopathy. Plasminogen activators are depressed in some of these patients, in whom inhibitors of plasminogen activators are elevated. Studies have shown low levels of tissue-type plasminogen activator and elevated levels of plasminogen inhibitor in patients with lupus nephritis that is associated with glomerular capillary deposition of fibrin or thrombus formation. Because these alterations in plasma levels of tissue plasminogen activator and 2-antiplasmin would be expected to retard fibrinolysis, they were corrected by

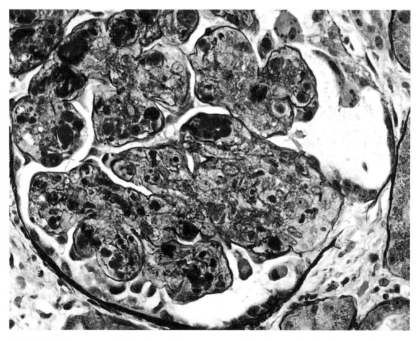

FIG. 1.272 Lupus nephritis. One of the most prominent vascular lesions seen in association with diffuse or focal lupus nephritis is the presence of intracapillary thrombi. There is also endocapillary proliferation. This is associated with the presence of antiphospholipid antibodies or lupus anticoagulant (Jones, ×400).

administration of the fibrinolytic agent ankyroid to patients with lupus glomerulonephritis. Thus, it is proposed that the disorder in fibrinolysis predisposes some patients with SLE to renal microvascular thrombi. Others have confirmed the association of glomerular thrombi with the presence of antiphospholipid antibodies in some, but not all, of these patients. Patients with this lupus anticoagulant in their serum are subject to glomerular thrombosis, which might be independent of the presence of glomerular inflammation. In such patients, the glomerular thrombosis sometimes is the primary pathogenic event and likely causes the progression of renal disease without participation of the accompanying immune responses.

Necrotizing vasculitis with vascular necrosis and leukocyte infiltration is a rare finding, but it appears to be a marker of poor prognosis in patients with lupus nephritis (Fig. 1.273a). The

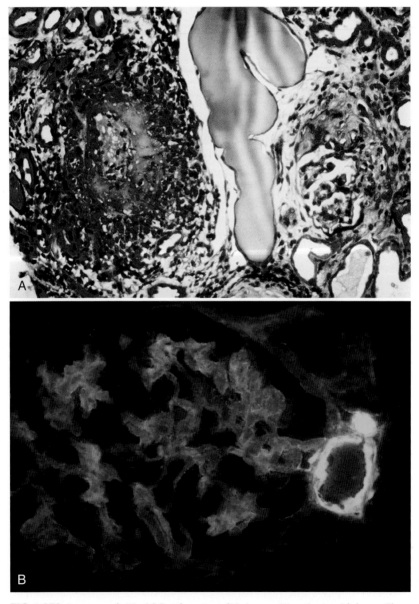

FIG. 1.273 Lupus nephritis. (a) Rarely, a vasculitis is seen in patients with lupus. The vasculitis resembles that of microscopic polyarteritis and shows transmural necrosis associated with an inflammatory infiltrate (Masson trichrome, ×200). (b) Immunofluorescence of these vessels often reveals deposition of immunoglobulins (anti-IgG immunofluorescence, ×400).

lesions can resemble the necrotizing arteriolitis that is seen with malignant hypertension and hemolytic uremic syndrome or a true vasculitis characterized by fibrinoid necrosis of small arteries and arterioles surrounded by an inflammatory infiltrate of the vessel wall.

Immunofluorescence microscopy sometimes reveals immune complex deposition in the vessel wall without any light microscopic reaction (Fig. 1.273b). These lesions, so-called bland lupus vasculopathy, which are reported in as many as 10% of patients with lupus nephritis, do not appear to impact significantly on prognosis. When the massive vascular deposits are associated with fibrinoid material, encroaching on and narrowing the lumen, the term lupus vasculopathy is used. This lesion is distinct from lupus vasculitis in that there is no inflammatory component. Nephrosclerotic lesions with intimal fibroplasia and hyaline arteriolar sclerosis can also be encountered in biopsies of patients with SLE, particularly in hypertensive patients. These lesions also are a major comorbid factor, contributing not only to the progression of renal failure but possibly also having an adverse effect on patient survival. Renal venous thrombosis is another vascular complication of lupus nephritis, but it is seen almost exclusively in patients with membranous lupus nephritis complicated by nephrotic syndrome.

Tubulointerstitial Disease

Interstitial inflammation, fibrosis, and tubular epithelial changes frequently are encountered in lupus nephritis (Fig. 1.274). Severe active tubulointerstitial nephritis most commonly is seen in patients with class III or IV, focal or diffuse LN, glomerular lesions. Although in most instances the interstitial inflammation is composed of lymphocytes and plasma cells, granulocytes and eosinophils also frequently are found and probably reflect the more active lesion. Immunofluorescence microscopy occasionally reveals granular peritubular deposits or, rarely, a linear deposition, the latter suggesting an antitubular basement membrane antibody. Granular tubular basement membrane deposits are accompanied by electron-dense deposits by

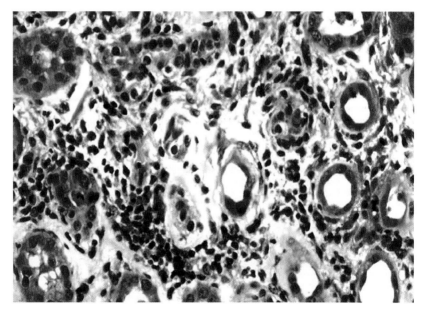

FIG. 1.274 Lupus nephritis. A tubular interstitial nephritis in which there is evidence of tubulitis with lymphocytes invading the tubular epithelium sometimes accompanies the glomerular lesion. Eosinophils are often prominent in the infiltrate. The tubular interstitial disease in some instances progresses independently of the glomerular disease and can in and of itself lead to end-stage kidney disease (hematoxylin and eosin, ×400).

Lupus Nephritis Key Diagnostic Findings

- Immune complexes, usually full house staining by immunofluorescence
- Immune complex deposits and tubuloreticular inclusions by electron microscopy
- Variable location of deposits results in variable injury patterns

---

Differential Diagnosis of Lupus Nephritis

- Other immune complex diseases must be excluded, with the following guidelines:
- IgA nephropathy is considered when deposits are IgA dominant or codominant.
- Postinfectious glomerulonephritis is considered with dominance of C3, usually with absence of C1q, with hump-type deposits.
- Cryoglobulinemic glomerulonephritis often has IgM dominance of deposits, whereas lupus nephritis is IgG dominant in nearly all cases. Cryoglobulinemic glomerulonephritis also may have a clonal component and PAS-positive cryo-plugs by light microscopy.

Notes: Tubuloreticular inclusions (a.k.a reticular aggregates) are common in lupus nephritis, but not seen in the above. Of note, some patients with lupus nephritis may also have concomitant cryoglobulins and injury related to these deposits.

---

electron microscopy. Linear antitubular basement membrane staining shows no corresponding deposits by electron microscopy. In most instances, the presence of interstitial disease without immune deposits suggests that several different mechanisms may be involved in the pathogenesis of this component of lupus nephritis. Of interest is the observation that tubular interstitial disease may progress independently of glomerular disease in some patients. It has been suggested that the infiltrate of T cells and monocytes may be an important determinant of the pathogenesis and progression of chronic injury in lupus nephritis by mediating interstitial injury.

Assessment of Severity and Chronicity

Several studies have emphasized the importance of using semiquantitative biopsy analyses to assess the activity and severity of lupus nephritis. Disease activity has been related to the presence of necrosis, cellular crescent formation, endocapillary and mesangial cellular proliferation, glomerular leukocytic infiltration, so-called hyaline thrombi (i.e., massive subendothelial deposits bulging into the capillary lumen), and glomerular and interstitial inflammation (Table 1.7). Chronicity has been graded according to the degree of glomerulosclerosis and fibrosis as well as the amount of interstitial scarring and tubular atrophy. The ISN/RPS 2003 classification does not require the use of a formal activity or chronicity index. It does include that the diagnostic line should identify the proportion of glomeruli with active and chronic lesions, fibrinoid necrosis, and crescents; also state the extent of tubulointerstitial fibrosis; and specify the presence of any extraglomerular vascular lesions. Although some authors have questioned the value of these indices and their reproducibility, such an approach has been useful in studies of large groups of patients. Recent studies have suggested that quantification may be of value in assessing the prognosis for individual patients. Because application of these indices is both observer and institution dependent, variations can occur between institutions. Within an institution, however, where greater standardization for the application of criteria can be accomplished, these indices are of value in following patients, particularly those who undergo serial or repeat biopsies.

The clinical value of renal biopsy in lupus nephritis appears to be well established. Some still question its usefulness, whereas others recommend it for every patient, even in the absence of clinical and laboratory data indicating renal involvement. On the other hand, most investigators agree that it is impossible to predict the types of severity and activity of renal lesions from any combination of clinical and laboratory findings alone. Further advances are needed in the treatment of severe lupus nephritis both to reduce the current mortality rate of 10-20% after 10 years and to decrease the development of renal insufficiency during dialysis, which occurs in nearly 25% of patients. Close collaboration between the clinical nephrologist and the renal pathologist is most important in making appropriate therapeutic decisions in the application of new strategies. To the extent that findings from renal biopsy provide a rationale for the use of potentially toxic drugs, the procedure appears to be more than worthwhile. This team approach will help to reduce the current mortality rate and to decrease the development of renal insufficiency requiring dialysis.

Etiology/Pathogenesis

SLE is an autoimmune syndrome characterized by autoantibodies to nuclear constituents. An important factor in determining glomerular damage is autoimmunity to double-stranded (ds) DNA and nucleosomes. In situ binding of anti-dsDNA antibodies initiates the inflammatory changes present in lupus nephritis. These autoantibodies colocalize with nucleosome-binding anti-dsDNA/-histone/-transcription factor antibodies derived from apoptotic cells and are not directed to intrinsic glomerular structures. The patterns of the different classes of lesions of lupus nephritis correspond to the experimental lesions produced by immune complex deposition in animal models. The pathogenesis varies with the class of the lesion. The generation of relatively small numbers of stable immune complexes of intermediate size with antibodies having high affinity and high avidity accumulate in the mesangium as a result of the mesangial clearing system for removal of macromolecules. The relatively small number of complexes, which is characteristic of minimal mesangial and mesangial proliferative LN, Class I and II, respectively, prevents the mesangial system from becoming overloaded and allows the complexes to be sequestered in the mesangium, where they are subject to degradation and removal rather than remaining at sites where they could initiate an inflammatory response. Fibronectin is an important component of the mesangial matrix, and given its capacity to interact with aggregates of immunoglobulins and immune complexes in the circulation, its presence in the mesangium may play a role in this type of localization, particularly when IgA antibodies are present.

Immune complexes localized to the subendothelial region as seen in focal and diffuse LN, Class III and IV, respectively, have access to plasma inflammatory mediators initiating the severe glomerulonephritis that is seen in these forms of lupus nephritis. Large numbers of intermediate-size complexes or large complexes that are formed by high-affinity antibodies likely overcome the mesangial ability to clear these macromolecules. As a result, these complexes accumulate in a paramesangial subendothelial location, and then ultimately in the peripheral capillary loops. The nature of the antigen and antibody also may contribute to the predominance of subendothelial localization in this class. Characteristics of certain antibodies, such as cationic charge, could permit binding of complexes that contain such antibodies to negative charges provided by nucleosomes generated from apoptotic glomerular cells, thus accounting for the nephrotropism. If the complexes are large and highly cationic, they will bind and fix to the closest anionic charges that are encountered at the subendothelial location. Following the initial binding of what might only be a small population of nephrotropic antibodies, activation of inflammatory cytokines can increase the permeability of the capillary wall, thus allowing other complexes to deposit.

The pathogenetic mechanism leading to the membranous pattern of Class V lupus nephritis likely results from in situ formation of immune complexes. This suggests an immune response that is characterized by the presence of small, unstable, circulating immune complexes formed by low-avidity and low-affinity antibodies in the presence of antigen excess. Under such conditions, complexes may disassociate with the antigen or antibody lodging in the glomerular capillaries. Subsequently, complexes are formed in situ attaching to the target protein, which has been planted in the outer aspect of the GBM. Of particular importance is that nucleosomes, apoptotic chromatin either derived from the circulation or from local glomerular cells, provide anionic sites in the GBM to facilitate in situ deposition of autoantibodies. Because such epimembranous deposits also are sequestered from access to circulating inflammatory mediators, an inflammatory component with cellular infiltration is not present.

Selected Reading

Kashgarian, M., 2002. Lupus Nephritis: Pathology, Pathogenesis, Clinical Correlations and Prognosis. In: Wallace, D.J., Hahn, B.H. (Eds.), Dubois's Lupus Erythematosus, sixth ed. Lippincott Williams & Wilkins, pp. 1061-1076.

Markowitz, G.S., D'Agati, V.D., 2009. Classification of lupus nephritis. Current Opinion in Nephrology and Hypertension 18, 220-225.

Schwartz, M.M., Korbet, S.M., Lewis, E.J.; Collaborative Study Group, 2008. The prognosis and pathogenesis of severe lupus glomerulonephritis. Nephrology Dialysis Transplantation 23, 1298-1306.

Weening, J.J., D'Agat, I.V., Schwartz, M.M., et al., on behalf of the International Society of Nephrology and Renal Pathology Society Working Group on the Classification of Lupus Nephritis, 2004. The classification of glomerulonephritis in systemic lupus erythematosus revisited. Kidney International 65, 521-530.

HENOCH–SCHÖNLEIN PURPURA

Henoch–Schönlein purpura is a form of IgA nephropathy with prominent extrarenal involvement. The clinical picture is that of an acute nephritis and is associated with the presence of purpuric lesions of the skin, arthritis, and gastrointestinal hemorrhage. It is the most common form of systemic vasculitis in children. It is a multiorgan systemic vasculitis that is immune complex–mediated by IgA-rich immune complexes. Although largely a disease of children, reports of Henoch–Schönlein purpura have encompassed the entire age range. Clinical manifestations of Henoch–Schönlein purpura mimic those of systemic vasculitis of various types. Classically, patients present with palpable purpura, arthralgia, abdominal pain with gastrointestinal bleeding, and renal disease. Renal manifestations range from mild, with only microscopic hematuria, to severe, with acute renal failure.

The pathologic lesions of Henoch–Schönlein purpura are similar to that of other immune complex–mediated diseases. The lesions associated with Henoch–Schönlein purpura are varied and range from a pure mesangial proliferative glomerulonephritis to a focal segmental necrotizing glomerulonephritis to a diffuse crescentic glomerulonephritis and a pattern similar to that of membranoproliferative glomerulonephritis (Figs. 1.275-1.283). The variety of

---

Key Diagnostic Features of Henoch–Schlönlein Purpura

- IgA dominant or codominant deposits by immunofluorescence, frequent IgG and occasional IgM
- Mesangial and subendothelial deposits by electron microscopy
- Variable light microscopic pattern, frequently with crescents

Note: The morphologic appearance of Henoch–Schönlein purpura nephritis overlaps with IgA nephropathy. However, there more often may be crescents, perhaps reflecting in part a bias to biopsy patients with more aggressive course.

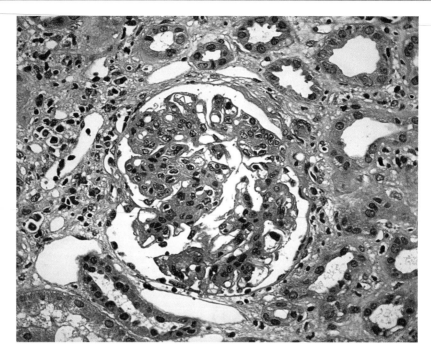

FIG. 1.275 Henoch–Schönlein purpura. The glomerulus shows evidence of lobular accentuation, mesangial hypercellularity, and focal thickening of the peripheral capillary walls (hematoxylin and eosin, ×400).

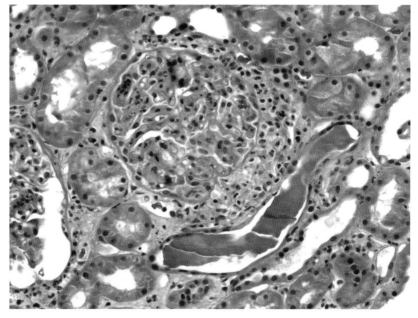

FIG. 1.276 Henoch–Schönlein purpura. The glomerulus shows evidence of lobular accentuation, mesangial hypercellularity, and focal thickening of the peripheral capillary walls and segmental necrosis (hematoxylin and eosin, ×400).

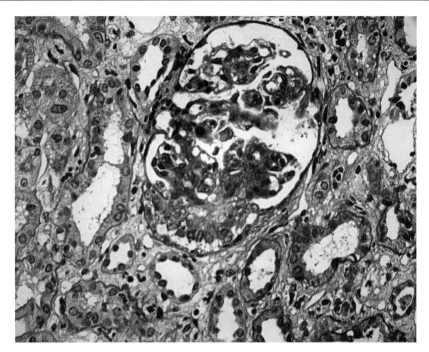

FIG. 1.277 Henoch–Schönlein purpura. The glomerulus demonstrates moderate diffuse mesangial proliferation with an early epithelial crescent (periodic acid Schiff, ×400).

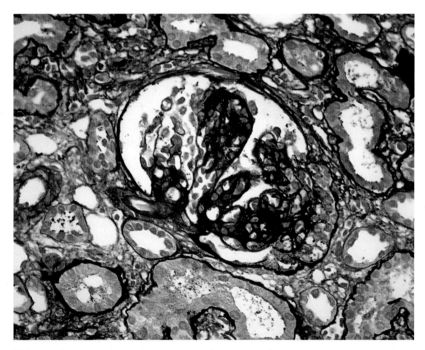

FIG. 1.278 Henoch–Schönlein purpura. There is an adhesion to Bowman's capsule, early crescent formation and an increase in mesangial matrix. The pattern is segmental (Jones, ×400).

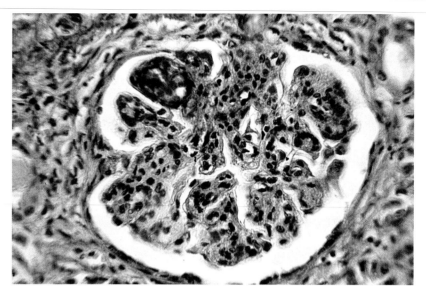

FIG. 1.279 Henoch–Schönlein purpura. There is segmental necrosis with accumulation of fibrinoid material. The remainder of the glomerulus shows mesangial hypercellularity and an increase in matrix (trichrome, ×400).

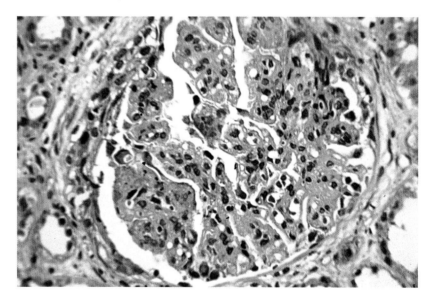

FIG. 1.280 Henoch–Schönlein purpura. A later stage demonstrates more extensive mesangial sclerosis in addition to the continued presence of fragmented red blood cells and leukocytes within the capillary lumina (trichrome, ×400).

lesions seen in Henoch–Schönlein purpura is similar to that seen in lupus glomerulonephritis. Immunofluorescence microscopy is characterized by the deposition of IgA in glomeruli and depending on the severity of the lesion, the pattern of the lesion may range from a mesangial distribution to a peripheral capillary distribution (Figs. 1.284, 1.285). A feature that distinguishes Henoch–Schönlein purpura from other forms of IgA nephropathy is the

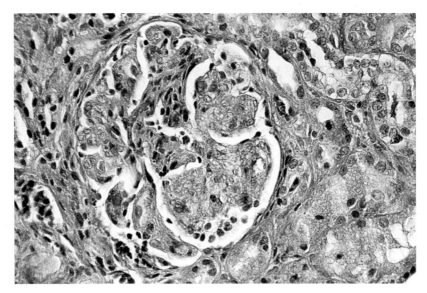

FIG. 1.281 Henoch–Schönlein purpura. Segmental sclerosis is prominent with loss of the normal architecture. The remainder of the glomerulus appears to have somewhat less hypercellularity (trichrome, ×400).

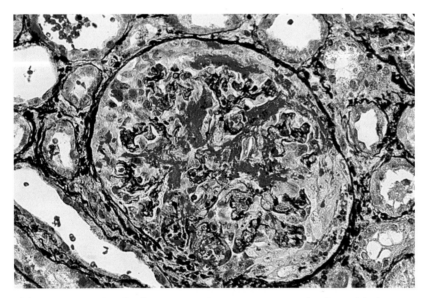

FIG. 1.282 Henoch–Schönlein purpura. A more severe example where global glomerular necrosis is present with abundant fibrin within Bowman's space (Jones, ×400).

frequent presence of deposits of IgG and occasionally IgM. Complement components and fibrinogen coexist with the immunoglobulins. Electron microscopy is also varied. Abundant mesangial electron-dense deposits are the most characteristic finding but subendothelial and subepithelial deposits with mesangial interposition are also present in severe cases (Figs. 1.286-1.289).

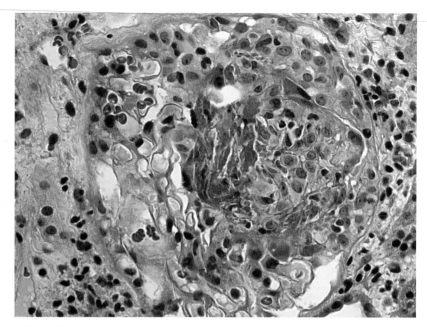

FIG. 1.283 Henoch–Schönlein purpura. A more severe example where global glomerular necrosis is present with abundant fibrin within Bowman's space and a small cellular crescent (Jones, ×400).

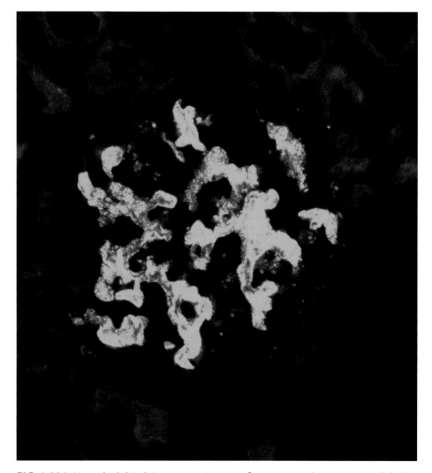

FIG. 1.284 Henoch–Schönlein purpura. Immunofluorescence demonstrates global and diffuse mesangial and segmented capillary loop deposition of IgA (anti-IgA immunofluorescence, ×400).

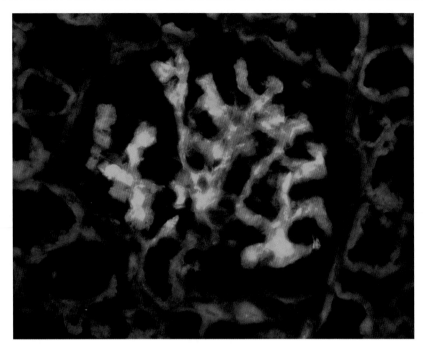

FIG. 1.285 Henoch–Schönlein purpura. IgG is also present in a similar global and diffuse mesangial and segmental capillary loop pattern (anti-IgG immunofluorescence).

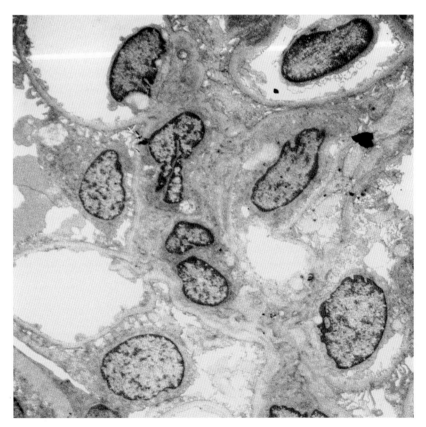

FIG. 1.286 Henoch–Schönlein purpura. Electron microscopy reveals an increase in mesangial cellularity with the presence of mesangial deposits. The capillary lumina are occluded by the presence of numerous leukocytes (transmission electron microscopy, ×3000).

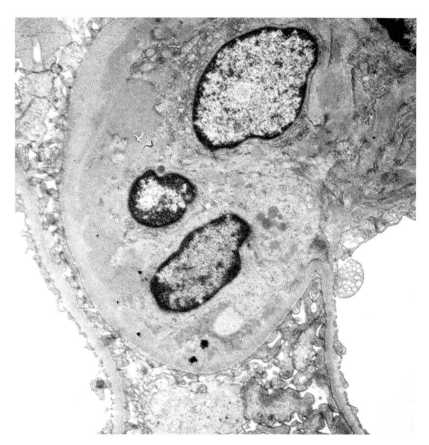

FIG. 1.287 Henoch–Schönlein purpura. The endothelial cells are swollen and there are subendothelial and mesangial electron-dense deposits corresponding to the IgA, IgG deposits seen on immunofluorescence (transmission electron microscopy, ×5000).

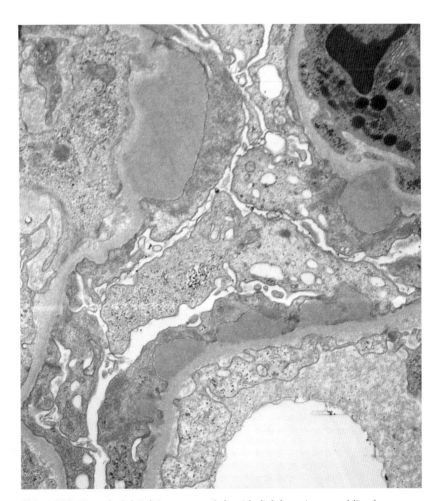

FIG. 1.288 Henoch–Schönlein purpura. Subepithelial deposits resembling humps are also occasionally seen. The capillary lumen on the top right demonstrates a leukocyte, which has stripped the endothelium away from the basement membrane (transmission electron microscopy, ×5000).

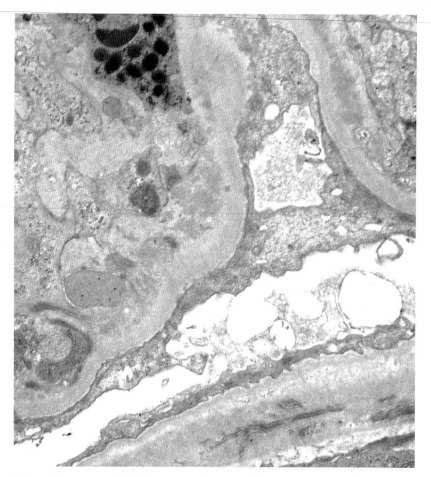

FIG. 1.289 Henoch–Schönlein purpura. Mesangial deposits are universally present. In this image, a leukocyte can be seen in the mesangial area (top left) as well as the presence of subendothelial deposits in the capillary loops with endothelial cell swelling. There is also segmental effacement of the podocyte foot processes (transmission electron microscopy, ×5000).

Etiology/Pathogenesis

Henoch–Schönlein purpura is an immune complex disease characterized by the presence of immune complexes of IgA antibody and exogenous antigens. Exogenous antigens from food, drugs, and infections have all been implicated. Mucosal infections of the upper respiratory tract and gastrointestinal tract have been of special interest as these are the sites of IgA-mediated immunity.

Selected Reading

Gardner-Medwin, J.M., Dolezalova, P., Cummins, C., et al., 2002. Incidence of Henoch-Schönlein purpura, Kawasaki disease, and rare vasculitidis in children of different ethnic origins. Lancet 360, 1197-1202.

Pillebout, E., Thervet, E., Hill, G., et al., 2002. Henoch-Schönlein purpura in adults: Outcome and prognostic factors. Journal of the American Society of Nephrology 13, 1271-1278.

MIXED CONNECTIVE TISSUE DISEASE

Mixed connective tissue disease (MCTD) is an overlap syndrome carrying features of SLE, progressive systemic sclerosis (PSS), and polymyositis. Serologically, it is distinguished from SLE and PSS by high-titer antinuclear antibodies and antibodies to a saline-extractable nuclear antigen that is ribonuclease sensitive. Clinical features include a variety of systemic manifestations, similar to SLE and PSS. Renal manifestations are relatively uncommon. The clinical manifestations of renal involvement are variable in degrees of proteinuria, including a full-blown nephrotic syndrome. A few patients have marked hypertension and microangiopathic hemolytic anemia.

The most common pattern of renal pathology in MCTD is a membranous nephropathy (Figs. 1.290-1.294). As in lupus, there are usually mesangial deposits and some degree of mesangial proliferation. Immunofluorescence studies typically reveal granular capillary staining for IgG and C3 and occasionally IgA and IgM (Fig. 1.295). Less commonly, the renal lesion is a diffuse mesangial proliferative glomerulonephritis (Figs. 1.296, 1.297). Rarely, a few cases demonstrate subendothelial deposits and have a more diffuse membranoproliferative pattern (Figs. 1.298-1.300). The renal findings essentially parallel those in lupus with a more prominent involvement of membranous lesions. Vascular lesions are similar to those of systemic sclerosis (Fig. 1.301).

Etiology/Pathogenesis

Mixed connective tissue disease is an autoimmune disease with prominent development of antibodies to ribonuclear proteins. The etiology and pathogenesis of the renal lesions are essentially similar to that of lupus nephritis (see section on SLE).

Text continued on page 241

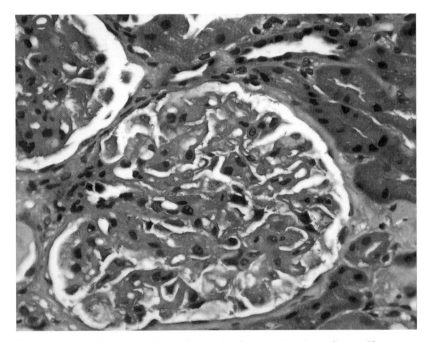

FIG. 1.290 Membranous nephropathy in mixed connective tissue disease. The pattern is similar to that seen in lupus with lobular accentuation and diffuse thickening of the basement membranes (hematoxylin and eosin, ×400).

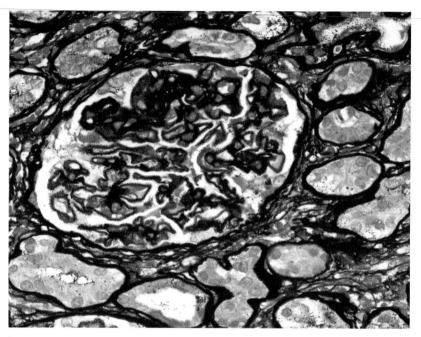

FIG. 1.291 Membranous nephropathy in mixed connective tissue disease. Silver methenamine stain demonstrates thickening of the capillary walls and a typical spike and dome appearance (Jones, ×400).

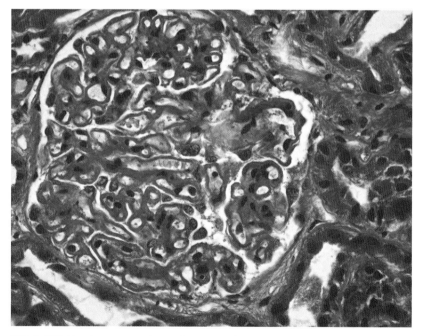

FIG. 1.292 Membranous nephropathy in mixed connective tissue disease. Trichrome stain demonstrates diffuse thickening and the presence of eosinophilic deposits in the glomerular basement membranes (trichrome, ×400).

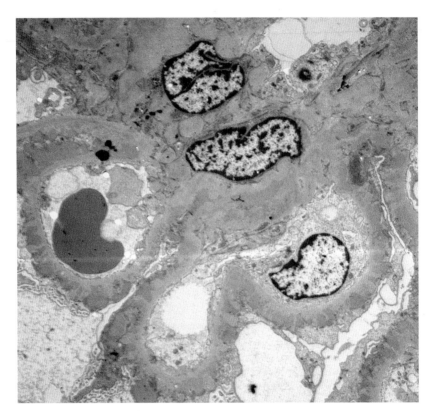

FIG. 1.293 Membranous nephropathy in mixed connective tissue disease. Electron micrograph demonstrates diffuse thickening of the glomerular basement membrane with patent capillary loops. Numerous subepithelial and intramembranous deposits are present (transmission electron microscopy, ×3000).

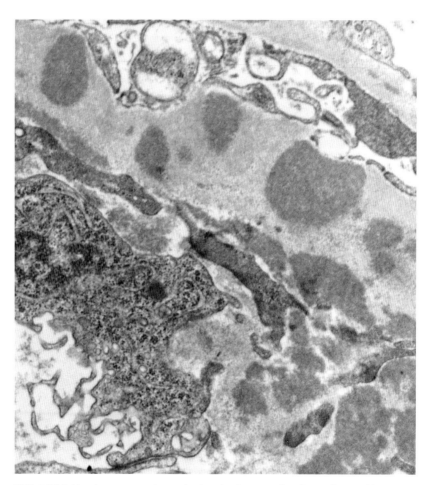

FIG. 1.294 Membranous nephropathy in mixed connective tissue disease. Numerous subepithelial and occassional intramembranous and mesangial electron-dense deposits are present (transmission electron microscopy, ×10,000).

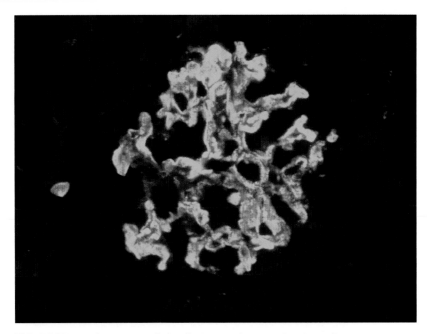

FIG. 1.295 Membranous nephropathy in mixed connective tissue disease. Immunofluorescence studies typically reveal a peripheral granular staining for IgG and occassionally IgM and IgA (anti-IgM immunofluorescence, ×400).

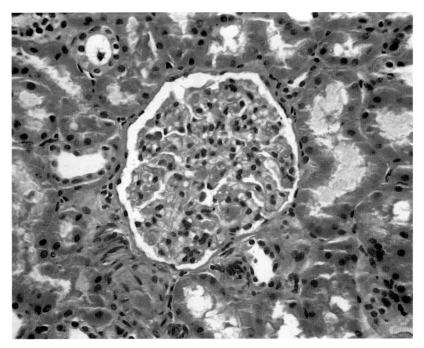

FIG. 1.296 Mesangial proliferative glomerulonephritis in mixed connective tissue disease. There is diffuse mesangial hyperplasia, peripheral capillary loops are well preserved, and leukocytic infiltration is not prominent (HPS, ×200).

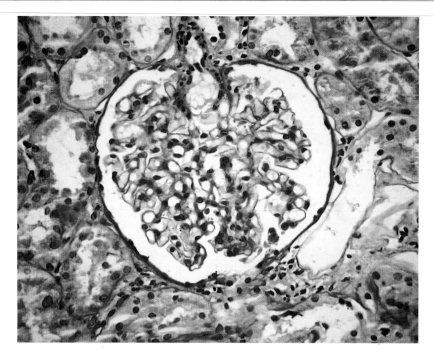

FIG. 1.297 Mesangial proliferative glomerulonephritis in mixed connective tissue disease. There is mild increase in mesangial cellularity and matrix (periodic acid Schiff, ×200).

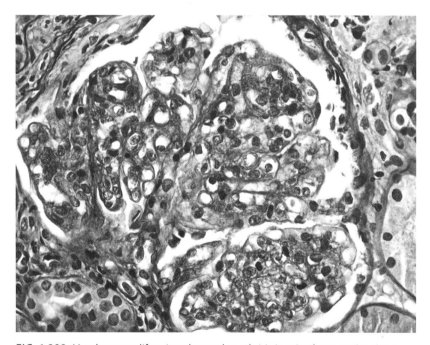

FIG. 1.298 Membranoproliferative glomerulonephritis in mixed connective tissue disease. The pattern here is similar to that seen in systemic lupus erythematosus with lobular accentuation, increase in mesangial cellularity and matrix and double contours and cellular interposition of the peripheral capillary loops (periodic acid Schiff, ×400).

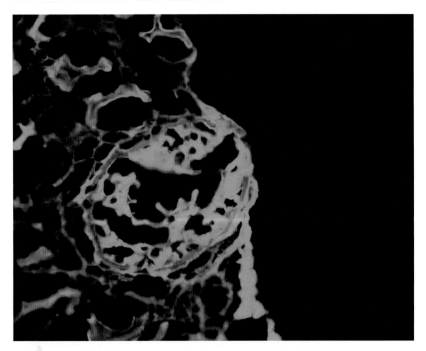

FIG. 1.299 Membranoproliferative glomerulonephritis in mixed connective tissue disease. Immunofluorescence demonstrates the presence of immunoglobulins in a mesangial and peripheral capillary pattern (anti-IgG immunofluorescence, ×200). *MPGN*, membranoproliferative glomerulonephritis.

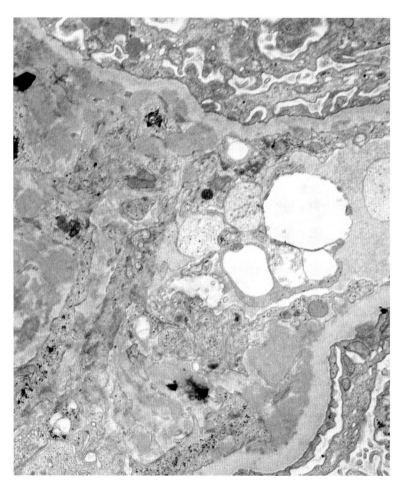

FIG. 1.300 Membranoproliferative glomerulonephritis in mixed connective tissue disease. Electron microscopy demonstrates mesangial deposits and paramesangial and subendothelial deposits (transmission electron microscopy, ×5000). *MPGN,* membranoproliferative glomerulonephritis.

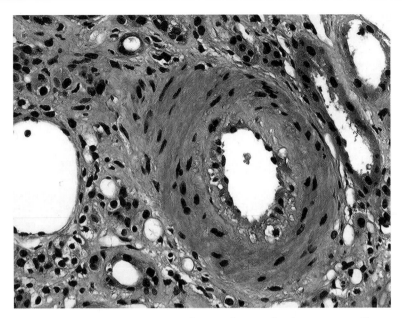

FIG. 1.301 Mixed connective tissue disease. The vascular changes are similar to those of systemic sclerosis with concentric hyperplasia of the media of this interlobular artery (hematoxylin and eosin, ×400).

Selected Reading

Cohen, A.H., Weiss, M.A., 1986. Renal pathology forum. American Journal of Nephrology 6, 51-56.

Kobayashi, S., Nagase, M., Kimura, M., et al., 1985. Renal involvement in MCTD. American Journal of Nephrology 5, 282-291.

MIXED CRYOGLOBULINEMIA

Three types of cryoglobulinemic disease (Types I, II, and III) have been described. Type I is composed of monoclonal antibodies due to an underlying plasma cell dyscrasia, including monoclonal IgM, and is described elsewhere. Mixed cryoglobulinemia is of two types. Type II or essential mixed cryoglobulinemia contains both a polyclonal IgG (which may either act as an antigen or be directed against an antigen) and a monoclonal IgM rheumatoid factor directed against the IgG. Most cases are due to chronic infection with hepatitis C virus and less frequently infection with hepatitis B virus and Epstein–Barr virus. Type III is also a mixed cryoglobulinemia in which both components of the cryoglobulin are polyclonal and are often secondary to chronic inflammatory and autoimmune diseases as well as in patients with hepatitis C infection.

By light microscopy, the pattern is identical to that seen in Type I membranoproliferative glomerulonephritis (Figs. 1.302-1.305). The glomeruli are enlarged, have lobular accentuation, and have varying degrees of leukocytic infiltration. Double contours of the peripheral capillaries can be seen, and capillary lumina contain eosinophilic deposits that correspond to the circulating cryoglobulins (Fig. 1.306). They are often referred to as hyaline thrombi or cryo-plugs, and stain strongly positive for PAS due to the frequent presence of IgM, a glycated immunoglobulin (PAS stains glycoproteins strongly). There are no distinguishing morphologic features to separate Type III mixed cryoglobulinemia from the other forms. Immunofluorescence microscopy demonstrates the presence of IgM and IgG as well as complement components. In cryoglobulin-related glomerulonephritis, IgM may be more

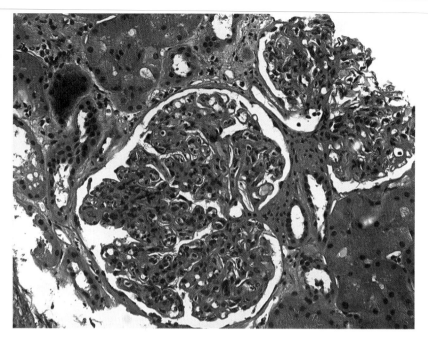

FIG. 1.302 Mixed cryoglobulinemia. There is lobular accentuation of the glomerular architecture with an increase in mesangial cellularity and matrix. The capillaries are pushed to the periphery and double contours and cellular interposition of the capillaries can be identified (hematoxylin and eosin, ×400).

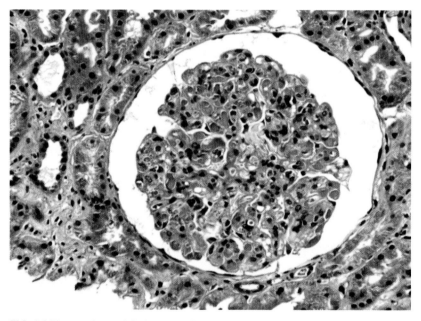

FIG. 1.303 Mixed cryoglobulinemia. Glomerulus from the biopsy of a patient with cryoglobulinemia. There is lobular accentuation of the glomerular architecture with an increase in mesangial cellularity and matrix. The capillaries show hyaline thrombi (cryoplugs) within capillary lumina (hematoxylin and eosin, ×400).

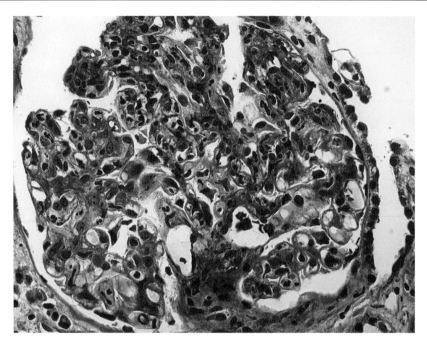

FIG 1.304 Mixed cryoglobulinemia. Trichrome stain shows the lobular accentuation, evidence of mesangialization with capillaries filled with leukocytes. Hyaline thrombi (cryoplugs) area also seen within some capillary lumina (trichrome stain, ×400).

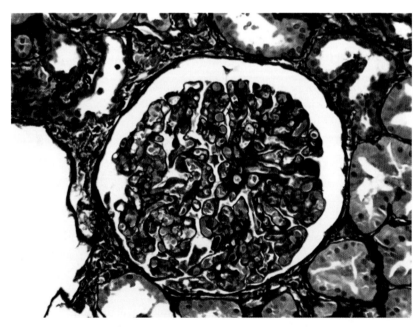

FIG. 1.305 Mixed cryoglobulinemia. Silver stain shows the lobular accentuation, and evidence of capillaries filled with hyaline thrombi (cryoplugs) within capillary lumina (Silver stain, ×400).

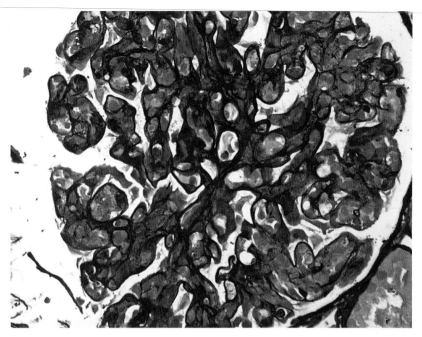

FIG. 1.306 Mixed cryoglobulinemia. Silver stains show evidence of reduplication of the capillary basement membrane due to interposed mesangial cells and monocytes (Jones, ×400).

Key Diagnostic Features of Mixed Cryoglobulinemic Glomerulonephritis

- Mesangial or membranoproliferative features by light microscopy
- Periodic acid Schiff (PAS)–positive cryo-plugs
- IgM, often clonal, deposits by immunofluorescence, often with lesser IgG
- Vague fibrillary or occasionally microtubular substructure of deposits by electron microscopy

Note: Not all cases of cryoglobulinemic glomerulonephritis will display all or any of these features.

---

prominent than other IgGs. When a monoclonal component is present, there may be predominance of either kappa or lambda (Figs. 1.307-1.310). Electron microscopy reveals a pattern similar to that seen with Type I membranoproliferative glomerulonephritis (Figs. 1.311-1.314). One distinguishing feature seen in cryoglobulinemia is the presence of organized deposits. Deposits have a crystalline structure or vague short fibrillary substructure, and sometimes a tubular configuration (Figs. 1.315-1.317). Once again, there are no distinguishing features to separate out Type III cryoglobulinemia on a morphologic basis, and the diagnosis of the specific type of cryoglobulin is made on analysis of the serum cryoglobulins.

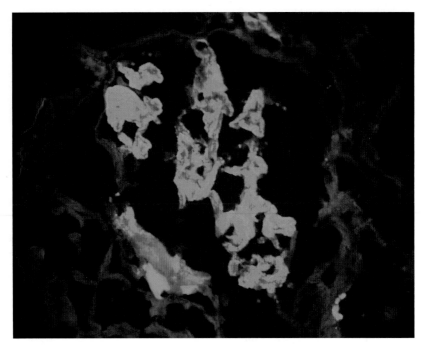

FIG. 1.307 Mixed cryoglobulinemia. Immunofluorescence demonstrates the presence of IgM in a peripheral capillary and mesangial pattern. The peripheral capillary pattern is markedly granular (anti-IgM immunofluorescence, ×400).

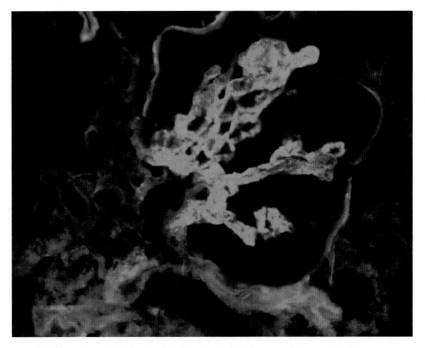

FIG. 1.308 Mixed cryoglobulinemia. Immunofluorescence microscopy also demonstrates the presence of IgG. Complement is present in a similar pattern (anti-IgG immunofluorescence, ×400).

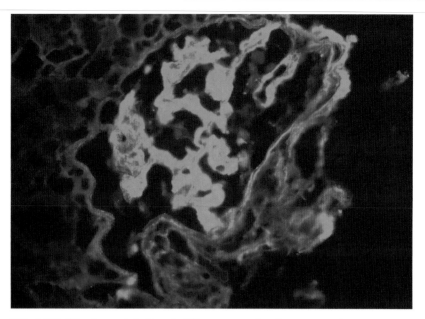

FIG. 1.309 Mixed cryoglobulinemia. When a monoclonal component is present, either dominant kappa or lambda chain staining is seen in a similar peripheral pattern (anti-kappa immunofluorescence, ×400).

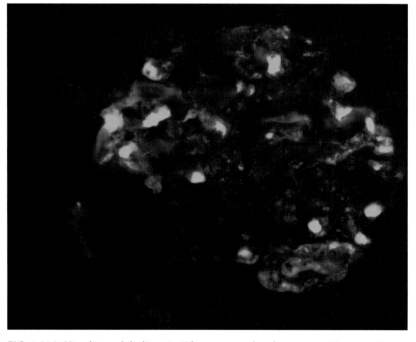

FIG. 1.310 Mixed cryoglobulinemia. When a monoclonal component is present, either kappa or lambda chain staining is seen in a similar peripheral pattern. Cryoplugs are prominent (anti-kappa immunofluorescence, ×400).

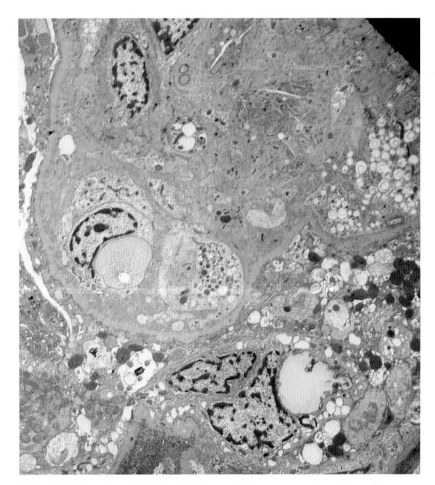

FIG. 1.311 Mixed cryoglobulinemia. Electron microscopy reveals evidence of interposition of mesangial cells and monocytes of the peripheral capillary loops with the presence of abundant subendothelial deposits. The capillary lumina are filled with leukocytes (transmission electron microscopy, ×3000).

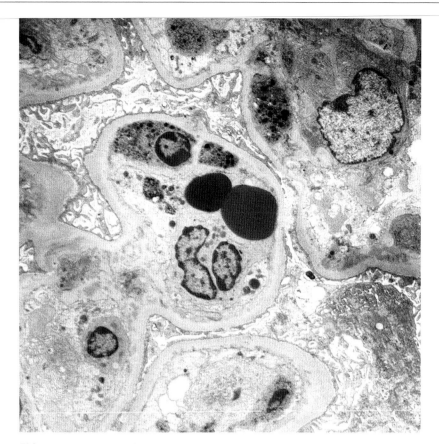

FIG. 1.312 Mixed cryoglobulinemia. Leukocytic infiltration with occlusion of the capillary lumen is prominent (transmission electron microscopy, ×3000).

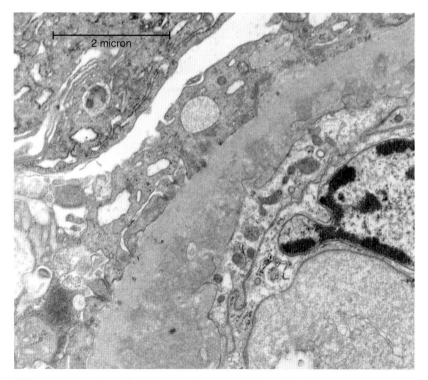

FIG. 1.313 Mixed cryoglobulinemia. There is marked endothelial cell swelling and the subendothelial deposits have an irregular organized appearance (transmission electron microscopy, ×8000).

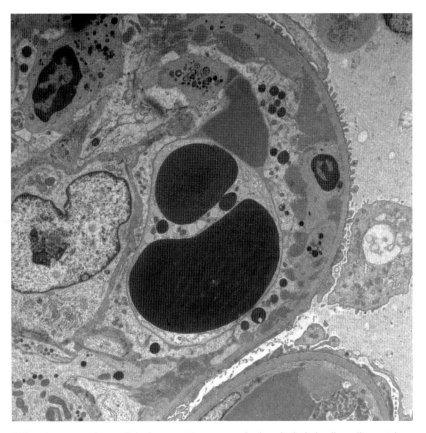

FIG. 1.314 Mixed cryoglobulinemia. There is marked endothelial cell swelling with subendothelial deposits and leukocytes filling the lumen (transmission electron microscopy, ×4000).

Differential Diagnosis of Mixed Cryoglobulinemic Glomerulonephritis

- This entity must be distinguished from postinfectious glomerulonephritis, lupus nephritis, and glomerulonephritis associated with lupus-like conditions. When key diagnostic features (see above) are absent, this distinction may be difficult.
- However, cryoglobulinemic glomerulonephritis does not show reticular aggregates, as is typical of lupus nephritis, and lupus nephritis deposits are typically IgG dominant.
- Postinfectious glomerulonephritis is distinguished by dominant C3 with lesser IgG and hump-type deposits by electron microscopy.

Etiology/Pathogenesis

The pathogenesis of the renal lesions is similar to that of the other types of cryoglobulin-associated disease but is distinguished by the presence of antibodies that are polyclonal specific for an antigen associated with a monoclonal or polyclonal rheumatoid factor IgM. Mixed cryoglobulins have been described in a variety of connective tissue diseases, infections, and malignancies. The link with hepatitis C infection has emerged in the last several years.

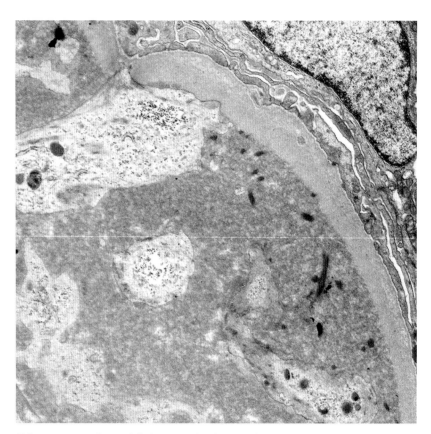

FIG. 1.315 Mixed cryoglobulinemia. The "hyaline thrombi" or so-called "cryoplugs" seen on light microscopy consist of large subendothelial deposits bulging into the capillary lumen with an organized tubular appearance by electron microscopy. Occassional dark fibrin tactoids are also present (transmission electron microscopy, ×12,000).

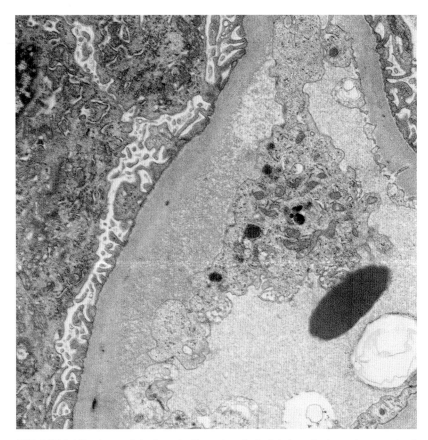

FIG. 1.316 Mixed cryoglobulinemia. The subendothelial deposits have the organized appearance characteristic of cryoglobulinemia (transmission electron microscopy, ×6000).

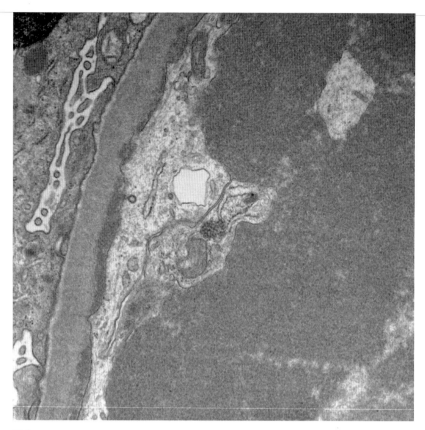

FIG. 1.317 Mixed cryoglobulinemia. The subendothelial deposits have the organized appearance characteristic of cryoplugs. A reticular aggregate is also seen in the endothelial cytoplasm (transmission electron microscopy, ×8000).

Selected Reading

Brouet, J.C., Clauvel, J.P., Danon, F., et al., 1974. Biological and clinical significance of cryoglobulins. American Journal of Medicine 57, 775-788.

D'Amico, G., Colasanti, G., Ferrario, F., et al., 1989. Renal Involvement in mixed cryoglobulinemia. Kidney International 35, 1004-1014.

Sinico, R.A., Winearls, C.G., Sabadini, E., et al., 1988. Identification of glomerular immune complexes in cryoglobulinemia glomerulonephritis. Kidney International 34, 109-116.

ANTI-GBM ANTIBODY–MEDIATED GLOMERULONEPHRITIS

Patients with anti-GBM antibody–mediated glomerulonephritis typically present with rapidly progressive glomerulonephritis. Patients may have isolated renal disease and inconspicuous or absent pulmonary symptoms. The antibody cross-reacts in some patients with alveolar basement membranes and thus causes pulmonary hemorrhage. The occurrence of RPGN and pulmonary hemorrhage is called Goodpasture syndrome. When the cause is anti-GBM antibodies, the term *Goodpasture disease* should be used. Men are affected more commonly than women. The disease occurs at any age, but is more common in adults aged 20-40 years. A flu-like illness may precede the onset of Goodpasture disease.

By light microscopy, the glomeruli show breaks of the GBM due to fibrinoid necrosis (Figs. 1.318-1.320). In very early disease, crescents may not be apparent. This early stage is typically seen in patients who present with severe, life-threatening lung disease, who undergo renal biopsy for more specific and sensitive diagnosis of Goodpasture disease than possible by lung

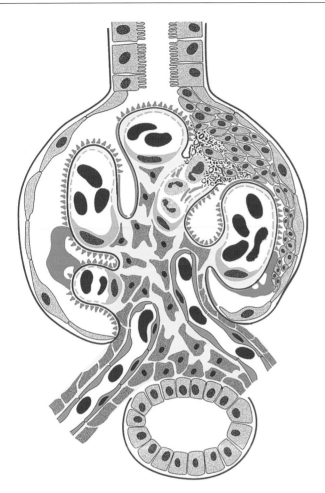

FIG. 1.318 Anti-GBM antibody–mediated disease. There is segmental necrosis with a break of the glomerular basement membrane, and fibrinoid necrosis and polymorphonuclear leukocytes in this area, with a cellular crescent developing in response to this GBM break. The remainder of the glomerulus is unremarkable without proliferation and without deposits. Differentiation from other causes of crescentic glomerulonephritis without evident proliferation by light microscopy is made by immunofluorescence, which demonstrates linear staining for IgG in anti-GBM antibody–mediated disease. *GBM,* glomerular basement membrane.

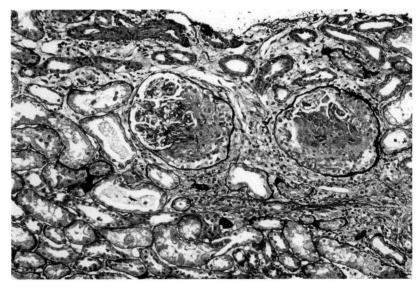

FIG. 1.319 Anti-GBM antibody–mediated glomerulonephritis. There is evident segmental necrosis in both glomeruli, with uninvolved segments of the glomeruli showing no proliferation or evidence of immune complexes. There is early cellular crescent formation (Jones silver stain, ×100). *GBM,* glomerular basement membrane.

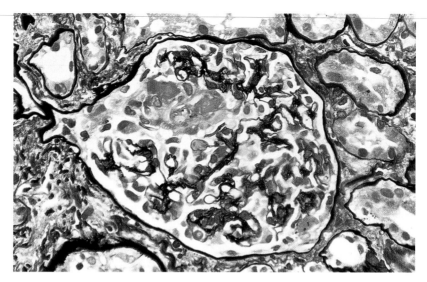

FIG. 1.320 Anti-GBM antibody–mediated glomerulonephritis. Early segmental fibrinoid necrosis is present, with glomerular basement membrane rupture. There is not yet a cellular crescentic reaction. The remaining portion of the glomerulus shows no proliferation or evidence of immune complexes (Jones silver stain, ×400). *GBM*, glomerular basement membrane.

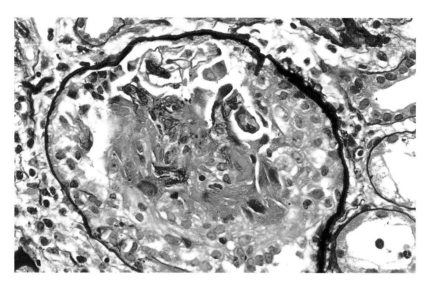

FIG. 1.321 Anti-GBM antibody–mediated glomerulonephritis. There is fibrinoid necrosis with karyorrhexis and ruptured fragments of GBM, with a small remaining intact portion of the glomerulus at the top. There is surrounding cellular crescent formation, and periglomerular inflammatory infiltrate (Jones silver stain, ×400). *GBM*, glomerular basement membrane.

biopsy. Cellular crescents develop consequent to the GBM breaks (Fig. 1.321). The GBM shows ischemic corrugation with ruptures, with no apparent deposits or proliferation (Fig. 1.322). With ongoing disease, Bowman's capsule ruptures, and there is periglomerular fibrosis and organization of the cellular crescent to a fibrocellular and ultimately fibrous crescent (Fig. 1.323). The interstitium shows lymphoplasmacytic infiltrate particularly around crescentic glomeruli with Bowman's capsule rupture and interstitial fibrosis and tubular atrophy developing. A granulomatous or giant cell reaction may even be present. Although fibrinoid necrosis

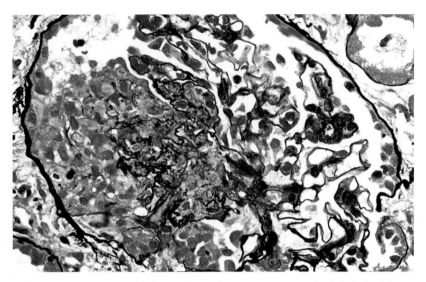

FIG. 1.322 Anti-GBM antibody–mediated glomerulonephritis. The right half of the glomerulus is completely preserved, while the left half shows glomerular basement membrane ruptures, with corrugation and cellular crescent (Jones silver stain, ×400). *GBM,* glomerular basement membrane.

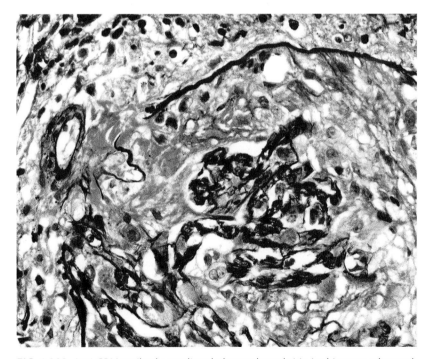

FIG. 1.323 Anti-GBM antibody–mediated glomerulonephritis. In this more advanced lesion, there is corrugation and rupture of glomerular basement membrane with early fibrocellular organization of the crescent and rupture of Bowman's capsule with corresponding fibrinoid necrosis and surrounding periglomerular inflammation (Jones silver stain, ×400). *GBM,* glomerular basement membrane.

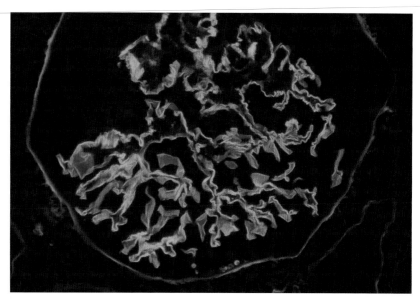

FIG. 1.324 Anti-GBM antibody–mediated glomerulonephritis. Linear glomerular basement membrane staining with IgG is diagnostic of this disease in this setting (anti-IgG immunofluorescence, ×400). *GBM,* glomerular basement membrane.

Key Diagnostic Features of Anti-GBM Antibody–Mediated Glomerulonephritis

- Crescents and segmental glomerular necrosis
- Linear staining of glomerular basement membranes by immunofluorescence for IgG and C3
- Absence of deposits by electron microscopy

---

may extend from the glomerular tuft to the arteriole at the hilum, the interlobular and larger arteries do not show vasculitic lesions.

Immunofluorescence microscopy is diagnostic, revealing strong, linear GBM staining for IgG (Fig. 1.324). C3 is positive in nearly all cases, but is usually weaker than IgG and may be discontinuous or even granular (Fig. 1.325). Very rare cases of other immunoglobulin anti-GBM antibodies have been described, with case reports of linear IgA or IgM in apparent anti-GBM antibody–mediated glomerulonephritis. Occasionally, anti-GBM antibodies may cross-react with tubular basement membranes, resulting in linear tubular basement membrane staining (Fig. 1.326). This may contribute to an interstitial nephritis.

By electron microscopy, no deposits are detected (Fig. 1.327). This may reflect the uniform distribution of the antigen, the non-collagenous (NC1) domain of alpha 3(IV) collagen, and/or that these uniformly distributed deposits have the same density as the GBM. IgG antibody has been identified along the lamina interna of the GBM by immunoelectron microscopy. Breaks in the GBM may be detected by electron microscopy (Fig. 1.328), along with fibrin tactoids reflecting the segmental fibrinoid necrosis.

Etiology/Pathogenesis

Anti-GBM antibody–mediated glomerulonephritis is due to the development of autoantibody against the noncollagenous C-terminal (NC1) domain of alpha 3(IV) collagen. The antibody to GBM cross-reacts with lung basement membrane, giving rise in some patients to combined

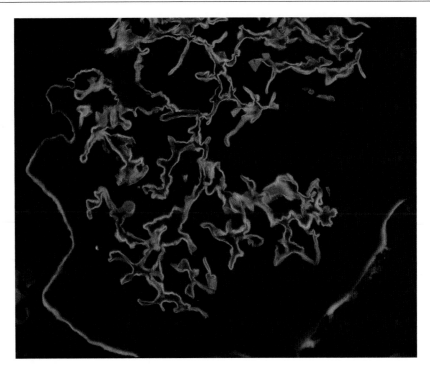

FIG. 1.325 Anti-GBM antibody–mediated glomerulonephritis. Linear staining for C3 typically accompanies the IgG staining in cases of anti-GBM antibody–mediated glomerulonephritis, a useful but not pathognomonic feature to distinguish from the linear accentuation and staining with IgG that may occur in diabetic nephropathy (anti-C3 immunofluorescence, ×400). *GBM,* glomerular basement membrane.

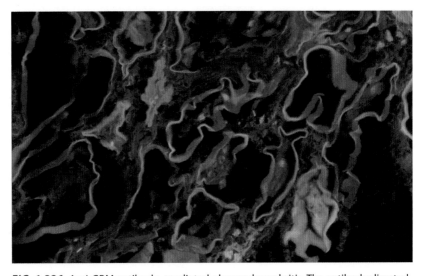

FIG. 1.326 Anti-GBM antibody–mediated glomerulonephritis. The antibody directed against the GBM may sometimes cross-react with the tubular basement membrane, as in this case, and may then be causal in an associated interstitial nephritis and tubular injury (anti-IgG immunofluorescence, ×400). *GBM,* glomerular basement membrane.

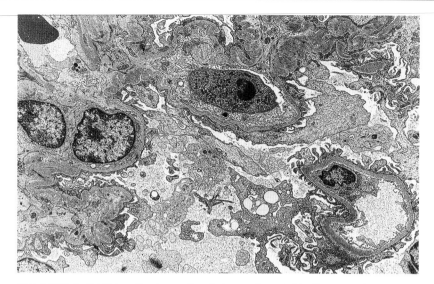

FIG. 1.327 Anti-GBM antibody–mediated glomerulonephritis. Electron microscopy shows no discrete immune complexes since the antigen, the noncollagenous domain of α3 collagen, is a diffusely distributed integral part of the type IV collagen of the glomerular basement membrane. Only mild foot process effacement and segmental corrugation are present in this glomerulus (transmission electron microscopy, ×6000). *GBM,* glomerular basement membrane.

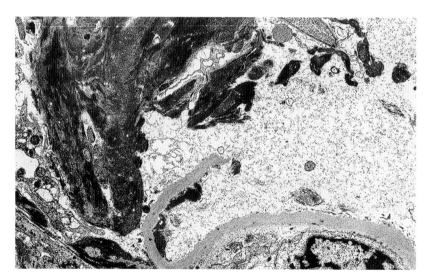

FIG. 1.328 Anti-GBM antibody–mediated glomerulonephritis. Electron microscopy may sometimes demonstrate the glomerular basement membrane breaks also seen by light microscopy, as demonstrated here. There are associated fibrin tactoids (transmission electron microscopy, ×8000). *GBM,* glomerular basement membrane.

pulmonary and renal lesions. A similar histologic pattern may occur in renal transplants in some patients with Alport syndrome, who develop autoantibodies against normal type IV collagen in the transplanted kidney (see Alport syndrome). Recent studies show that a conformational change in the alpha 3 (IV) collagen is found in Goodpasture's disease and is thus postulated to cause the immune response. The events that trigger this conformational change are unknown. The rare development of anti-GBM antibody–mediated glomerulonephritis in some patients with membranous nephropathy, resulting in superimposed crescents, suggests that immune deposits can rarely be such a trigger. The development of disease sometimes is preceded by a flu-like illness or hydrocarbon or solvent exposure, suggesting the possibility that alveolar antigens may have become exposed and caused an autoimmune response. Anti-GBM antibody–mediated glomerulonephritis can rarely recur in the transplant, usually when antibody titers remain high (Fig. 1.329).

Interestingly, the appellation Goodpasture's syndrome by Drs Stanton and Tange did not meet with Dr Goodpasture's approval, in that he deduced that the young man whom he

---

Differential Diagnosis of Anti-GBM Antibody–Mediated Glomerulonephritis

Linear positivity of GBMs by IF:
- Linear accentuation of GBMs for IgG may be seen in diabetic injury. In anti-GBM antibody–mediated glomerulonephritis, there is associated necrotizing, crescentic injury, and often C3 staining of GBM, features that are absent in diabetic nephropathy.
- Linear GBM staining is also present in monoclonal immunoglobulin deposition disease, most commonly light chain deposition disease (LCDD). In LCDD, there is typically mesangial expansion, often nodular, and accompanying tubular basement membrane staining with monoclonal light chain, with corresponding amorphous deposits by EM.

Crescentic lesions:
- Immune complex disease may have crescents, and are diagnosed by disease-specific IF and EM findings.
- Pauci-immune necrotizing crescentic glomerulonephritis (often antineutrophil cytoplasmic antibody–associated) has little or no IF staining, and no significant deposits by EM. By LM, crescentic lesions tend to vary more in stage of activity vs chronicity than in anti-GBM glomerulonephritis.

EM, electron microscopy; *GBM,* glomerular basement membrane; *IF,* immunofluorescence; *LM,* light microscopy.

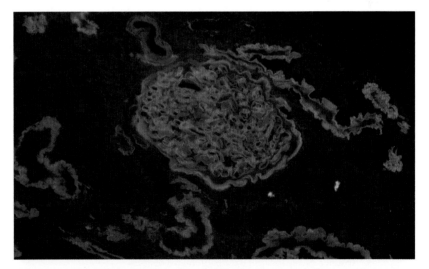

FIG. 1.329 Anti-GBM antibody–mediated glomerulonephritis. When antibody titers persist at time of transplantation, this disease may occasionally recur in the transplant, as in this case, where linear anti-GBM antibody staining was associated with mild glomerular injury. Note the associated linear tubular basement membrane staining (anti-IgG immunofluorescence, ×200). *GBM,* glomerular basement membrane

described with pulmonary-renal syndrome and also additional systemic vasculitis during the 1919 influenza epidemic did not have anti-GBM antibody–mediated disease.

Selected Reading

Couser, W.G., 1988. Rapidly progressive glomerulonephritis: classification, pathogenetic mechanisms, and therapy. American Journal of Kidney Disease 11, 449-464.

Goodpasture, E.W., 1919. The significance of certain pulmonary lesions in relation to the etiology of influenza. Australasian Journal of Medical Science 158, 863-870.

Levy, J.B., Lachmann, R.H., Pusey, C.D., 1996. Recurrent Goodpasture's disease. American Journal of Kidney Disease 27, 573-578.

Pedchenko, V., Bondar, O., Fogo, A.B., et al., 2010. Molecular architecture of the Goodpasture autoantigen in anti-GBM nephritis. New England Journal of Medicine 363, 343-354.

Saus, J., Wieslander, J., Langeveld, J.P., et al., 1988. Identification of the Goodpasture antigen as the alpha 3(IV) chain of collagen IV. Journal of Biology and Chemistry 263, 13374-13380.

Savage, C.O., Pusey, C.D., Bowman, C., et al., 1986. Antiglomerular basement membrane antibody mediated disease in the British Isles 1980-4. British Medical Journal 292, 301-304.

Stanton, M.C., Tange, J.D., 1958. Goodpasture's syndrome (pulmonary haemorrhage associated with glomerulonephritis). Australasian Annals of Medicine 7, 132-144.

Wilson, C.B., Dixon, F.J., 1973. Anti-glomerular basement membrane antibody-induced glomerulonephritis. Kidney International 3, 74-89.

Diseases Associated with the Nephritic Syndrome or RPGN: Pauci-Immune- or Non-Immune-Mediated

INTRODUCTION

Rapidly progressive glomerulonephritis is a variant of the acute nephritic syndrome in which patients initially present with acute glomerulonephritis associated with a rapid onset of severe acute renal failure. The onset of the disease is characterized by oliguria, advancing azotemia, proteinuria of varying amounts, hematuria with cellular casts, and hypertension, which is sometimes in the malignant range. The nephrotic syndrome is occasionally present. *Extrarenal organ involvement is common.* In a few patients, renal function eventually stabilizes at an impaired level after several weeks, but in most patients, progression to end-stage renal insufficiency occurs. The clinical pathologic entity can be divided into three subgroups. These include patients with postinfectious immune complex glomerulonephritis of a severe nature and patients with an antibody to GBMs. These are discussed elsewhere in this atlas. The third group has been termed pauci-immune in that antibody deposition is not present and no

---

Key Diagnostic Features of Pauci-immune Necrotizing Crescentic Glomerulonephritis

- Glomerular necrosis, crescents
- Absence of endocapillary proliferative lesions
- Absence of significant IF findings or EM deposits.

Note: Occasional IF positivity and EM densities may be found.
EM, electron microscopy; IF, immunofluorescence.

definite relationship to a particular antigen has been identified, although 80% of patients in this group have the presence of an ANCA directed against either myeloperoxidase or serine protease in their serum. Pauci-immune glomerulonephritis with positive serum ANCA encompasses four subgroups. These include patients with renal involvement alone, patients with renal and systemic involvement by microscopic polyangiitis, patients with granulomatosis with polyangiitis (GPA, also called Wegener granulomatosis) (Fig. 1.330) and patients with Churg–Strauss syndrome. The histopathology is similar in all forms of pauci-immune glomerulonephritis.

Key Differential Diagnosis of Pauci-immune Necrotizing Crescentic Glomerulonephritis

- Anti-GBM glomerulonephritis is distinguished by linear anti-GBM staining with IgG by IF
- Occasionally, subacute bacterial endocarditis may have limited deposits and it may be difficult to distinguish this lesion from antineutrophil cytoplasmic antibody–associated pauci-immune glomerulonephritis. Hump-type deposits, or dominant C3 and IgM by IF would favor subacute bacterial endocarditis–associated glomerulonephritis.

GBM, glomerular basement membrane; *IF,* immunofluorescence.

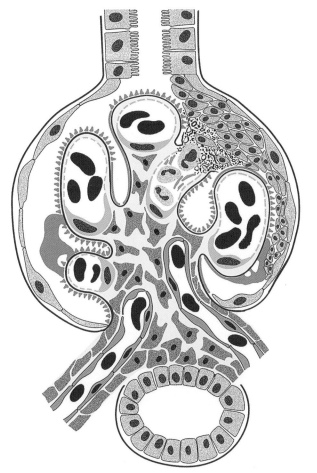

FIG. 1.330 Pauci-immune crescentic glomerulonephritis. There is segmental necrosis with a break of the GBM, and fibrinoid necrosis and polymorphonuclear leukocytes in this area, with a cellular crescent developing in response to this GBM break. The remainder of the glomerulus is unremarkable without proliferation and without deposits. *GBM,* glomerular basement membrane.

GRANULOMATOSIS WITH POLYANGIITIS (WEGENER)/ MICROSCOPIC POLYANGIITIS

Light microscopy demonstrates the presence of a necrotizing glomerulonephritis accompanied with an active interstitial nephritis (Figs. 1.331-1.333). Vascular necrosis may also be present with a transmural vasculitis (Figs. 1.334, 1.335). Glomerular necrosis may be focal and segmental or diffuse and global (Figs. 1.336, 1.337). Glomerular necrosis is uniformly accompanied by crescents. The crescents may be cellular or fibrous depending on the stage of evolution of the glomerular lesion (Fig. 1.338). The crescents consist of accumulations of cells derived from the parietal epithelium and infiltrating monocytes in Bowman's space and they appear to be initiated by the deposition of fibrin across gaps or disruptive lesions of the glomerular capillary with extrusion of fibrin into Bowman's space. As the crescents mature, fibroblasts with collagen begin to replace the cells and become fibroepithelial, and finally fibrous crescents are formed. Segmental areas of necrosis of the glomerular capillaries are usually present as well as areas of glomerular capillary collapse and focal increases in mesangial matrix. The necrosis and inflammation may extend through Bowman's capsule and form a granulomatous glomerulonephritis (Fig. 1.339). The light microscopic picture is similar in all three types of pathogenic mechanisms that are better characterized on the basis of immuno-fluorescence and electron microscopy. However, immune complex–related crescentic disease typically shows mesangial or endocapillary proliferation, depending on the underlying condition, whereas the pauci-immune disease does not show significant proliferation of uninvolved glomeruli or segments thereof. Of note, granulomas do not typically occur in the kidney in granulomatosis with polyangiitis (GPA, also called Wegener's granulomatosis), but rather are present in bronchioles. Thus, microscopic polyangiitis and GPA appear identical in the kidney and must be distinguished based on clinical criteria. Inflammation and necrosis of arterioles and venules may be present but is often not seen in the limited sampling present in renal

Text continued on page 267

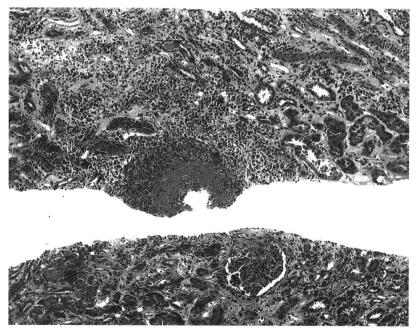

FIG. 1.331 Granulomatosis with polyangiitis (Wegener). There is a diffuse interstitial infiltrate with marked tubular epithelial changes. An artery shows necrosis within the wall. The glomeruli show focal necrosis with adhesion and crescent formation (hematoxylin and eosin, ×100).

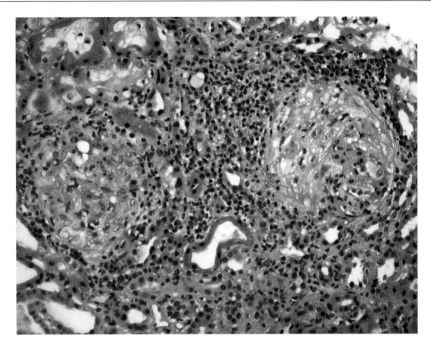

FIG. 1.332 Granulomatosis with polyangiitis (Wegener). Two glomeruli demonstrating glomerular necrosis and crescents with dense inflammatory reaction extending into the interstitium with a granulomatous appearance (hematoxylin and eosin, ×200).

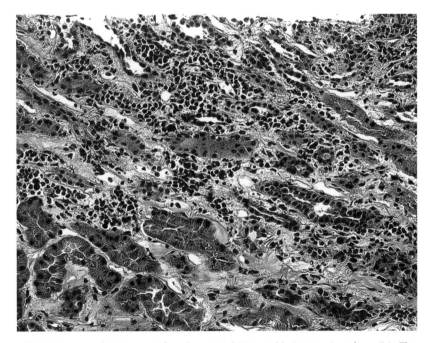

FIG. 1.333 Granulomatosis with polyangiitis (Wegener)/microscopic polyangiitis. The interstitial inflammatory infiltrate consists of mononuclear cells and has an abundant eosinophilic component with tubulitis (hematoxylin and eosin, ×200).

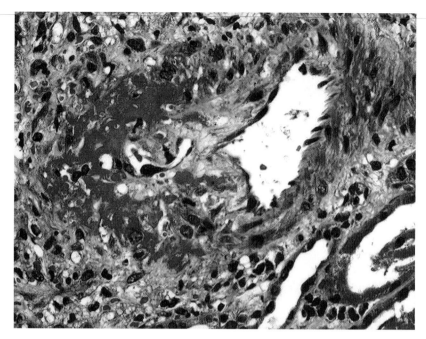

FIG. 1.334 Granulomatosis with polyangiitis (Wegener)/microscopic polyangiitis. Artery showing focal transmural necrosis extending into the interstitium with a granulomatous interstitial infiltrate (trichrome, ×200).

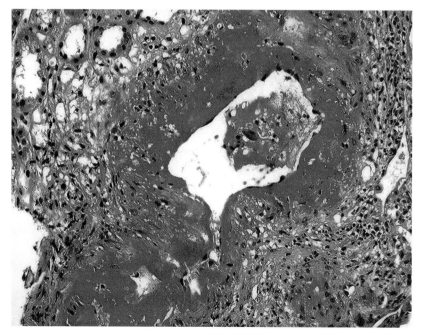

FIG. 1.335 Granulomatosis with polyangiitis (Wegener)/microscopic polyangiitis. Artery with transmural necrosis involving the vessels circumferentially with a significant inflammatory infiltrate with mixed polymorphonuclear leukocytes and mononuclear cells (hematoxylin and eosin, ×200).

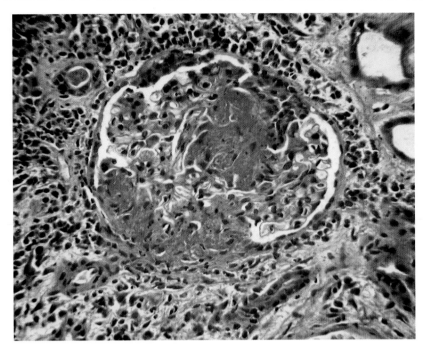

FIG. 1.336 Granulomatosis with polyangiitis (Wegener)/granulomatosis/microscopic polyangiitis. Glomerulus demonstrating focal and segmental necrosis with adhesion to Bowman's capsule and proliferation of parietal epithelium (HPS, ×400).

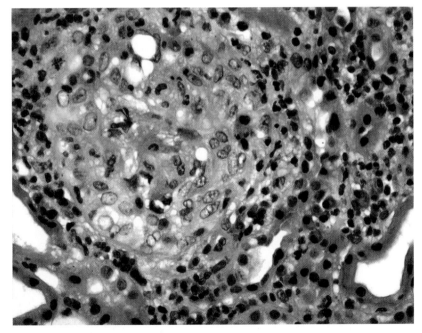

FIG. 1.337 Granulomatosis with polyangiitis (Wegener)/microscopic polyangiitis. A globally necrotic glomerulus with total obliteration of the architecture and infiltration with numerous leukocytes (hematoxylin and eosin, ×400).

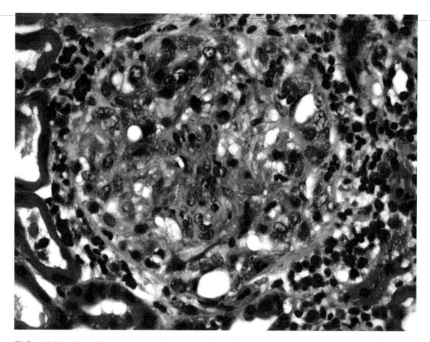

FIG. 1.338 Granulomatosis with polyangiitis (Wegener)/microscopic polyangiitis. Trichrome stain demonstrates the residual portions of the glomerulus and the entire Bowman's space is filled with proliferating epithelial cells and infiltrating monocytes (trichrome, ×400).

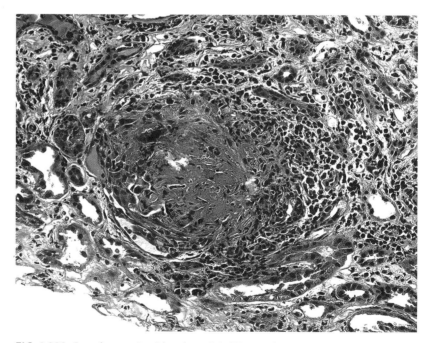

FIG. 1.339 Granulomatosis with polyangiitis (Wegener)/microscopic polyangiitis. A glomerulus with global necrosis surrounded by a granulomatous inflammatory infiltrate (hematoxylin and eosin, ×400).

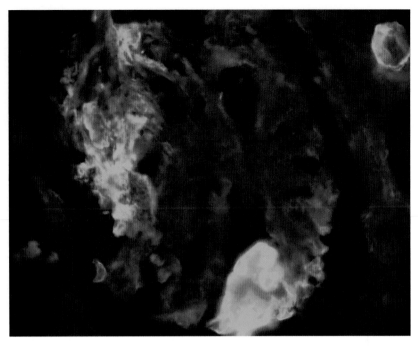

FIG. 1.340 Granulomatosis with polyangiitis (Wegener)/microscopic polyangiitis. Immunofluorescence reveals that the crescent is associated with abundant fibrin deposition (antifibrin immunofluorescence, ×400).

biopsies. Involvement of larger arteries is more characteristic of classical polyarteritis nodosa (see below).

By immunofluorescence, the findings are variable. No specific immunoglobulin deposition is identified by immunofluorescence microscopy. Complement components and fibrinogen may be present focally and are usually seen in association with the crescents (Figs. 1.340-1.342). This relative lack of immunoglobulin deposition has given rise to the term *pauci-immune*.

Electron microscopy findings are also variable. Patients with pauci-immune disease do not demonstrate electron-dense deposits. In most instances, fibrin deposition is prominent and is often associated with breaks within the capillary wall and the basement membrane (Figs. 1.343-1.345). Electron microscopy is also helpful in separating primary forms of crescentic glomerulonephritis from the miscellaneous immune complex–associated diseases described elsewhere, which also can display crescents by light microscopy.

Etiology/Pathogenesis

The role of ANCA in the pathogenesis of glomerulonephritis is still incompletely understood. In vivo and in vitro studies indicate that the pathogenesis of ANCA-associated glomerulonephritis involves activation of neutrophils and monocytes via the binding of ANCA to target antigens on or near the surface of neutrophils and monocytes. Experimental studies in mice have produced lesions similar to those in humans by injection of anti-myeloperoxidase IgG alone in immune-deficient animals. The most convincing evidence is the clinical association of these antibodies with crescentic glomerulonephritis and small vessel vasculitis.

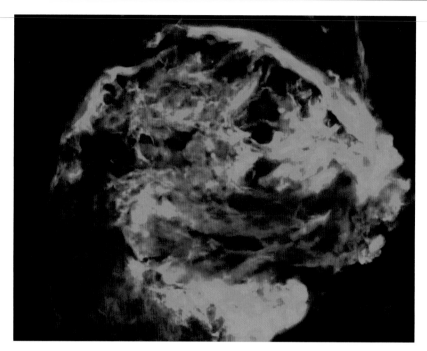

FIG. 1.341 Granulomatosis with polyangiitis (Wegener)/microscopic polyangiitis. Fibrin deposition is also present in a segmental fashion in the capillaries (antifibrin immunofluorescence, ×400).

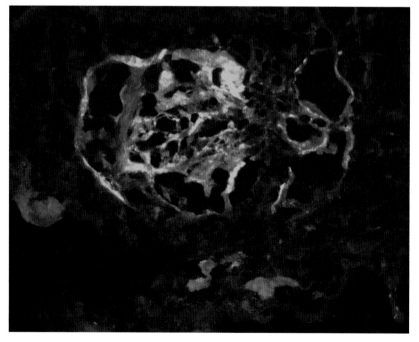

FIG. 1.342 Granulomatosis with polyangiitis (Wegener)/microscopic polyangiitis. Complement is also occasionally seen in association with necrosis and fibrin deposition (anti-C3 immunofluorescence, ×400).

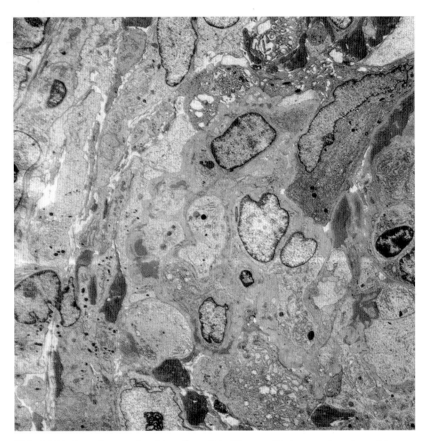

FIG. 1.343 Granulomatosis with polyangiitis (Wegener)/microscopic polyangiitis. Electron microscopy reveals the crescent to consist of a variety of cell types including mononuclear cells and epithelial cells (transmission electron microscopy, ×4000).

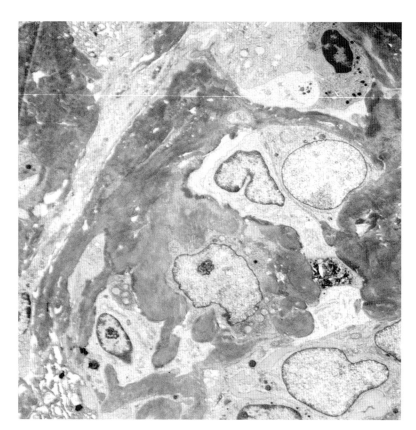

FIG. 1.344 Granulomatosis with polyangiitis (Wegener)/microscopic polyangiitis. Abundant fibrin tactoids are also interspersed with the cells of the crescent (transmission electron microscopy, ×3000).

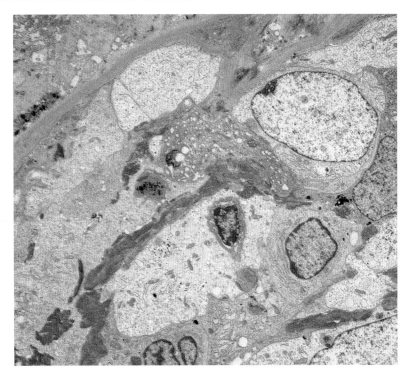

FIG. 1.345 Granulomatosis with polyangiitis (Wegener)/microscopic polyangiitis. There is endothelial cell swelling associated with accumulation of fibrin within the capillary lumen, and numerous leukocytes are also present (transmission electron microscopy, ×3000).

Selected Reading

Berden, A.E., Ferrario, F., Hagen, E.C., et al., 2010 Oct. Histopathologic classification of ANCA-associated glomerulonephritis. Journal of the American Society of Nephrology 21, 1628-1636.

Falk, R.J., Jennette, J.C., 2010 May. ANCA disease: where is this field heading? Journal of the American Society of Nephrology 21, 745-752.

Falk, R.J., Gross, W.L., Guillevin, L., et al., 2011. "Granulomatosis with polyangiitis (Wegener's)": an alternative name for "Wegener's granulomatosis." A joint proposal of the American College of Rheumatology, the American Society of Nephrology, and the European League Against Rheumatism. Journal of the American Society of Nephrology 22, 587-588.

Jennette, J.C., Falk, R.J., 2008 Jan. New insight into the pathogenesis of vasculitis associated with antineutrophil cytoplasmic autoantibodies. Current Opinion in Rheumatology 20, 55-60.

POLYARTERITIS NODOSA

This is a rare disease, which primarily affects medium-size arteries with "blow-out," pseudoaneurysmal, vasculitic lesions, which give rise to the nodose appearance of these vessels. Organs affected include the heart, liver, kidney, and mesenteric arteries. Radiographic studies show typical beaded appearance. In the kidney, large vessels show a transmural vasculitis (Fig. 1.346). Glomeruli are not affected. There are no immune complexes by immunofluorescence or electron microscopy. There are associated hemorrhagic infarcts related to the large vessel lesions.

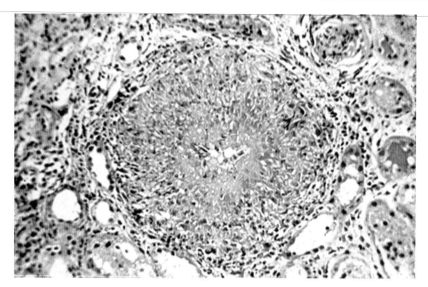

FIG. 1.346 Polyarteritis nodosa. Periarteritis involving an intrarenal artery. There is a transmural inflammatory infiltrate, which extends into the interstitium (trichrome, ×200).

Etiology/Pathogenesis

Polyarteris nodosa has been associated with illicit drug exposure, hepatitis B infection, and chronic infectious diseases. The precise etiology is not known.

Selected Reading

Jennette, J.C., Falk, R.J., 2007 Jan. Nosology of primary vasculitis. Current Opinion in Rheumatology 19, 10-16.

CHURG–STRAUSS SYNDROME

Clinically, patients have asthma and eosinophilia, and often have pulmonary-renal syndrome or only rapidly progressive glomerulonephritis. Renal lesions are similar but tend to be milder than those seen in granulomatosis with polyangiitis or microscopic polyangiitis. Glomeruli may also show varying mesangial proliferation, and there may not even be a crescentic component. There are no immune complexes by either immunofluorescence or electron microscopy. Despite the eosinophilia, there may not be prominent eosinophils in the renal inflammatory infiltrate, and indeed, this finding is not a required criterion to make the diagnosis of Churg–Strauss syndrome. Specific diagnosis rests on clinicopathologic criteria.

Etiology/Pathogenesis

The etiology is unknown. ANCAs are detected in about 40-60% of patients. The presence of allergic rhinitis, asthma, positive skin tests, and eosinophilia suggests hypersensitivity with heightened Th2 immunity.

Selected Reading

Churg, J., Strauss, L., 1951. Allergic granulomatosis, allergic angiitis, and periarteritis nodosa. American Journal of Pathology 27, 277-301.

Tsurikisawa, N., Saito, H., Tsuburai, T., et al., 2008. Differences in regulatory T cells between Churg–Strauss syndrome and chronic eosinophilic pneumonia with asthma. Journal of Allergy and Clinical Immunology 122, 610-616.

Diseases of the Basement Membrane

ALPORT SYNDROME

Classical Alport syndrome is inherited in an X-linked dominant pattern and is the most common form of Alport syndrome (85% of cases). Rare autosomal forms exist. The common underlying defect is an inability to form the α3, 4,5 (IV) collagen heterotrimer. The X-linked form is due to mutation of alpha 5 type IV collagen. The overall incidence of Alport syndrome in the USA is between 1:5000 and 1:10,000. Hematuria is the initial renal presentation of disease in childhood, although some proteinuria may also be present. Other manifestations of Alport syndrome in affected men include hearing loss and ocular defects. The organs affected reflect the sites where the α3, 4,5 (IV) collagen is critical for function (see below). Diminished hearing is detected in late childhood, and gradual deafness develops in about 55% of adult males. Ocular defects occur in up to one third of patients. Anterior lenticonus is the most common eye defect. Nephrotic syndrome may develop in as many as 30%-40% of patients with severe disease because of more extensive abnormality of the mutated type IV collagen. Chronic kidney disease develops in 30%-40% of patients. Female carriers of X-linked classic Alport syndrome have hematuria and may develop progressive renal disease. Males and females both can develop chronic kidney disease when Alport syndrome is caused by rare autosomal mutations of type IV collagen genes (alpha 3 or 4 type IV collagen chains, see below).

Light microscopy is unremarkable in the early stage in males with X-linked disease, and in carrier females (Fig. 1.347). At later stages, secondary, nonspecific glomerulosclerosis, interstitial fibrosis and prominent interstitial foam cells are typical in males with X-linked disease, or in either gender with autosomal disease (Fig. 1.348-1.351). These foam cells are not specific for this disease and are found in numerous proteinuric states.

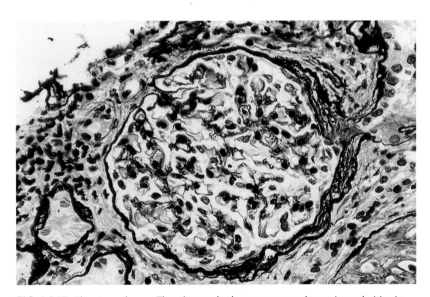

FIG. 1.347 Alport syndrome. The glomerular basement membrane irregularities in Alport syndrome are not detectable by light microscopy. Early in the course, the glomeruli may be unremarkable. In this case, there is early periglomerular fibrosis (Jones silver stain, ×200).

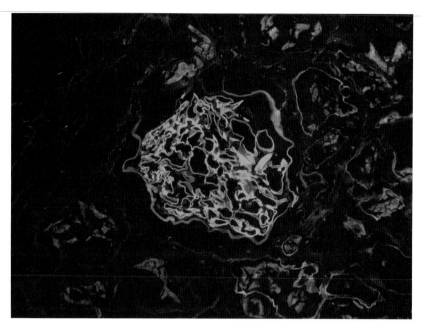

FIG. 1.348 Normal kidney immunofluorescence for alpha 5 (IV) collagen. The normal control tissue shows strong, continuous staining for alpha 5 type IV collagen of the glomerular basement membrane and focal tubular basement membrane, and Bowman's capsule (anti–alpha 5 type IV collagen immunofluorescence, ×200).

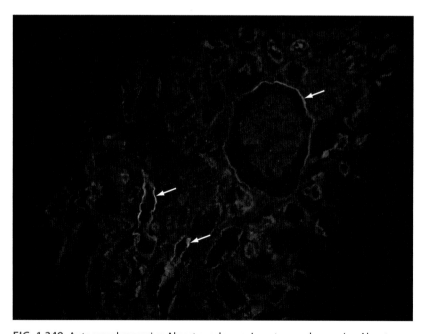

FIG. 1.349 Autosomal recessive Alport syndrome. In autosomal recessive Alport, there is a mutation of alpha 3 or alpha 4 type IV collagen, and thus the normal alpha 3,4,5 heterotrimer of the glomerular basement membrane is not formed, and there is no staining for alpha 5 type IV collagen in the glomerular basement membrane. However, because alpha 5 (IV) collagen is not itself mutated, it is still expressed as part of other alpha 5,5,6 heterotrimers in Bowman's capsule and in some tubular basement membranes (arrows) (anti–alpha 5 type IV collagen immunofluorescence, ×200).

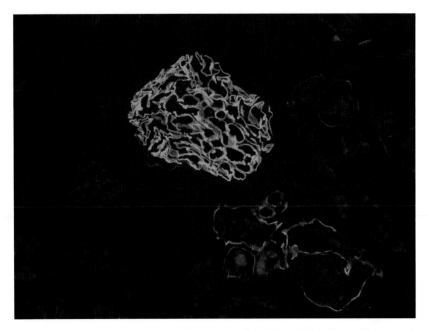

FIG. 1.350 Normal kidney immunofluorescence for alpha 3 (IV) collagen. The normal control tissue shows strong, continuous staining for alpha 3 type IV collagen of the glomerular basement membrane and focal tubular basement membrane (anti–alpha 3 type IV collagen immunofluorescence, ×200).

FIG. 1.351 Autosomal recessive Alport syndrome. In autosomal recessive Alport, there is a mutation of alpha 3 or alpha4 type IV collagen, and thus the normal alpha 3,4,5 heterotrimer of the glomerular basement membrane is not formed, and there is no staining for alpha 3 type IV collagen in the glomerular basement membrane. Because alpha 3 (IV) collagen is mutated, it is also not expressed or stained elsewhere (anti –alpha 3 type IV collagen immunofluorescence, ×200).

Standard immunofluorescence may show only nonspecific trapping of IgM. Immunofluorescence for type IV collagen molecules in either skin or kidney biopsy is useful for diagnosis. Type IV collagen organizes in heterotrimers composed of various combinations of alpha 1-6 collagen chains. The epidermal basement membrane normally contains alpha 1, alpha 2, alpha 5, and alpha 6(IV) collagen, but not alpha 3 or alpha 4(IV) collagen. Skin biopsy staining to demonstrate the absence of alpha 5(IV) collagen has therefore been suggested as a tool to distinguish patients with X-linked Alport syndrome from those with other causes of hematuria. In the kidney, the GBM contains alpha 3, 4, 5 (IV) heterotrimers, while Bowman's capsule and the distal tubule contain alpha 1, 1, 2 and 5, 5, 6 heterotrimers. In kidney biopsies, about 70%-80% of males with X-linked Alport lack staining of GBM, distal tubular basement membrane, and Bowman's capsule for alpha 5(IV) chains. Alpha 3 and alpha 4(IV) collagen staining is also lacking in the GBM in patients with classic Alport syndrome, because the molecular defect in alpha 5(IV) collagen results in defective incorporation of the alpha 3 and alpha 4 chains. In autosomal recessive Alport, the kidney GBMs also show no expression of alpha 3, 4, or 5(IV) collagen, because a defect in any one of the molecules of the heterotrimer prevents its formation.

However, in contrast to X-linked cases, autosomal recessive cases show strong expression of alpha 5 in Bowman's capsule, distal tubular basement membrane, and skin, reflecting the normal incorporation of the nonmutated alpha 5(IV) collagen in the alpha 5, 5, 6(IV) heterotrimers of these basement membranes. Female heterozygotes for X-linked Alport syndrome frequently show mosaic staining of GBM and distal TBM for alpha 3, alpha 4, and alpha 5(IV) chains, and skin mosaic staining for alpha 5(IV) (Fig. 1.352). Patients with autosomal dominant Alport have not been studied immunohistochemically.

Thus, the coabsence of alpha 3 and alpha 5(IV) collagen in the GBM is a major diagnostic clue to the diagnosis of Alport syndrome. As alpha 3 or alpha 4(IV) collagens are not normally expressed in the skin, autosomal recessive Alport cannot be diagnosed by this approach.

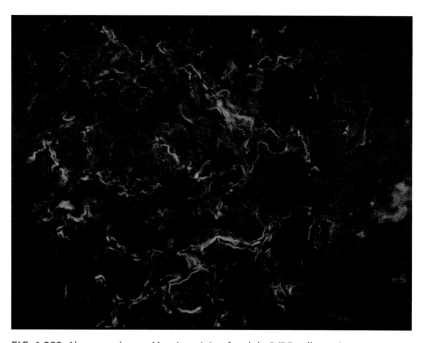

FIG. 1.352 Alport syndrome. Mosaic staining for alpha5 (IV) collagen is present along the glomerular basement membrane, strongly supporting a heterozygous carrier state of X-linked Alport syndrome. By electron microscopy, this female patient showed only diffuse thinning of the glomerular basement membrane (anti-alpha 5(IV) collagen immunofluorescence, ×400).

Key Diagnostic Features of Alport Syndrome

- Thin or basket-weaving appearance of glomerular basement membrane by electron microscopy

---

Key Differential Diagnosis of Alport Syndrome

- Consideration of a morphologic diagnosis of thin GBMs and its differential requires that extensive thinning must be present, that is, greater than 50% of GBM.
- Thin GBMs are found early in Alport or in carriers of Alport, and might also be seen in benign familial hematuria. Some of these patients are carriers for autosomal recessive Alport, and clinically manifest so-called benign familial hematuria.
- Differential of irregular, possible basket-weaving appearance of GBMs:
  - Irregular areas of GBMs may also be seen in, for example, chronic immune complex diseases due to resorbed deposits, in patients with Frasier syndrome, in patients with Pierson syndrome.
  - Chronic immune complex disease with resorbed immune deposits may be distinguished from Alport by immunofluorescence positivity for deposits or clinical history.
  - Frasier syndrome, due to WT-1 mutation, presents with FSGS lesions and may have irregular basket-weaving appearance of GBMs, but is distinguished from Alport by normal collagen IV staining. Pierson syndrome, due to laminin beta 2 mutation, typically has associated systemic abnormalities (microcoria), and shows normal collagen IV staining, but abnormally decreased or lacking laminin beta 2 staining, with unusual irregular blebs on the outer aspect of the GBM by electron microscopy.

GBM, glomerular basement membrane.

However, the sensitivity and specificity of skin or renal biopsy immunofluorescence studies in the diagnosis of Alport syndrome have not been proven, and occasional patients with Alport syndrome clinically and by renal biopsy showed normal alpha 5(IV) collagen pattern of skin or kidney immunofluorescence staining. About 20% of male classic Alport patients and affected homozygous autosomal recessive Alport patients show faint or even normal staining of the GBM for alpha 3 and alpha 5(IV) collagen. This is thought to reflect a mutation that still leaves intact the epitope recognized by the commercially available antibodies. Thus, an apparent normal staining pattern in either skin or kidney does not definitively rule out Alport syndrome.

By electron microscopy, the diagnostic lesion in established Alport consists of irregular thinned and thickened areas of the GBMs with splitting and irregular multilaminated appearance of the lamina densa, with thin fibrils amid irregular lucent thickened areas of the lamina densa, with short stubs of fibrils at right angles to the GBM, resulting in a "basket weaving" pattern (Figs. 1.343-1.356). In between these lamina, granular, mottled material is present. At early stages of disease, that is, in children or carriers, the basement membrane shows only thinning rather than thickening (Fig. 1.353). Of note, some kindreds with typical Alport syndrome clinically have only manifested basement membrane thinning as a morphologic change, even at advanced stages. Ultrastructural features do not strictly correlate with type of mutation, in that some patients with major gene rearrangements had no significant lesions, and varying ultrastructural abnormalities were present even within the same kindred. Thus, normal thickness and appearance GBM by electron microscopy without areas of thinning and/or basket weaving rules out Alport. Thin GBM may represent early stage of Alport in an affected patient, Alport carrier female for X-linked Alport, or so-called benign familial hematuria (most are carriers for autosomal recessive Alport, see below).

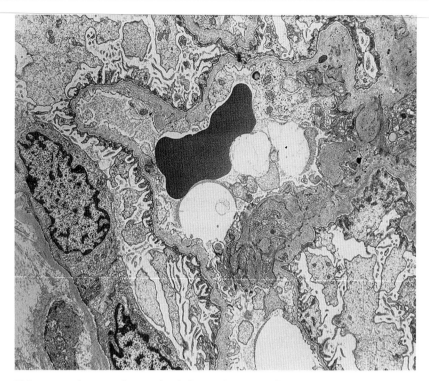

FIG. 1.353 Alport syndrome. The definitive diagnosis of Alport syndrome is made by electron microscopy. Early in the course, there is only thinning of the GBM, with segments of irregular thickening due to a loose, mottled, so-called basket-weaving appearance of the glomerular basement membrane. There is only minimal effacement of the overlying foot processes (transmission electron microscopy, ×3000).

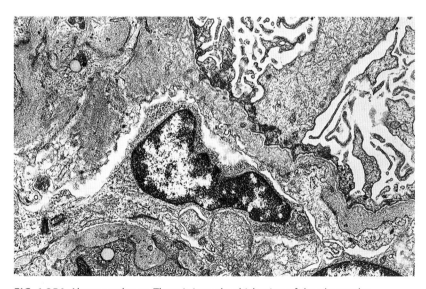

FIG. 1.354 Alport syndrome. There is irregular thickening of the glomerular basement membrane with a loose, basket-woven appearance. The overlying foot processes are blunted and partially effaced (transmission electron microscopy, ×17,125).

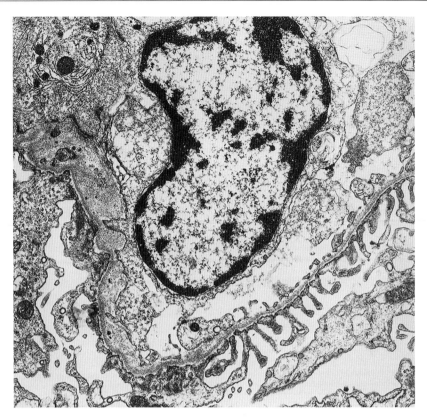

FIG. 1.355 Alport syndrome. Alternating areas of extreme thinning of the glomerular basement membrane (~120 nm) with thick, irregular areas with basket weaving are shown (transmission electron microscopy, ×7000).

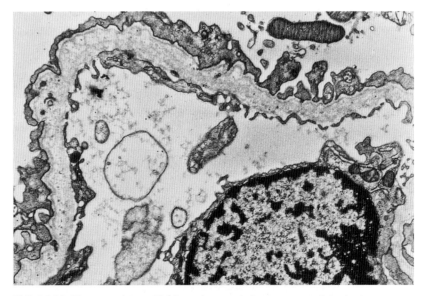

FIG. 1.356 Alport syndrome. The irregular mottled appearance of the basket-weaving lesion is illustrated. There are no immune deposits, and overlying foot processes are only partially effaced. The lamellated appearance is highly characteristic of Alport syndrome, but may be seen to very minor degree in small areas in other scarring conditions (transmission electron microscopy, ×9750).

Etiology/Pathogenesis

The alpha 5(IV) collagen chain (COL4A5) gene is mutated in classic, X-linked Alport syndrome. Rare mutations of alpha 3 or alpha 4 type IV collagen genes (COL4A3 or COL4A4) cause autosomal recessive Alport syndrome, or very rarely autosomal dominant Alport syndrome.

The organs involved reflect sites where these collagen chains are normally highly expressed and are necessary for function and structure. Alpha 3, alpha 4, and alpha 5(IV) collagen chains are normally highly expressed in the kidney, lens of the eye, and cochlea of the ear and organize as the alpha 3, 4, 5(IV) heterotrimer of the GBM. The abnormal alpha 5(IV) collagen prevents incorporation of alpha 3(IV) and alpha 4(IV) into these heterotrimers. In situ hybridization and immunostaining reveal normal mRNA transcription of COL4A3 and COL4A4 and normal alpha 3(IV) staining in podocytes in Alport patients, implicating events downstream to transcription, RNA processing, and protein synthesis in the absent staining in X-linked Alport patients.

Each Alport kindred reported thus far has presented its own unique mutation. The rate of progression to end stage and deafness are mutation dependent. Large deletions, nonsense mutations, or mutations that changed the reading frame were associated with 90% risk of end-stage renal disease before age 30 years in affected males with X-linked Alport, with only 50% risk for patients with missense and 70% risk for those with splice site mutations. Risk for hearing loss before age 30 years was 60% in patients with missense mutations, versus 90% risk for all other mutations. Transplantation in patients with Alport syndrome has shed additional light on the molecular basis for this disease. Some patients with Alport receiving kidney transplants, probably about 5%–10%, develop antibodies to the normal GBM in the transplant (Fig. 1.357). These antibodies may cross-react with the tubular basement membrane (Fig. 1.358). Occurrence of this posttransplant anti-GBM disease appears more frequent in patients with more extensive deletion of the COL4A5 gene. The antibody binding results in a necrotizing, crescentic lesion, usually resulting in loss of the graft (Figs. 1.359, 1.360).

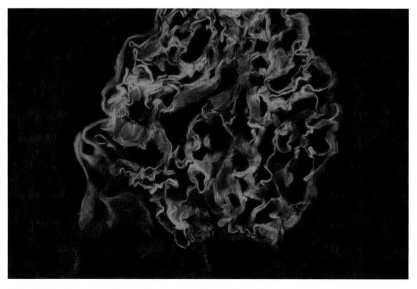

FIG. 1.357 Alport syndrome. In some patients with Alport syndrome receiving a transplant, there is an antibody response to the normal type IV collagen of the transplanted kidney resulting in anti-GBM antibody–mediated glomerulonephritis with linear staining for IgG by immunofluorescence, as in this case (anti-IgG immunofluorescence, ×400). *GBM,* glomerular basement membrane.

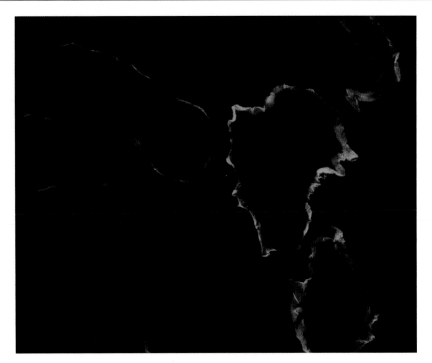

FIG. 1.358 Alport syndrome. The anti-GBM antibody developing against the transplant in some patients with Alport may also cross-react with tubular basement membranes, and thus give rise to a tubulitis. This tubulitis must be distinguished from acute rejection, by correlating with glomerular findings and clinical course (anti-IgG immunofluorescence, ×400). *GBM,* glomerular basement membrane.

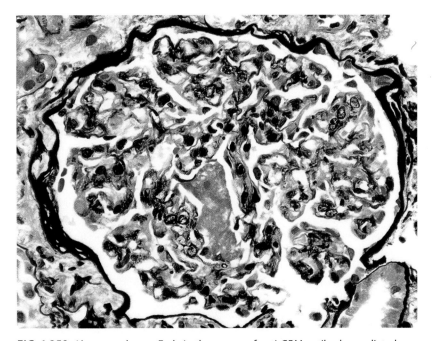

FIG. 1.359 Alport syndrome. Early in the course of anti-GBM antibody–mediated glomerulonephritis occurring in the Alport patient posttransplant, there may only be subtle, very early segmental fibrinoid necrosis and glomerular basement membrane breaks as shown here. Immunofluorescence is key in evaluating this lesion and making the correct diagnosis (see Figs. 1.351 and 1.352) (Jones silver stain, ×400). *GBM,* glomerular basement membrane.

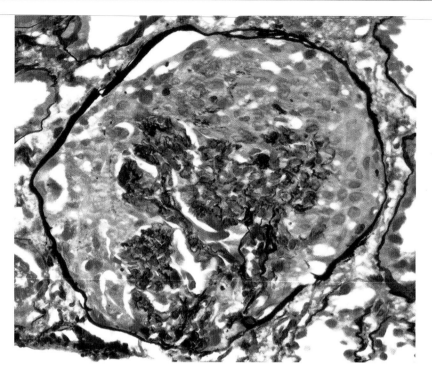

FIG. 1.360 Alport syndrome. The early necrotizing lesion shown in Figure 1.359 does, with time, give rise to a frank crescentic glomerulonephritis, associated with linear immunofluorescence, as in this case (Jones silver stain, ×200).

Selected Reading

Bodziak, K.A., Hammond, W.S., Molitoris, B.A., 1994. Inherited diseases of the glomerular basement membrane. American Journal of Kidney Disease 23, 605-618.

Churg, J., Sherman, R.L., 1973. Pathologic characteristics of hereditary nephritis. Archives of Pathology 95, 374-379.

Ding, J., Kashtan, C.E., Fan, W.W., et al., 1994. A monoclonal antibody marker for Alport syndrome identifies the Alport antigen as the α5 chain of type IV collagen. Kidney International 45, 1504-1506.

Gubler, M.C., 2008. Inherited diseases of the glomerular basement membrane. Nature Clinical Practice Nephrology 2008. 4, 24-37.

Haas, M., 2009. Alport syndrome and thin glomerular basement membrane nephropathy: a practical approach to diagnosis. Archives of Pathology Laboratory Medicine 133, 224-232.

Jais, J.P., Knebelmann, B., Giatras, I., et al., 2000. X-linked Alport syndrome: natural history in 195 families and genotype-phenotype correlations in males. Journal of the American Society of Nephrology 11, 649-657.

Kashtan, C.E., 2000. Alport syndromes: phenotypic heterogeneity of progressive hereditary nephritis. Pediatric Nephrology 14, 502-512.

Kashtan, C.E., Gubler, M.C., Sisson-Ross, S., et al., 1998. Chronology of renal scarring in males with Alport syndrome. Pediatric Nephrology 12, 269-274.

Kashtan, C.E., Segal, Y., 2011. Genetic disorders of glomerular basement membranes. Nephron Clinical Practice 118, c9-c18.

Lemmink, H.H., Nillesen, W.N., Mochizuki, T., et al., 1996. Benign familial hematuria due to mutation of the type IV collagen α4 gene. Journal of Clinical Investigation 98, 1114-1118.

Liapis, H., Gokden, N., Hmiel, P., et al., 2002. Histopathology, ultrastructure, and clinical phenotypes in thin glomerular basement membrane disease variants. Human Pathology 33, 836-845.

Mazzucco, G., Barsotti, P., Muda, A.O., et al., 1998. Ultrastructural and immunohistochemical findings in Alport's syndrome: a study of 208 patients from 97 Italian families with particular emphasis on COL4A5 gene mutation correlations. Journal of the American Society of Nephrology 9, 1023-1031.

Nakanishi, K., Yoshikawa, N., Iijima, K., et al., 1996. Expression of type IV collagen α3 and α4 chain mRNA in X-linked Alport syndrome. Journal of the American Society of Nephrology 7, 938-945.

Pirson, Y., 1999. Making the diagnosis of Alport's syndrome. Kidney International 56, 760-775.

THIN BASEMENT MEMBRANE LESIONS

Thin GBMs underlie the condition of "benign familial hematuria" in most kindreds. This term has been used to distinguish these families from Alport syndrome since affected individuals have been thought to have a benign prognosis. However, morphology alone does not allow one to make specific prognostic inferences. Kindreds may show autosomal dominant or apparent autosomal recessive inheritance; many are carriers of autosomal recessive Alport (see below). The clinical manifestation is that of hematuria, either macroscopic or microscopic, intermittent or continuous. This lesion is common and is present in 20-25% of patients biopsied for persistent isolated hematuria in some series. The lesion may also coexist with other glomerular disease, commonly diabetic nephropathy changes (alternating very thin and thick GBM), or IgA nephropathy. Occasionally patients with thin basement membranes have nephrotic range proteinuria, with five of eight reported cases in one series showing superimposed FSGS lesions.

Light microscopy shows no specific lesion, and standard immunofluorescence studies are negative (Figs. 1.361, 1.362). The diagnosis of thin basement membranes is thus based on morphometric measurements from electron microscopic examination, revealing marked and extensive thinning of the lamina densa of the GBMs (Figs. 1.363, 1.364). Thinning should

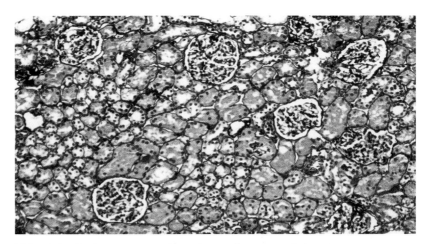

FIG. 1.361 Thin basement membrane lesion. There are no light microscopic abnormalities in thin basement membrane lesion. This lesion is common, and may therefore be found superimposed on other diseases, such as IgA nephropathy or diabetic nephropathy. When occurring with diabetic nephropathy, there are alternate segments of thick and very thin GBM with very sudden transition (Jones silver stain, ×100). *GBM,* glomerular basement membrane.

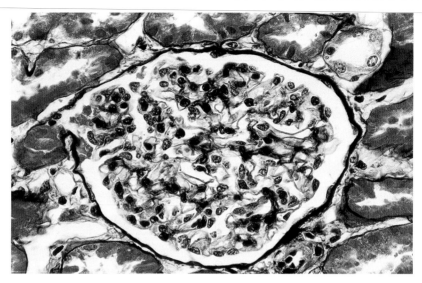

FIG. 1.362 Thin basement membrane lesion. The thin glomerular basement membrane cannot be detected by light microscopic examination (Jones silver stain, ×200).

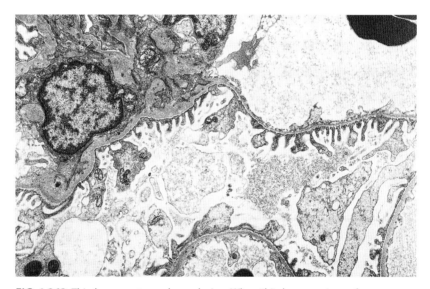

FIG. 1.363 Thin basement membrane lesion. When thin basement membranes are associated with benign familial hematuria, a carrier state of Alport or early in the course of Alport, the lesion is diffuse and global. Very segmental areas of thinning may occur nonspecifically (transmission electron microscopy, ×9750).

involve most loops to consider this diagnosis, as small segmental areas of thinning are non-specific and nondiagnostic. Diagnosis of thinning must be made by comparison to age-matched controls, because the GBM thickness normally increases with age. Normal thickness in adults in one series was 373 ± 42 nm in men versus 326 ± 45 nm in women. Glomerular basement membrane thickness <250 nm has been used as a cutoff in many series. In children, the diagnosis of thin basement membranes must be made with special care, establishing normal age-matched controls within each laboratory. In our laboratory, we found a range of GBM thickness in normal children from approximately 110 nm at age 1 year, to 222 ± 14 nm in 7-year-olds.

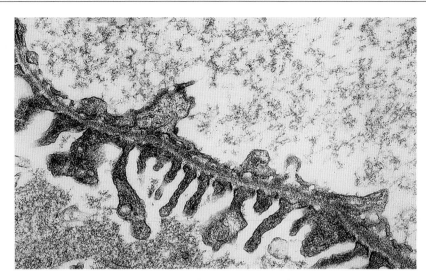

FIG. 1.364 Thin basement membrane lesion. Diagnosis of thin basement membrane is made specifically by measurements of the electron microscopic images and must be compared with the normal for age, as GBM thickness normally increases from childhood to adulthood. However, the relative thickness of the base of the intact foot process versus the GBM gives an approximate guide to the GBM thickness. In the adult, the normal GBM is 2-3 times the thickness of the base of the normal foot process of the podocyte (transmission electron microscopy, ×20,250). *GBM,* glomerular basement membrane.

Etiology/Pathogenesis

Mutation of the α4 or α3 type IV collagen gene segregates with hematuria many patients with "benign familial hematuria." One patient described had electron microscopic changes typical of Alport syndrome by renal biopsy at age 5 years, that is, areas of lamellation alternating with areas of thinning. This boy's parents both had microscopic hematuria and family histories of benign hematuria without progression in any members. In contrast, the boy developed proteinuria at age 16 years. This patient likely inherited one mutant allele from each parent, resulting in full-blown Alport syndrome. Thus, carriers of autosomal recessive Alport syndrome with mutation in one allele of either COL4A4 or COL4A3 present clinically as "benign familial hematuria/thin basement membrane disease." In contrast, patients with homozygosity or compound heterozygosity for mutations in the α3 or α4 chains develop Alport syndrome.

Furthermore, benign familial hematuria may not be entirely benign. Some patients with thin basement membranes on renal biopsies showed increased global sclerosis, and later increased hypertension and late onset of renal insufficiency. However, these patients were not defined molecularly and were presumed to not have Alport based on absence of hearing or eye abnormalities. Renal disease also developed over the follow-up in some relatives. It is possible that a second process, such as arterionephrosclerosis, was also present in these families, or that this represents a part of a continuum of basement membrane abnormalities. These observations further reiterate that the finding of thin basement membranes alone does not allow one to predict a "benign" process.

Selected Reading

Badenas, C., Praga, M., Tazon, B., et al., 2002. Mutations in the COL4A4 and COL4A3 genes cause familial benign hematuria. Journal of the American Society of Nephrology 13, 1248-1254.

Buzza, M., Wang, Y.Y., Dagher, H., et al., 2001. COL4A4 mutation in thin basement membrane disease previously described in Alport syndrome. Kidney International 60, 480-483.

Cosio, F.G., Falkenhain, M.E., Sedmak, D.D., 1994. Association of thin glomerular basement membrane with other glomerulopathies. Kidney International 46, 471-474.

Deltas, C., 2009. Thin basement membrane nephropathy: is there genetic predisposition to more severe disease? Pediatric Nephrology 24, 877-879.

Haas, M., 2009. Alport syndrome and thin glomerular basement membrane nephropathy: a practical approach to diagnosis. Archives of Pathology & Laboratory Medicine 133, 224-232.

Hisano, S., Kwano, M., Hatae, K., et al., 1991. Asymptomatic isolated microhaematuria: natural history of 136 children. Pediatric Nephrology 5, 578-581.

Kashtan, C.E., Segal, Y., 2011. Genetic disorders of glomerular basement membranes. Nephron Clinical Practice 118, c9-c18.

Lemmink, H.H., Nillesen, W.N., Mochizuki, T., et al., 1996. Benign familial hematuria due to mutation of the type IV collagen a4 gene. Journal of Clinical Investigation 98, 1114-1118.

Longo, I., Porcedda, P., Mari, F., et al., 2002. COL4A3/COL4A4 mutations: from familial hematuria to autosomal-dominant or recessive Alport syndrome. Kidney International 61, 1947-1956.

Matsumae, T., Fukusaki, M., Sakata, N., et al., 1994. Thin glomerular basement membrane in diabetic patients with urinary abnormalities. Clinical Nephrology 42, 221-226.

Nieuwhof, C.M.G., de Heer, F., de Leeuw, P., et al., 1997. Thin GBM nephropathy: Premature glomerular obsolescence is associated with hypertension and late onset renal failure. Kidney International 51, 1596-1601.

Pierides, A., Voskarides, K., Athanasiou, Y., et al., 2009. Clinico-pathological correlations in 127 patients in 11 large pedigrees, segregating one of three heterozygous mutations in the COL4A3/ COL4A4 genes associated with familial haematuria and significant late progression to proteinuria and chronic kidney disease from focal segmental glomerulosclerosis. Nephrology Dialysis Transplantation 24, 2721-2729.

Tiebosch, A.T.M.G., Frederik, P.M., van Breda Vriesman, P.J.C., et al., 1989. Thin-basement-membrane nephropathy in adults with persistent hematuria. New England Journal of Medicine 320, 14-18.

Yoshiokawa, N., Matsuyama, S., Iijima, K., et al., 1988. Benign familial hematuria. Archives of Pathology & Laboratory Medicine 112, 794-797.

NAIL-PATELLA SYNDROME

Nail-patella syndrome is inherited in autosomal dominant fashion, and occurs in approximately 22/1,000,000. Patients show hypoplastic or absent patellae, dystrophic fingernails and toenails, and abnormalities of bones in the elbow and iliac horns. Additional abnormalities include vasomotor and neurologic disturbances. Renal disease occurs in less than one half of affected patients and is quite variable, even within a given kindred. End-stage renal disease develops in ~10% of patients; only half of these patients manifest proteinuria, microhematuria, edema, and hypertension. The disease has not been reported to recur in the transplant.

The light microscopic appearance is normal at early stages, with glomerulosclerosis developing as disease advances, with associated tubulointerstitial fibrosis. Immunofluorescence studies do not show immune complexes. The renal biopsy diagnosis is made at the ultrastructural level. Glomerular basement membranes are thickened with irregular lucent areas with intervening clear zones and rarefied areas, resulting in a moth-eaten appearance. Some areas contain coarse fibrils that appear like cross-banded collagen (Fig. 1.365). Collagen fibrils are usually in the mid portion of the GBM but may occasionally be present in the subepithelial or

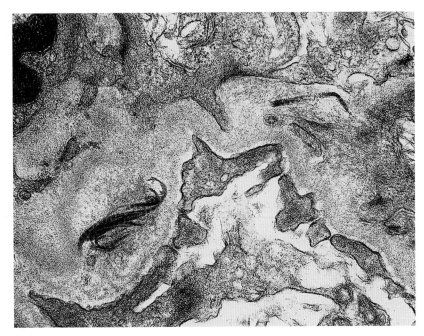

FIG. 1.365 Nail-patella syndrome. Light microscopy is nonspecific, and the diagnosis is made by electron microscopy, which shows mottled, moth-eaten areas of the glomerular basement membrane, and banded collagen within the glomerular basement membrane (transmission electron microscopy, ×8000).

Key Diagnostic Features of Nail-Patella Syndrome

- Mottled, moth-eaten areas of glomerular basement membrane
- Banded collagen

Note: Occasional banded collagen may be associated with glomerulosclerosis in any condition.

---

subendothelial area, and rarely in the mesangium. Staining with phosphotungstic acid enhances these collagen bundles.

Etiology/Pathogenesis

The gene mutated in nail-patella syndrome, LMX1B on chromosome 9, has now been identified. The gene encodes a LIM-homeodomain transcription factor. Mice null-mutated for the LMX1B gene develop a phenotype remarkably similar to human nail-patella syndrome, and have markedly decreased α3 and α4 collagen type IV expression in their GBM. These knockout mice also have abnormal podocytes lacking typical slit diaphragms. CD2AP and podocin – two key components of the slit diaphragm – were markedly reduced, although other podocyte genes such as nephrin, synaptopodin, ZO1, alpha-3 integrin, and specific laminins were preserved. Thus, the LMX1b gene product plays an integral part in foot process development and integrity, pointing to important interactions of the podocyte and the underlying GBM. Understanding of correlation between aspects of the phenotype and specific mutations are emerging: family history of nephropathy and mutation of the homeodomain of the gene are both associated with higher risk of renal disease in an individual with this syndrome.

Selected Reading

Bongers, E.M., Huysmans, F.T., Levtchenko, E., et al., 2005. Genotype-phenotype studies in nail-patella syndrome show that LMX1B mutation location is involved in the risk of developing nephropathy. European Journal of Human Genetics 13, 935-946.

Chen, H., Lun, Y., Ovchinnikov, D., et al., 1998. Limb and kidney defects in LmX1b mutant mice suggest an involvement of LMX1B in human nail patella syndrome. Nature Genetics 19, 51-55.

Gubler, M.C., 2008. Inherited diseases of the glomerular basement membrane. Nature Clinical Practice Nephrology 4, 24-37.

Kashtan, C.E., Segal, Y., 2011. Genetic disorders of glomerular basement membranes. Nephron Clinical Practice 118, c9-c18.

Lemley, K.V., 2009. Kidney disease in nail-patella syndrome. Pediatric Nephrology 24, 2345-2354.

McIntosh, I., Dreyer, S.D., Clough, M.V., et al., 1998. Mutation analysis of LMX1B gene in nail-patella syndrome patients. American Journal of Human Genetics 63, 1651-1658.

Miner, J.H., Morello, R., Andrews, K.L., et al., 2002. Transcriptional induction of slit diaphragm genes by LmX1b is required in podocyte differentiation. Journal of Clinical Investigation 109, 1065-1072.

Morello, R., Zhou, G., Dreyer, S.D., et al., 2001. Regulation of glomerular basement membrane collagen expression by LMX1B contributes to renal disease in nail patella syndrome. Nature Genetics 27, 205-208.

Morita, T., Laughlin, L.O., Kawano, K., et al., 1973. Nail-patella syndrome. Light and electron microscopic studies of the kidney. Archives of Internal Medicine 131, 271-277.

Taguchi, T., Takebayashi, S., Nishimura, M., et al., 1988. Nephropathy of nail-patella syndrome. Ultrastructural Pathology 12, 175-183.

Glomerular Involvement with Bacterial Infections

SUBACUTE BACTERIAL ENDOCARDITIS

Subacute bacterial endocarditis (SBE) may result in glomerulonephritis regardless of the causative organisms (e.g., *Streptococcus viridans*, Enterococci, *Streptococcus aureus*). Patients have hematuria and proteinuria and may occasionally have acute nephritic or nephrotic syndrome. There is often associated hypocomplementemia, fever, rash, weakness, and enlarged spleen.

By light microscopy, there is typically a focal segmental proliferative glomerulonephritis, often with crescents (Figs. 1.366-1.370). In some patients, there may be more diffuse and global endocapillary proliferation, or minimal proliferation with a crescentic necrotizing lesion dominating. Crescents often occur along with the proliferative lesions (Fig. 1.371). Infiltrating cells are typically monocytes/macrophages, rather than PMNs as seen in acute postinfectious glomerulonephritis or shunt nephritis. Segmental thrombosis and necrosis may also be present, and with chronicity organize as segmental scars and adhesions. There is proportional

---

Key Diagnostic Features of Subacute Bacterial Endocarditis–Associated Glomerulonephritis

- Variable proliferation by light microscopy, +/− crescents
- Variable immunofluorescence positivity, IgG/IgM and C3 mesangial and occasionally subendothelial deposits by electron microscopy

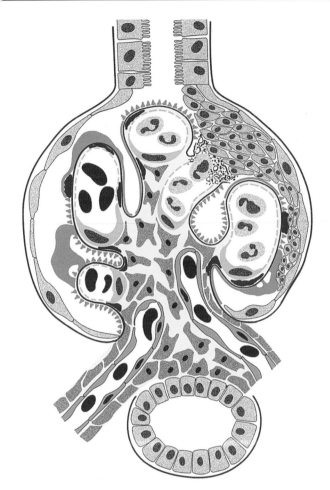

FIG. 1.366 Subacute bacterial endocarditis-associated glomerulonephritis. There is focal segmental proliferative glomerulonephritis, often with crescents, with predominant mesangial deposits and occasional subendothelial deposits associated with endocapillary proliferation, with only rare subepithelial deposits.

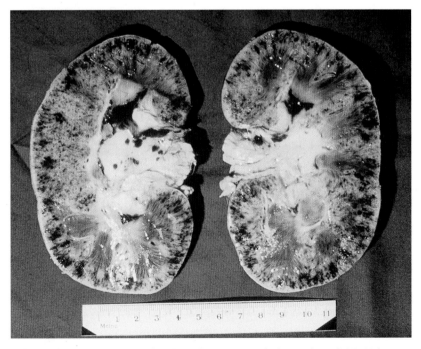

FIG. 1.367 Subacute bacterial endocarditis-associated glomerulonephritis. Kidney lesions may result from embolization of portions of the valve vegetations, resulting in multiple infarcts due to occlusion of interlobular arteries and arterioles.

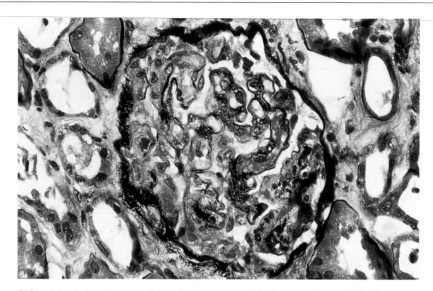

FIG. 1.368 Subacute bacterial endocarditis-associated glomerulonephritis. The glomeruli in subacute bacterial endocarditis show hypercellularity, often with a membranoproliferative pattern, but in a focal and segmental distribution. There is often coexistence of segmental sclerosis. This glomerulus shows widespread glomerular basement membrane reduplication and only rare polymorphonuclear leukocytes (Jones silver stain, ×400).

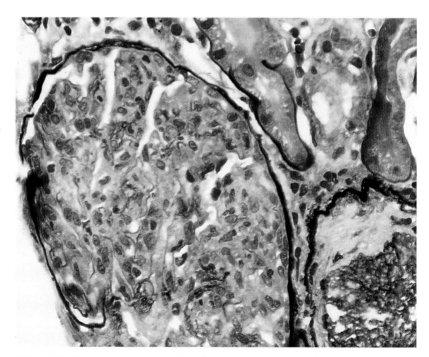

FIG. 1.369 Subacute bacterial endocarditis-associated glomerulonephritis. A global proliferative pattern is present in this glomerulus, with scattered polymorphonuclear leukocytes (same case as Fig. 1.368, Jones silver stain, ×400).

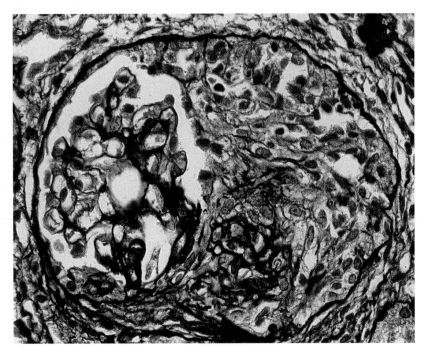

FIG. 1.370 Subacute bacterial endocarditis-associated glomerulonephritis. Crescents are often associated with proliferative lesion of subacute bacterial endocarditis. This glomerulus shows segmental proliferation and sclerosis with an associated fibrocellular crescent (Jones silver stain, ×400).

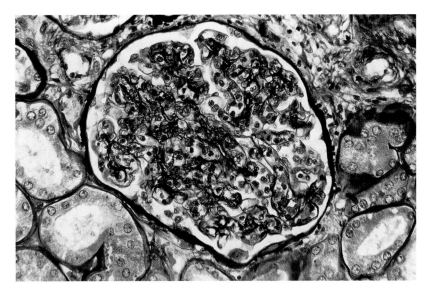

FIG. 1.371 Subacute bacterial endocarditis-associated glomerulonephritis. When the underlying valve lesion is not successfully treated, lesions may progress. In this case (same case as Fig. 1.368), the patient became septicemic and died weeks after renal biopsy. At autopsy, there was a diffuse proliferative glomerulonephritis with numerous polymorphonuclear leukocytes (Jones silver stain, ×400).

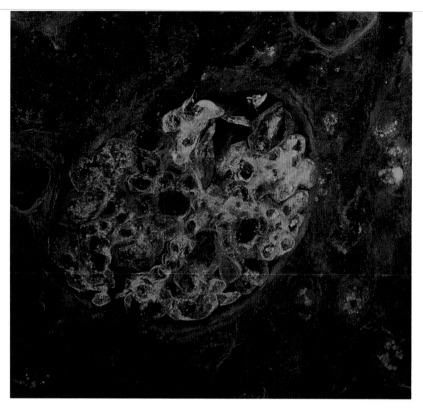

FIG. 1.372 Subacute bacterial endocarditis-associated glomerulonephritis. Immunofluorescence shows chunky deposits in the mesangial area, frequently extending to capillary loops, corresponding to subendothelial deposits in the diffuse, membranoproliferative forms of subacute bacterial endocarditis-associated glomerulonephritis. Deposits typically stain with IgG, IgM, C3, and C1q. This glomerulus (same case as Fig. 1.368) shows typical segmental accentuation of staining with mesangial and peripheral capillary loop deposits (anti-IgG immunofluorescence, ×200).

Key Differential Diagnosis of Subacute Bacterial Endocarditis–Associated Glomerulonephritis

- The proliferative form does not show specific morphologic features to distinguish it from glomerulonephritis caused by other chronic infections.
- Unlike typical poststreptococcal postinfectious glomerulonephritis, subepithelial deposits are rare.
- In cases with more limited deposits, it may be difficult to distinguish this lesion from antineutrophil cytoplasmic antibody–associated pauci-immune glomerulonephritis; presence of humps, strong C3/IgM suggest subacute bacterial endocarditis–associated glomerulonephritis.

---

tubulointerstitial fibrosis. Vessels do not show any specific lesions. By immunofluorescence, there are diffuse mesangial granular deposits of IgG, IgM, and C3, with rare other components (Figs. 1.372, 1.373). IgM dominance is typical in those cases with minimal proliferation. Endocapillary proliferation is associated with peripheral loop deposits. Electron microscopy shows the presence of mesangial deposits, with subendothelial deposits in those patients with endocapillary proliferation (Figs. 1.374, 1.375). Subepithelial deposits are rare.

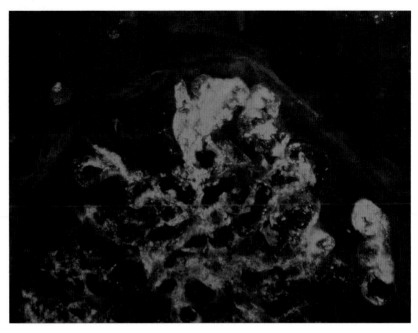

FIG. 1.373 Subacute bacterial endocarditis-associated glomerulonephritis. Chunky peripheral loop and mesangial deposits are evident in this case of subacute bacterial endocarditis-related glomerulonephritis. The smooth outer contours of some of the peripheral loop deposits correspond to their subendothelial location (anti-C3 immunofluorescence, ×400).

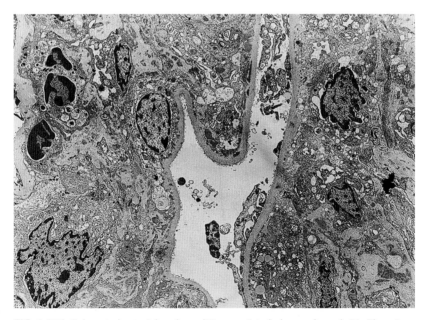

FIG. 1.374 Subacute bacterial endocarditis-associated glomerulonephritis. There is diffuse endocapillary proliferation and scattered mesangial and small subendothelial deposits. The lumens are filled with proliferating monocytes and occasional polymorphonuclear leukocytes along with resident endothelial and mesangial cells (transmission electron microscopy, ×3000).

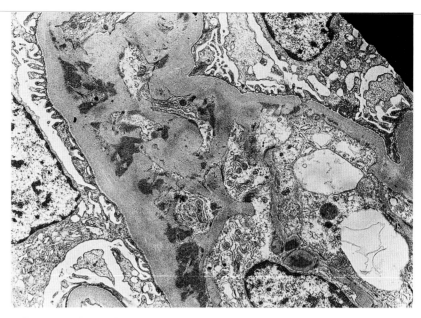

FIG. 1.375 Subacute bacterial endocarditis-associated glomerulonephritis. Scattered small to medium mesangial deposits are seen underneath the paramesangial glomerular basement membrane (transmission electron microscopy, ×14,000).

Etiology/Pathogenesis

Although renal cortical infarcts may occur because of emboli from the valve lesions, these do not play a role in the pathogenesis of the glomerulonephritis (Fig. 1.367). Patients with glomerulonephritis associated with SBE typically have circulating immune complexes that deposit in the kidney. Early lesions may resolve if the infection is eradicated with appropriate antibiotic treatment.

Selected Reading

Gutman, R.A., Striker, G.E., Gilliland, B.C., et al., 1972. The immune complex glomerulonephritis of bacterial endocarditis. Medicine (Baltimore) 51, 1-25.

Morel-Maroger, L., Sraer, J.D., Herreman, G., et al., 1972. Kidney in subacute endocarditis. Pathological and immunofluorescence findings. Archives of Pathology 94, 205-213.

Neugarten, J., Gallo, G.R., Baldwin, D.S., 1984. Glomerulonephritis in bacterial endocarditis. American Journal of Kidney Disease 5, 371-379.

SHUNT NEPHRITIS

Patients with nephritis due to infected shunts usually have coagulation-negative staphylococcus (*S. epidermidis*) infection. Deep visceral abscesses may give rise to a similar glomerulonephritis. Rarely, other bacteria may be involved. Patients typically exhibit anorexia, anemia, malaise, and fever, resulting from transient bacteremia. There may also be skin manifestations with purpura, arthralgias, hepatosplenomegaly, and lymphadenopathy. Renal signs include marked proteinuria, with more than half exhibiting nephrotic syndrome, with hematuria and edema.

By light microscopy, there is a diffuse proliferative glomerulonephritis that may show membranoproliferative features, with mesangial and endocapillary proliferation and GBM splitting (Figs. 1.376, 1.377). There are frequent intraglomerular PMNs (Figs. 1.378, 1.379). Pure mesangial proliferation is less common (Fig. 1.380). In some patients, there is only focal

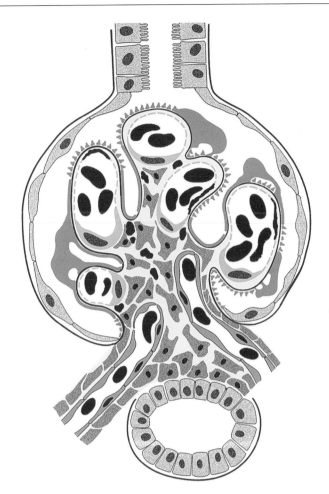

FIG. 1.376 Shunt nephritis. There is a diffuse proliferative glomerulonephritis, with mesangial and endocapillary proliferation and occasional glomerular basement membrane double contours, due to mesangial, subendothelial, and rare subepithelial immune complex deposits.

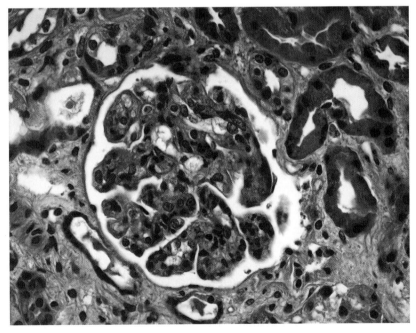

FIG. 1.377 Shunt nephritis. There typically are membranoproliferative features with predominant mesangial cells and macrophages, occasionally with scattered polymorphonuclear leukocytes (periodic acid Schiff, ×200).

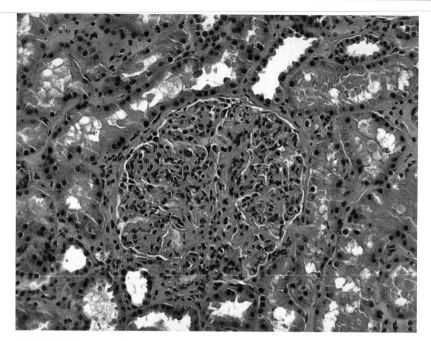

FIG. 1.378 Shunt nephritis. A predominant lobular pattern with numerous mononuclear cells and polymorphonuclear leukocytes is present in this case of shunt nephritis (hematoxylin and eosin, ×200).

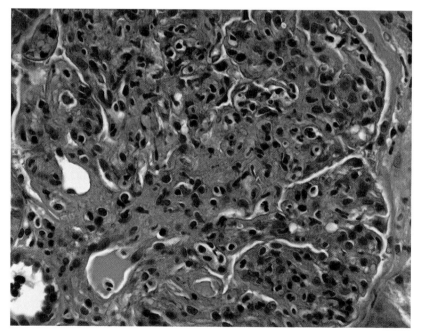

FIG. 1.379 Shunt nephritis. The marked lobular appearance is due to endocapillary proliferation with infiltrating mononuclear cells, including macrophages, and frequent polymorphonuclear leukocytes, in addition to proliferating mesangial cells. There is interposition and reduplication of the peripheral capillary wall, better seen on silver stain (hematoxylin and eosin, ×400).

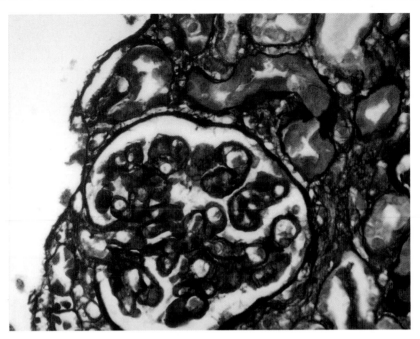

FIG. 1.380 Shunt nephritis. In some cases of shunt nephritis, there is only mesangial proliferation, with corresponding predominance of mesangial deposits by immunofluorescence and electron microscopy (Jones silver stain, ×200).

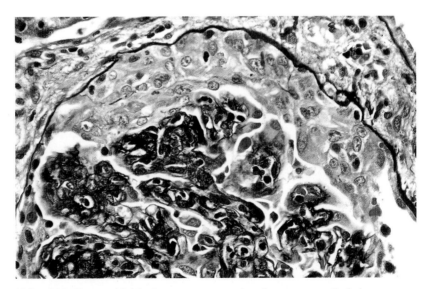

FIG. 1.381 Shunt nephritis. Crescents are occasionally present, particularly associated with proliferation. The underlying glomerulus shows endocapillary proliferation with frequent polymorphonuclear leukocytes, and segmental reduplication of the capillary wall (Jones silver stain, ×400).

segmental endocapillary proliferation. Crescents are not uncommon (Fig. 1.381). By immunofluorescence, there is coarse, chunky, prominent C3 and also C1q and C4 deposits, in addition to IgG and IgM (Figs. 1.382, 1.383). Deposits are present only in the mesangium in about half of patients, with some showing peripheral loop deposits corresponding to the common proliferative pattern found by light microscopy. When IgM is predominant, the possibility of a cryoglobulinemic response to the infection should be considered. By electron

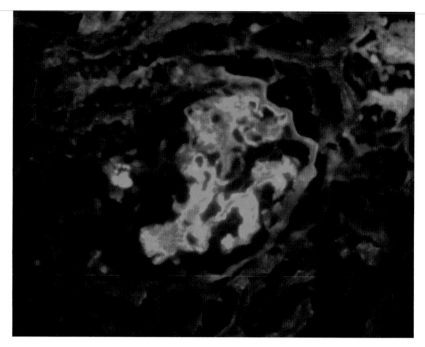

FIG. 1.382 Shunt nephritis. By immunofluorescence, there are chunky granular deposits of IgG, with very predominant C3 in mesangial areas and extending in an irregular, segmental distribution to peripheral loops (anti-IgG immunofluorescence, ×400).

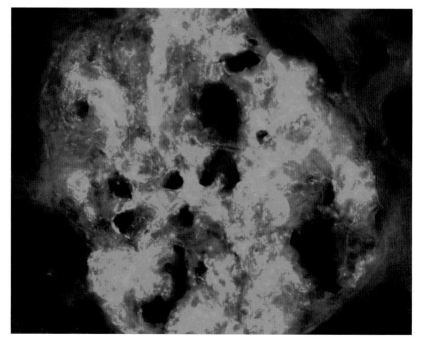

FIG. 1.383 Shunt nephritis. C3 is often very prominent in shunt nephritis, with chunky mesangial and peripheral loop deposits (same case as Figs. 1.378-1.382). There is strong, chunky to granular mesangial staining with segmental irregular chunky peripheral loop staining (anti-C3 immunofluorescence, ×400).

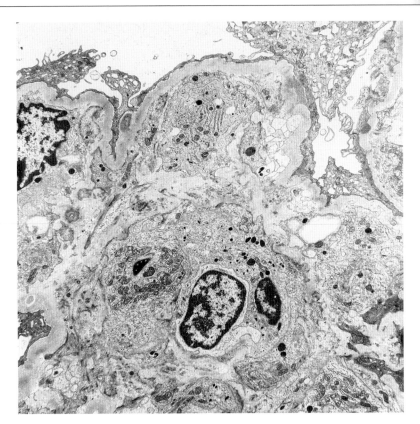

FIG. 1.384 Shunt nephritis. Marked endocapillary proliferation fills up the capillary lumen, with rare, scattered small mesangial, subendothelial, and small intramembranous deposits (transmission electron microscopy, ×3000).

microscopy, the deposits most frequently are localized in the mesangial and subendothelial areas, with rare intramembranous and subepithelial deposits (Figs. 1.384-1.386). Reduplication of the GBM due to interposition and subendothelial deposits is present.

Etiology/Pathogenesis

This glomerulonephritis may develop when ventriculoperitoneal, portocaval, or other shunts become infected – most commonly with *Streptococcus epidermidis* although other bacteria may also cause shunt nephritis. The nephritis is related to immune complex deposition, with marked activation of the classic complement pathway. Thus, the majority of patients have reduced complement levels. Colonization of the shunt is typically present. There may be low-grade bacteremia, but blood cultures may also be sterile, with identification of the pathogen only possible when the shunt is removed. Specific diagnosis and removal of the infected shunt allow recovery in patients, usually within months. Antibiotic therapy alone has not been as effective, although in some case this has also led to resolution of disease.

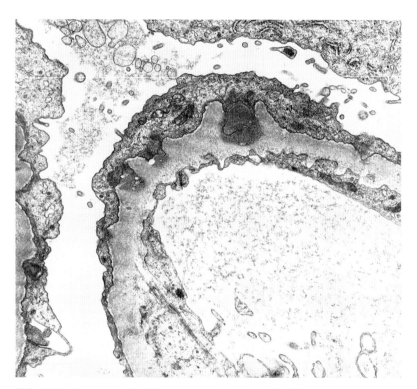

FIG. 1.385 Shunt nephritis. There may rarely be subepithelial or intramembranous deposits. Typical hump-shaped deposits, as in acute postinfectious glomerulonephritis, are not a typical feature of shunt nephritis (transmission electron microscopy, ×7000).

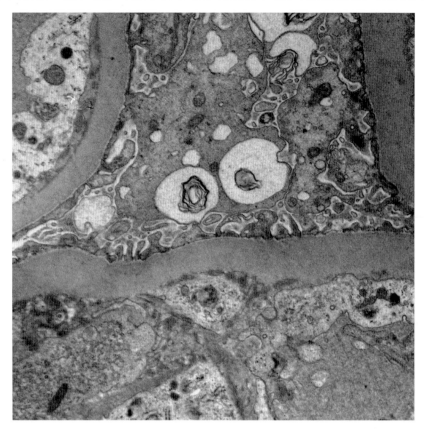

FIG. 1.386 Shunt nephritis. Small, sliver-like subendothelial deposits are present, along with marked endocapillary proliferation. There is extensive effacement of overlying foot processes (transmission electron microscopy, ×8000).

Selected Reading

Arze, R.S., Rashid, H., Morley, R., et al., 1983. Shunt nephritis: Report of two cases and review of literature. Clinical Nephrology 19, 48-53.

Beaufils, M., Morel-Maroger, L., Sraer, J.-D., et al., 1976. Acute renal failure of glomerular origin during visceral abscesses. New England Journal of Medicine 295, 185-189.

Dobrin, R.S., Day, N.K., Quie, P.G., et al., 1975. The role of complement, immunoglobulin and bacterial antigen in coagulase-negative staphylococcal shunt nephritis. American Journal of Medicine 59, 660-673.

Fukuda, Y., Ohtomo, Y., Kaneko, K., et al., 1993. Pathologic and laboratory dynamics following the removal of the shunt in shunt nephritis. American Journal of Nephrology 13, 78-82.

Rames, L., Wise, B., Goodman, J.R., et al., 1970. Renal disease with Staphylococcus albus bacteremia. A complication in ventriculoatrial shunts. Journal of the American Medical Association 212, 1671-1677.

Wakabayashi, Y., Kobayashi, Y., Shigematsu, H., 1985. Shunt nephritis: histological dynamics following removal of the shunt. Case report and review of the literature. Nephron 40, 111-117.

Vascular Diseases

Diabetic Nephropathy

Patients with diabetic nephropathy (DN) typically present with gradual progression of disease from microalbuminuria to proteinuria, usually about 15 years after onset of diabetes. Renal lesions are quite similar in type I and type II diabetes mellitus (DM), although the delay in clinical diagnosis of type II DM may give the appearance of shorter interval to DN in these patients. Patients with type I diabetes with DN have a high incidence of retinopathy, whereas only slightly more than half of those with type II diabetes have retinopathy. Type II diabetes and obesity are increasing epidemically worldwide, in adults as well as in children. Type II DM is particularly prevalent in some Native American Indian tribes, such as the Pima. DN only develops in about 30% of diabetic patients. Patients with the typical course of DN usually do not undergo renal biopsy. Thus, the biopsied diabetic patient is clinically atypical. Lesions other than DN, either alone, or superimposed on DN, are thus common in this biopsied population. DN also occurs in the transplant, either as recurrent disease or as a de novo lesion. DN develops more rapidly in this population than in native kidneys, with DN lesions present on average 6 years after transplant.

The earliest changes in diabetic patients' kidneys are renal enlargement, because of both hyperfiltration and hypertrophy. By light microscopy, glomerular hypertrophy, hyperplasia, and thickened glomerular basement membranes (GBMs) are present as early as 2-8 years after onset of diabetes in some patients. Mesangial volume expansion can be detected even earlier by morphometry from electron microscopic examinations (Fig. 2.1). Progressive increase in mesangial matrix and cellularity ensue and may culminate in diffuse increase in mesangial matrix or nodular glomerulosclerosis with associated hyaline in arterioles and occasionally in Bowman's capsule ("capsular drop") (Figs. 2.2-2.5). The nodules, so-called Kimmelstiel–Wilson nodules, have a lamellated appearance on silver stains (Figs. 2.6, 2.7). There often are

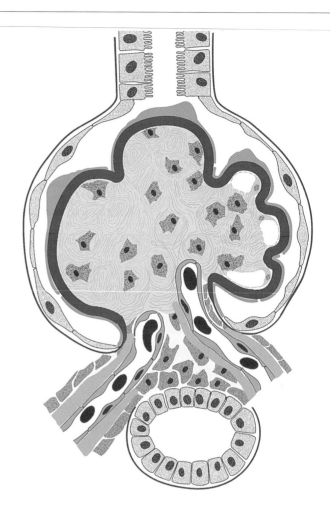

FIG. 2.1 Diabetic nephropathy. There is mesangial increase or nodular sclerosis, accompanied by hyalinosis of both afferent and efferent arterioles and thickening of the glomerular basement membrane lamina densa without deposits.

Key Diagnostic Features of Diabetic Nephropathy

- Mesangial expansion, may be nodular or diffuse
- Afferent and efferent arteriolar hyaline
- Glomerular basement membrane thickening
- No immune complexes

---

dilated capillary aneurysms surrounding the expanded Kimmelstiel–Wilson nodules, resulting from mesangiolysis and loss of tethering of the capillary walls of the GBM to the mesangium (Figs. 2.8-2.12). This repeated mesangiolysis with subsequent augmented mesangial matrix synthesis in a repair response gives rise to the laminated appearance. Occasionally, red blood cell fragments may be present in these nodules, thought to represent more severe localized microvascular injury.

The GBM is diffusely thickened without spikes or splitting on silver stains. Hyalinosis is common in DN, resulting from insudation of plasma proteins. The term *hyaline cap* (also called "fibrin cap") is used to describe hyalinosis in peripheral segments of the glomerular tuft. The term *capsular drop* is used to describe the appearance of hyaline material within Bowman's capsule. The latter lesion is quite rare, and highly specific, although not pathognomonic, for DN.

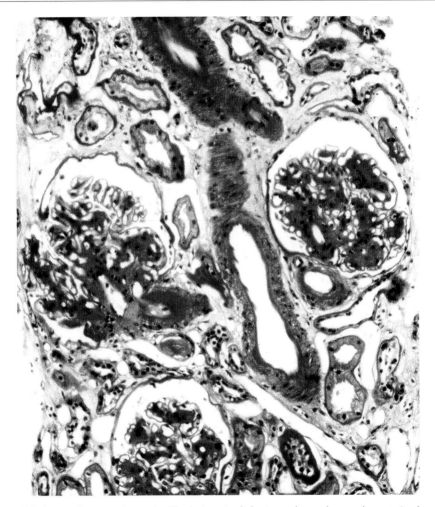

FIG. 2.2 Diabetic nephropathy. The lesions in diabetic nephropathy are characterized by arteriolar hyalinization, mesangial matrix expansion, and glomerular basement membrane thickening. There is also associated tubular interstitial fibrosis (periodic acid Schiff, ×100).

Diabetic Nephropathy: Key Differential Diagnosis of Nodular Sclerosis

- Nodular sclerosis may also be seen in light chain deposition disease or other monoclonal immunoglobulin associated disease – IF and EM demonstrate the light chain deposits along GBMs and tubular basement membranes.
- Amyloid is diagnosed by light chain IF staining in AL amyloid, and Congo red staining in all types of amyloid.
- Membranoproliferative glomerulonephritis may be lobular to nodular, but deposits are seen by IF and EM.
- Obesity-related glomerulopathy is characterized by marked glomerulomegaly, occasionally hilar-type focal segmental glomerulosclerosis, but without GBM thickening.
- Idiopathic nodular sclerosis is diagnosed by exclusion and may have morphologic appearance identical to diabetic nephropathy.

EM, electron microscopy; *IF,* immunofluorescence; *GBM,* glomerular basement membrane.

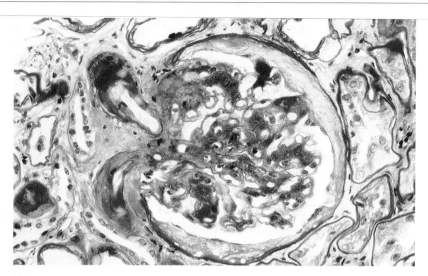

FIG. 2.3 Diabetic nephropathy. The arteriolar hyalinization in diabetes typically involves both afferent and efferent arterioles. The glomerulus shows diffuse mesangial matrix increase without formation of Kimmelstiel–Wilson nodules in this case. There is thickening of Bowman's capsule, and a small "capsular drop," that is, hyalin within Bowman's capsule at the 12 o'clock position (periodic acid Schiff, ×200).

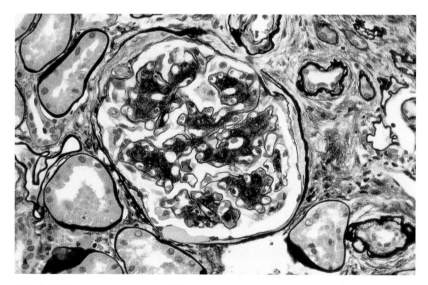

FIG. 2.4 Diabetic nephropathy. Diffuse mesangial matrix increase and basement membrane thickening are evident in this case of early diabetic nephropathy. A "capsular drop" is seen at the bottom of Bowman's capsule. There is moderate increase in mesangial matrix and cellularity, with surrounding tubulointerstitial fibrosis. There are no deposits, splitting, or irregularities of the basement membrane (Jones silver stain, ×200).

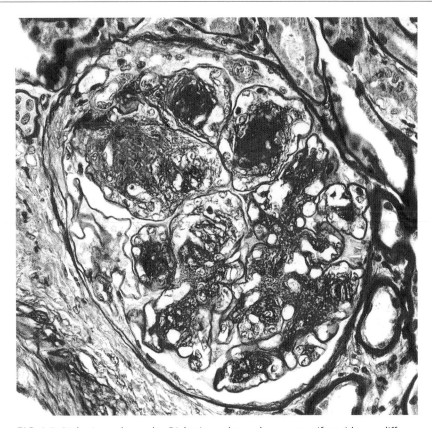

FIG. 2.5 Diabetic nephropathy. Diabetic nephropathy may manifest either as diffuse mesangial increase (as seen in Figs 2.3 and 2.4), or with nodular glomerulosclerosis as in this case. There are multiple nodules of mesangial matrix, surrounded by a small rim of intact capillaries. The glomerular basement membrane is prominent. The expanded nodules show a lamellated appearance, thought to be due to repeated injury with mesangiolysis and exuberant repair responses laying down increased matrix (periodic acid Schiff, ×200).

Overt DN is invariably accompanied by lesions of arterioles and arteries. Both afferent and efferent arterioles show hyalinosis in DN (Fig. 2.13). In contrast, arterionephrosclerosis (ANS) affects the afferent, but not the efferent, arteriole. Interlobular and larger arteries show arteriosclerosis in DN.

There is proportional tubulointerstitial fibrosis in DN. Recent studies have shown that increase in the cellular component of the interstitium precedes increase in matrix. Tubular basement membranes are thickened, and tubular atrophy and interstitial fibrosis occur in proportion to glomerulosclerosis (Fig. 2.7).

By immunofluorescence microscopy, there may be linear accentuation of GBMs, typically strongest for IgG (Fig. 2.14). Both kappa and lambda light chain usually stain, thus ruling out possible light chain deposition disease or light and heavy chain deposition disease, which has monoclonal light chain staining. Absence of accompanying C3 staining or crescents and the clinical history also aid in differentiating this staining from anti-GBM antibody–mediated glomerulonephritis. Albumin, used as a control IF stain, is also positive, showing the general "stickiness" of the altered GBM. There may also be linear accentuation with anti-IgG of Bowman's capsule and tubular basement membranes.

Electron microscopy confirms the diffuse GBM thickening due to widened lamina densa without immune complexes (Figs. 2.15, 2.16). The GBM may be several-fold normal thickness, up to 1200-1500 nm (normal in adult ~325-375 nm). Podocytes show effacement of

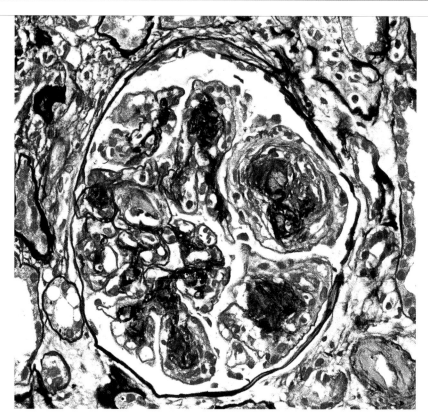

FIG. 2.6 Diabetic nephropathy. The lamellated appearance of the Kimmelstiel–Wilson nodule characteristic of the nodular sclerosis form of diabetic nephropathy is shown, along with arteriolar hyalinization and surrounding tubulointerstitial fibrosis (Jones silver stain, ×200).

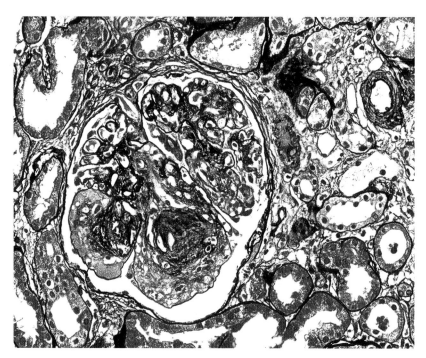

FIG. 2.7 Diabetic nephropathy. The large Kimmelstiel–Wilson nodules contain small red blood cell fragments and frayed, irregular mesangial matrix, evidence of early mesangiolysis (Jones silver stain, ×200).

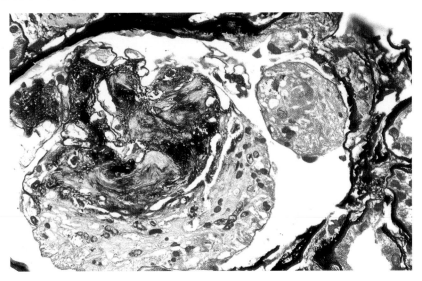

FIG. 2.8 Diabetic nephropathy. A large area of mesangial injury with red blood cell fragments and frayed, lucent-appearing mesangial matrix, indicative of mesangiolysis, are shown (Jones silver stain, ×400).

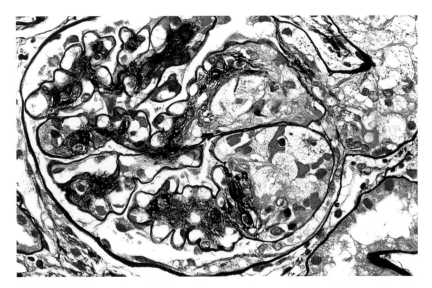

FIG. 2.9 Diabetic nephropathy. There is an area of mesangiolysis with foam cells with loss of matrix and breaks of attachments of the capillary loop. This loss of tethering of the mesangium is thought to give rise to microaneurysms. The glomerular basement membrane is also thickened, without evident deposits (Jones silver stain, ×400).

foot processes. The mesangial matrix is markedly expanded with lesser increase of mesangial cells without immune complexes. Areas of hyalinosis appear electron dense, are often present in sclerotic areas, often contain lipid, and should not be confused with immune complex–type deposits. Correlation with immunofluorescence and light microscopic findings is helpful in this regard. Superimposed, nondiabetic lesions are not uncommon and complete examination by immunofluorescence and electron microscopic should be done to investigate this possibility (Fig. 2.17). A recent schema to classify different levels of severity of this spectrum of morphologic alterations has been developed. This schema is not intended for diagnosis but rather

Text continued on page 314

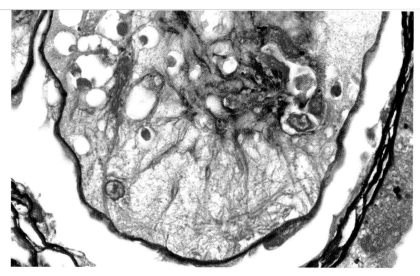

FIG. 2.10 Diabetic nephropathy. There is an area of mesangiolysis with fraying of the mesangium and loss of attachment of the mesangial area to the peripheral capillary loop. Red blood cell fragments are also present (Jones silver stain, ×1000).

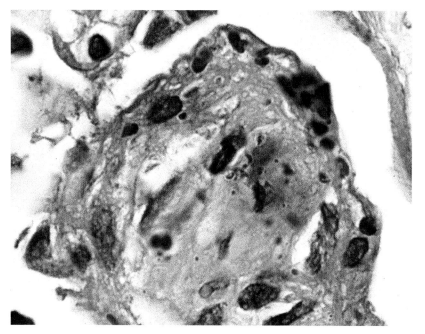

FIG. 2.11 Diabetic nephropathy. Numerous red blood cell fragments are present in this small Kimmelstiel–Wilson nodule. Red blood cell fragmentation has been associated with increased plasminogen-activator inhibitor-1 (PAI-1), and is associated with more severe disease. This is postulated to reflect local, more severe microvascular injury (hematoxylin and eosin, ×1000).

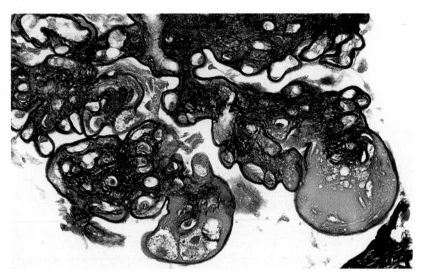

FIG. 2.12 Diabetic nephropathy. Insudation of plasma proteins may occur in any state where there is vascular injury and is often a prominent component of diabetic nephropathy. The term *fibrin cap* is often used for the presence of hyalinosis within the diabetic glomerulus. The glassy, smooth hyalin appearance of the insudated protein is evident, along with clear areas due to foam cells and lipid. The expanded mesangial matrix and thick glomerular basement membrane of diabetic nephropathy are evident (Jones silver stain, ×1000).

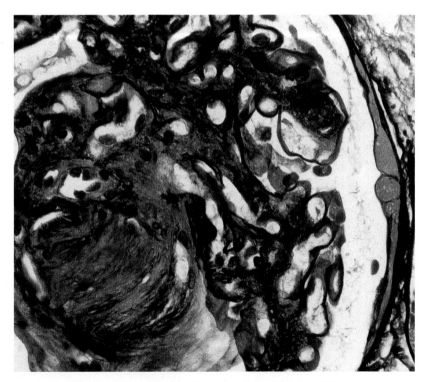

FIG. 2.13 Diabetic nephropathy. Insudation of plasma proteins within Bowman's capsule is a fairly rare, but characteristic, although not pathognomonic, lesion of diabetic nephropathy. This lesion, termed the "capsular drop," is associated in this case with thick basement membrane and a well-organized, lamellated Kimmelstiel–Wilson nodule on the right (Jones silver stain, ×400).

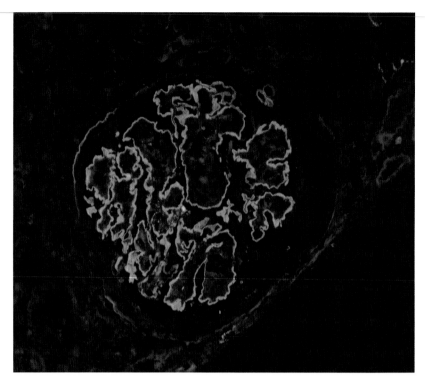

FIG. 2.14 Diabetic nephropathy. By immunofluorescence, there may be linear accentuation of the glomerular basement membrane in diabetic nephropathy. Differentiation from anti-GBM antibody–mediated glomerulonephritis is usually easy by correlation with clinical history, and light microscopic findings of nodular glomerulosclerosis in diabetic nephropathy versus crescents in anti-GBM antibody–mediated glomerulonephritis. In addition, C3 is often positive in a segmental, linear fashion in anti-GBM antibody–mediated glomerulonephritis but not in diabetic nephropathy (anti-IgG immunofluorescence, ×200).

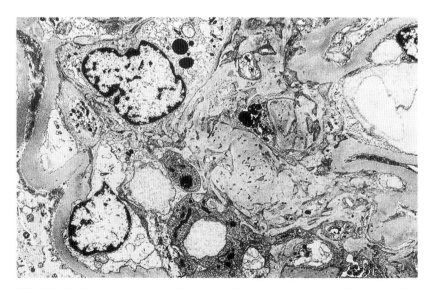

FIG. 2.15 Diabetic nephropathy. The mesangial matrix is expanded with increased mesangial cells without immune deposits. The glomerular basement membrane is usually several times normal in thickness because of a thickened lamina densa without deposits (transmission electron microscopy, ×5000).

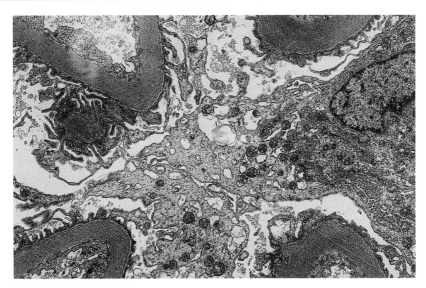

FIG. 2.16 Diabetic nephropathy. The markedly thickened glomerular basement membrane is illustrated here. Even without precise morphometric measurements, the increased thickness is apparent by examining the proportion of the glomerular basement membrane to the base of intact foot processes (transmission electron microscopy, ×6000).

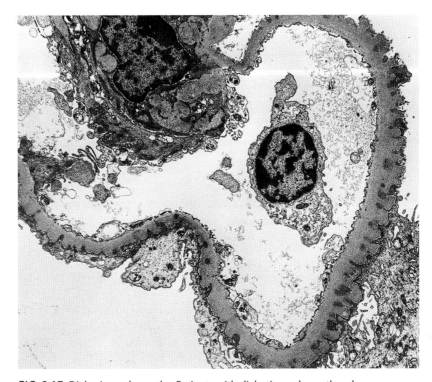

FIG. 2.17 Diabetic nephropathy. Patients with diabetic nephropathy who are biopsied typically have an unusual course of diabetic nephropathy and may occasionally have superimposed disease, as in this patient who had membranous glomerulonephritis with small subepithelial and intramembranous deposits, in addition to mesangial matrix expansion, lamina densa thickening, and arteriolar hyalinization related to their underlying diabetes mellitus. IgA nephropathy may also often be associated with diabetic nephropathy in biopsied diabetic patients (transmission electron microscopy, ×3000).

TABLE 2-1 Glomerular Classification of Diabetic Nephropathy

Class	Description	Inclusion Criteria
I	Mild or nonspecific LM changes and EM-proven GBM thickening	Biopsy does not meet any of the criteria mentioned below for class II, III, or IV GBM > 395 nm in female and >430 nm in male individuals 9 years of age and older
IIa	Mild mesangial expansion	Biopsy does not meet criteria for class III or IV Mild mesangial expansion in >25% of the observed mesangium
IIb	Severe mesangial expansion	Biopsy does not meet criteria for class III or IV Severe mesangial expansion in >25% of the observed mesangium
III	Nodular sclerosis (Kimmelstiel–Wilson lesion)	Biopsy does not meet criteria for class IV At least one convincing Kimmelstiel–Wilson lesion
IV	Advanced diabetic glomerulosclerosis	Global glomerular sclerosis in >50% of glomeruli Lesions from classes I through III

EM, electron microscopy; *GBM*, glomerular basement membrane; *LM*, light microscopy.

as a research tool for comparisons of progression and response to interventions in research settings (Table 2.1).

Biopsied diabetic patients are not typical, and lesions other than DN may frequently be encountered. On the other hand, the renal biopsy may show lesions of DN preceding clinical diagnosis of overt type II diabetes. Differential diagnosis is listed in the box titled "Key Diagnostic Features of Diabetic Nephropathy." Of note, obesity-related glomerulopathy is characterized by marked glomerulomegaly, occasionally hilar-type focal segmental glomerulosclerosis (FSGS), but without GBM thickening or nodular sclerosis, although vascular lesions may be present, related to hypertension.

Idiopathic nodular sclerosis is diagnosed by exclusion of other causes, and may have morphologic appearance and matrix content indistinguishable from DN. This morphologic lesion is loosely associated with smoking history.

Etiology/Pathogenesis

Diabetic nephropathy occurs in only 30-40% of patients with DN. Further, not all patients with DM who receive a kidney transplant develop recurrent DN in the transplant. Thus, multiple complex factors are involved with the pathogenesis of DN and are discussed in detail in "The Kidney."

In patients with type II DM who are carefully screened by clinical criteria to have DN as a cause of their proteinuria, renal biopsy done for clinical research studies indeed demonstrated lesions of DN similar to those in type I diabetes. In unscreened patients with type II DM biopsied for proteinuria, varying renal lesions, including various immune complex and other diseases were present in one-third of patients. Importantly, typical diabetic patients are not usually biopsied. Therefore, the finding of lesions other than or superimposed on DN is common in clinically indicated renal biopsies in diabetic patients.

Regression of mild DN lesions occurred in nondiabetic patients who inadvertently received kidney transplants with early DN lesions. In studies of patients who had their type I DM cured by pancreas transplant, regression of existing mild to moderate DN lesions was proven by repeat biopsies over a 10-year period. These important observations show the potential for modifying the course of DN. Current research is focused on the roles of intraglomerular hemodynamics and permselectivity defects, the renin–angiotensin system, advanced glycation end products, growth factors such as transforming growth factor-β, the plasmin/plasminogen activator system and matrix turnover, and cell proliferation, notably preserving or protecting podocytes from injury and loss.

Selected Reading

Bhalla, V., Nast, C.C., Stollenwerk, N., et al., 2003. Recurrent and de novo diabetic nephropathy in renal allografts. Transplantation 75, 66-71.

Chavers, B.M., Bilous, R.W., Ellis, E.N., et al., 1989. Glomerular lesions and urinary albumin excretion in type I diabetes without overt proteinuria. New England Journal of Medicine 320, 966-970.

Drummond, K., Mauer, M., 2002. The early natural history of nephropathy in type 1 diabetes: II. Early renal structural changes in type I diabetes. Diabetes 51, 1580-1587.

Fioretto, P., Steffes, M.W., Sutherland, D.E., et al., 1998. Reversal of lesions of diabetic nephropathy after pancreas transplantation. New England Journal of Medicine 339, 69-75.

Gambara, V., Mecca, G., Remuzzi, G., et al., 1993. Heterogeneous nature of renal lesions in type II diabetes. Journal of the American Society of Nephrology 3, 1458-1466.

Kambham, N., Markowitz, G.S., Valeri, A.M., et al., 2001. Obesity-related glomerulopathy: an emerging epidemic. Kidney International 59, 1498-1509.

Katz, A., Caramori, M.L., Sisson-Ross, S., et al., 2002, An increase in the cell component of the cortical interstitium antedates interstitial fibrosis in type 1 diabetic patients. Kidney International 61, 2058-2066.

Kimmelstiel, P., Wilson, C., 1936. Intercapillary lesions in glomeruli of kidney. American Journal of Pathology 12, 83-97.

Markowitz, G.S., Lin, J., Valeri, A.M., et al., 2002. Idiopathic nodular glomerulosclerosis is a distinct clinicopathologic entity linked to hypertension and smoking. Human Pathology 33, 826-835.

Mauer, S.M., Staffes, M.V., Ellis, E.N., et al., 1984. Structural-functional relationships in diabetic nephropathy. Journal of Clinical Investigation 74, 1143-1155.

Østerby, R., Gundersen, H.J., Horlyck, A., et al., 1983. Diabetic glomerulopathy: structural characteristics of the early and advanced stages. Diabetes 2, 79-82.

Schwartz, M.M., Lewis, E.J., Leonard-Martin, T., et al., 1998. Renal pathology patterns in type II diabetes mellitus: relationship with retinopathy. The Collaborative Study Group. Nephrology Dialysis Transplantation 13, 2547-2552.

Stokes, M.B., Holler, S., Cui, Y., et al., 2000. Expression of decorin, biglycan, and collagen type I in human renal fibrosing disease. Kidney International 57, 487-498.

Tervaert, T.W., Mooyaart, A.L., Amann, K., et al., 2010. Pathologic classification of diabetic nephropathy. Journal of the American Society of Nephrology 21, 556-563.

Thrombotic Microangiopathy/Thrombotic Thrombocytopenic Purpura

The thrombotic microangiopathies (TMAs) (Fig. 2.18) that involve the kidney consist of a heterogeneous group of disorders of different etiologies. Hemolytic uremic syndrome (HUS) and thrombotic thrombocytopenic purpura (TTP) are the classical diseases associated with TMA. Clinically, they are characterized by the triad of microangiopathic hemolytic anemia, thrombocytopenia, and acute renal failure. They may or may not have associated systemic involvement. Evidence of involvement of multiple organs may be present, including manifestations such as petechia, purpura, and intestinal bleeding, and neurologic symptoms such as aphasia, dysphasia, parasthenia, and visual problems, and even seizures and coma. Evidence

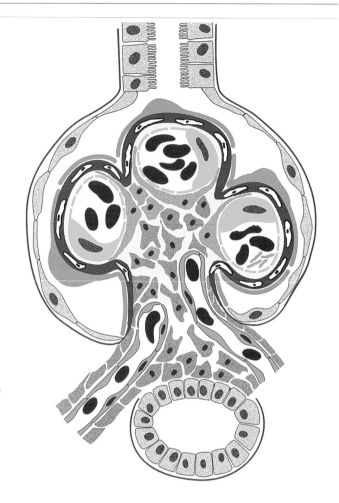

FIG. 2.18 Chronic thrombotic microangiopathy shows a split appearance of glomerular basement membrane by light microscopy, because of increased lamina rara interna, often with flocculent fibrin degradation products. Occasional fibrin tactoids may be seen by electron microscopy.

of renal involvement is present in a majority of patients with TMAs, which are described under the general rubric of HUS. Predominant central nervous system involvement with similar peripheral blood manifestations is seen in TTP. Glomerular capillary and large vessel thrombosis identical to that seen in HUS or TTP also occurs in lupus patients with circulating antiphospholipid antibodies. TMA also occurs in a wide range of diseases other than HUS/TTP, including autoimmune diseases, malignant hypertension, vascular rejection, and endothelial damage caused by drug toxicity.

The pathologic findings can be divided into those that affect the glomeruli and those that affect the arteries and arterioles. Furthermore, they can be analyzed as the lesions seen early after the onset of the disease and those that are prominent after the disease progresses. The lesions of the thrombotic microangiopathies can show a wide range of changes according both to the severity and duration of disease. The basic morphologic changes are similar in most cases regardless of the cause and relate to the presence of endothelial injury and the subsequent activation of the coagulation system.

In the early stages, glomeruli show thickening of the capillary walls caused by endothelial cell swelling and the accumulation of material between the endothelial cell and the underlying basement membrane (Figs. 2.19-2.21). By light microscopy the capillary walls show a double contour on silver stains (Fig. 2.22), and by electron microscopy this is demonstrated to correspond to acellular fibrillar material in the subendothelial region (Fig. 2.23). The term *bloodless glomeruli* has been used to characterize glomeruli in which the capillary loops are collapsed and that may contain fragmented red blood cells, fibrin, and platelet thrombi (Fig. 2.24).

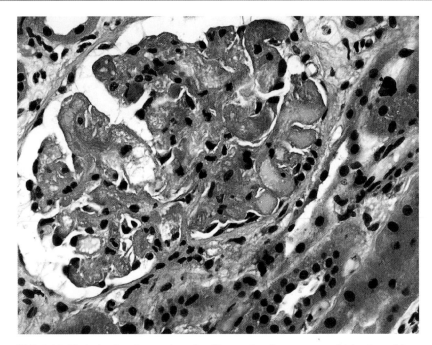

FIG. 2.19 Thrombotic microangiopathy. Glomerulus demonstrates thickening of the capillary walls caused by endothelial cell swelling and accumulation of material between the endothelial cell and the basement membrane. Microthrombi are also present (hematoxylin and eosin, ×400).

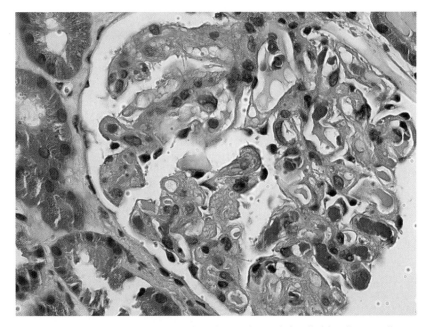

FIG. 2.20 Thrombotic microangiopathy. Glomerulus with focally bloodless capillaries caused by endothelial cell swelling and accumulation of material between the endothelial cell and the basement membrane. Microthrombi are also present (hematoxylin and eosin, ×400).

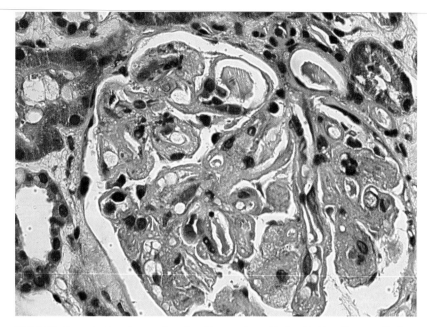

FIG 2.21 Thrombotic microangiopathy. Glomerulus with focally bloodless capillaries with endothelial cell swelling and accumulation of material between the endothelial cell and the basement membrane. Microthrombi are also present (trichrome, ×400).

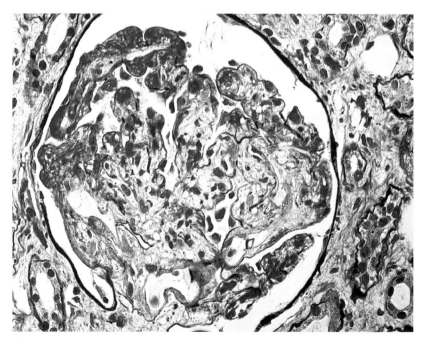

FIG. 2.22 Thrombotic microangiopathy. There is mesangiolysis and focal double contours of the peripheral capillary loops (Jones trichrome, ×400).

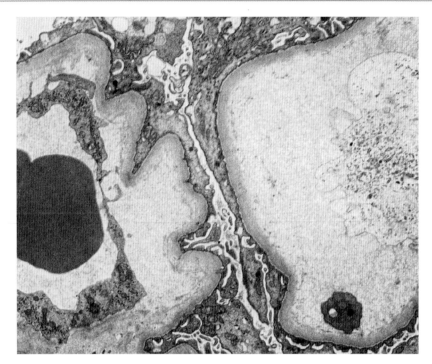

FIG. 2.23 Thrombotic microangiopathy. Electron microscopy demonstrates electron-lucent material separating the swollen endothelial cells from the basement membrane (transmission electron microscopy, ×5000).

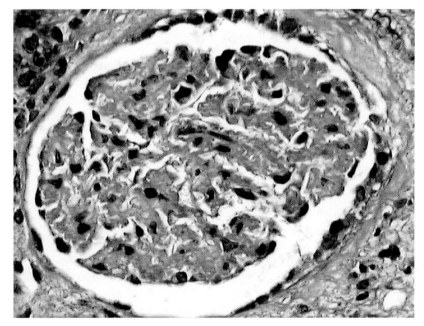

FIG. 2.24 Thrombotic microangiopathy. Trichrome stain demonstrates a "bloodless glomerulus" in which capillary loops are collapsed and occasionally contain fragmented red blood cells (trichrome, ×400).

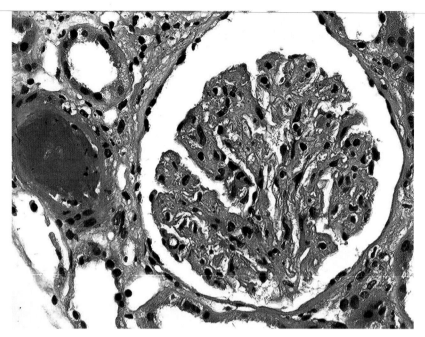

FIG. 2.25 Thrombotic microangiopathy. Fibrinoid necrosis of the afferent arteriole accompanies the characteristic collapsed and bloodless glomerulus (hematoxylin and eosin, ×400).

Key Diagnostic Features of Thrombotic Microangiopathy

- Intravascular fibrin thrombi in acute stage
- Double contours of glomerular basement membranes with variable proliferation and no immune complexes in chronic stage
- Mucoid change of arterioles in acute stage
- Intimal proliferation of arterioles in chronic stage

Fibrinoid necrosis in the afferent arteriole as it enters the glomerulus, associated with thrombosis, is also characteristic of the early phase (Fig. 2.25). Generally no increase in cellularity is seen. The mesangium may demonstrate loss of its architecture with apoptosis of mesangial cells, a process which has been termed *mesangiolysis* (Figs. 2.26, 2.27). Partial or complete dissolution of the mesangial matrix and cells results in the development of an aneurysmal dilatation of the capillaries (Fig. 2.28). Ischemic glomerular injury characterized by collapse of capillary loops and thickening and wrinkling of the capillary walls is prominent when there are severe acute vascular lesions, including thrombosis of arterioles and arteries (Figs. 2.29, 2.30). When necrosis of the glomerular capillaries occurs, small crescents may also be seen. As the lesion progresses, both a proliferative and sclerotic response can be seen individually and combined within the glomeruli (Fig. 2.31). Areas of mesangiolysis progress into sclerotic changes, proliferation of intrinsic glomerular cells can yield a membranoproliferative pattern that in some cases is indistinguishable by light microscopy from membranoproliferative glomerulonephritis type I (Fig. 2.32). Examination by immunofluorescence and electron microscopy allows correct classification as to the cause of the GBM splitting.

The acute arterial changes can range from mild with swelling of the endothelium to severe with evidence of fibrinoid necrosis of the media and thrombosis of the lumen (Fig. 2.33). As the disease progresses, there is myointimal proliferation with narrowing of the lumen, which involves the interlobular and arcuate arteries (Fig. 2.34). Myointimal cells have a swollen

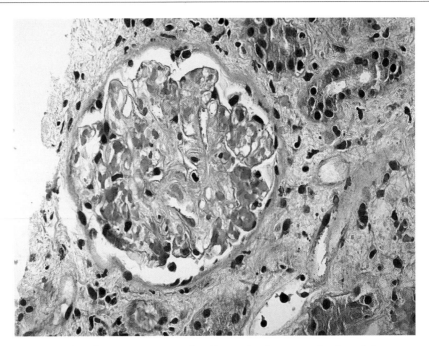

FIG. 2.26 Thrombotic microangiopathy. Glomerulus demonstrating loss of the normal architecture with apoptosis of mesangial cells, a process termed mesangiolysis (hematoxylin and eosin, ×400).

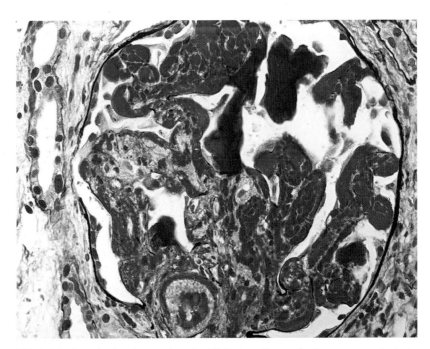

FIG. 2.27 Thrombotic microangiopathy. Trichrome silver stain demonstrates the lack of internal mesangial core with thrombosis of the peripheral capillaries (Jones trichrome, ×400).

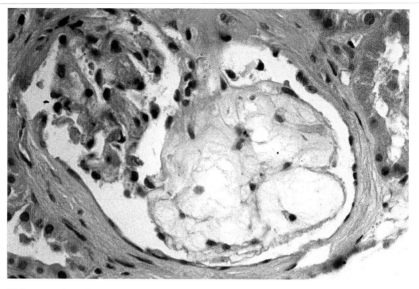

FIG. 2.28 Thrombotic microangiopathy. Glomerulus demonstrates aneurysmal dilatation of the capillaries following mesangiolysis (hematoxylin and eosin, ×400).

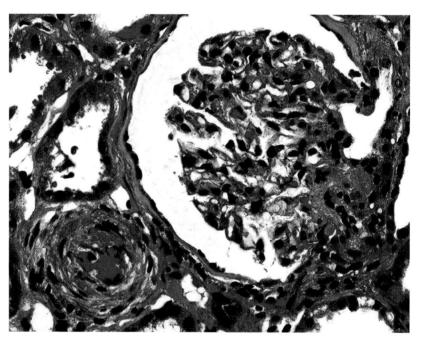

FIG. 2.29 Thrombotic microangiopathy. The afferent arterioles are also affected with evidence of fibrinoid necrosis and thrombosis (trichrome, ×400).

appearance. This lesion has been termed *mucoid intimal hyperplasia* and is highly characteristic for thrombotic microangiopathies. As the lesion advances, duplication of the internal elastic lamella occurs with permanent compromise of the vascular lumen. This phase is often associated with severe hypertension.

Tubular and interstitial changes are secondary to the glomerular and vascular lesions. There is often tubular collapse, occasionally associated with focal tubular necrosis. Patchy necrosis and true infarcts are also occasionally present in severe cases.

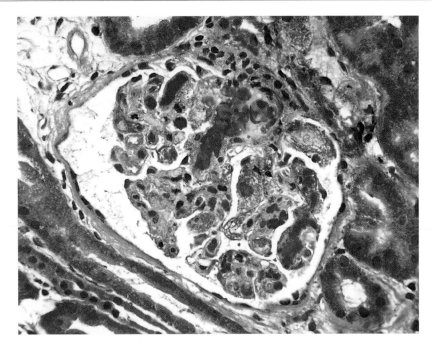

FIG. 2.30 Thrombotic microangiopathy. Thrombosis extends into the glomerular capillary loops from the afferent arteriole at the vascular pole (trichrome, ×400).

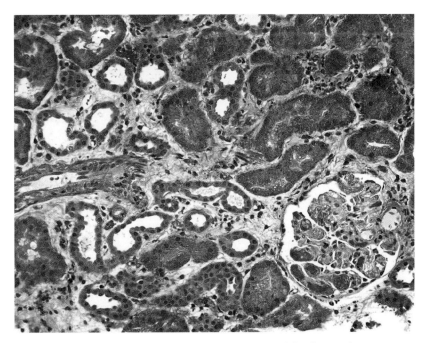

FIG. 2.31 Thrombotic microangiopathy. The later stage of the disease demonstrates interstitial fibrosis, tubular atrophy, and beginning glomerulosclerosis (trichrome, ×400).

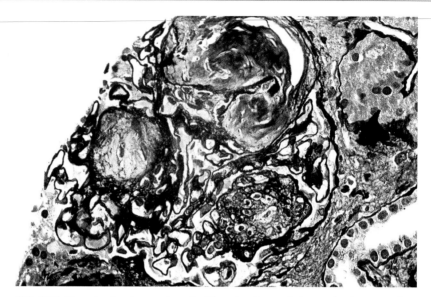

FIG. 2.32 Thrombotic microangiopathy. There is advanced glomerulosclerosis with nodularity mimicking lobular glomerulonephritis (Jones silver stain, ×400).

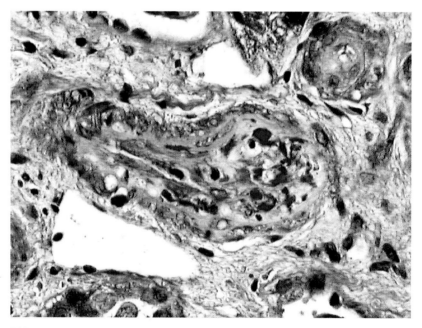

FIG. 2.33 Thrombotic microangiopathy. Arterial changes are present in more advanced cases with evidence of fibrinoid necrosis of the media and extravasation of red blood cells with mild intimal proliferation (trichrome, ×400).

Immunofluorescence microscopy demonstrates the deposition of fibrin or fibrinogen in the glomeruli and in the mesangium as well as within the vessel walls (Fig. 2.35). Occasionally, nonspecific deposition of other immunoglobulins and complement may be seen.

Electron microscopic findings are consistent with those seen by light microscopy and immunofluorescence. Early lesions demonstrate the separation of the endothelium from the basement membrane and the accumulation of subendothelial fibrillar material that corresponds to the presence of fibrinogen (Figs. 2.36-2.39). Thrombosis of the capillary lumina

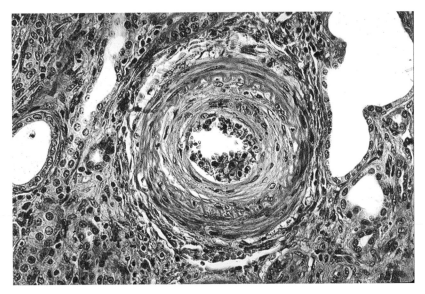

FIG. 2.34 Thrombotic microangiopathy. Cross section of the vessel demonstrating marked myointimal proliferation and narrowing of the lumen with foci of fibrinoid necrosis (hematoxylin and eosin, ×400).

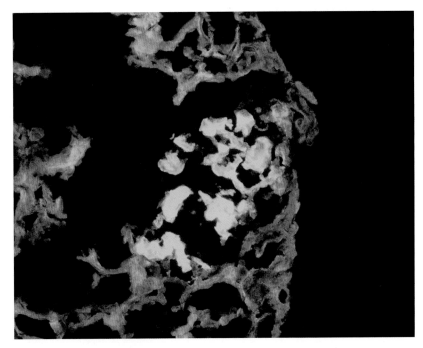

FIG. 2.35 Thrombotic microangiopathy. Immunofluorescence studies reveal diffuse deposition of fibrin throughout glomerular capillary loops (antifibrin immunofluorescence, ×200).

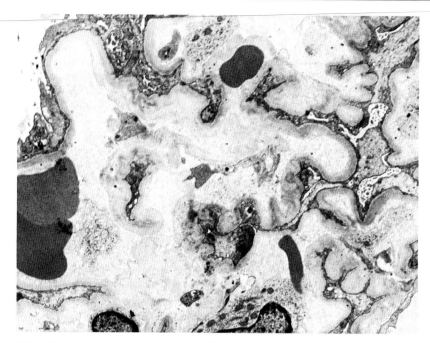

FIG. 2.36 Thrombotic microangiopathy. Electron micrograph demonstrates evidence of mesangiolysis with denudation of the endothelium from the basement membrane and loss of the mesangial architecture (transmission electron microscopy, ×3000).

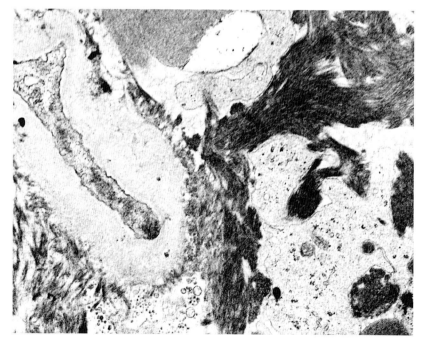

FIG. 2.37 Thrombotic microangiopathy. Electron micrograph demonstrates the presence of fibrin deposition within the capillary lumen and separating the endothelial cell from the basement membrane (transmission electron microscopy, ×5000).

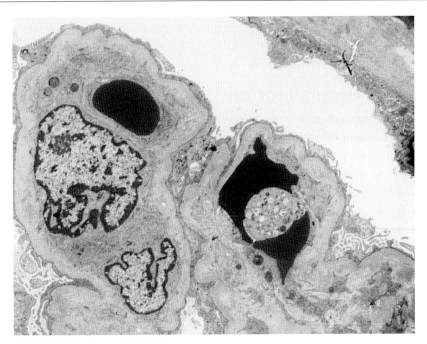

FIG. 2.38 Thrombotic microangiopathy. Electron micrograph demonstrates the presence of fragmented red blood cells within the capillary lumen and endothelial cell swelling and subendothelial fibrillar material (transmission electron microscopy, ×5000).

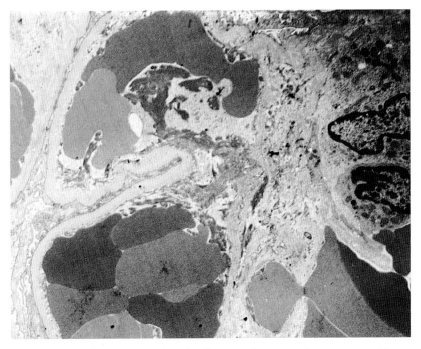

FIG. 2.39 Thrombotic microangiopathy. Electron micrograph demonstrates evidence of glomerular capillary thrombosis with fragmented red blood cells bound in a fibrin matrix (transmission electron microscopy, ×3000).

with fibrin tactoids is also occasionally seen as are accumulations of platelets. Endothelial cells in the glomeruli, arteries, and arterioles show swelling and separation from the underlying structures and evidence of apoptosis.

Etiology/Pathogenesis

Hemolytic uremic syndrome can be divided into individuals who present with diarrhea or those in whom diarrhea is not associated. Non-diarrhea-associated disease can be further classified as sporadic or familial. Diarrhea-associated disease is secondary to infection with *Escherichia coli* 0157.H7 and more recently associated with *E. coli* 0104.H4. Pathogenic factors for *E. coli* 0157 and 0104 are the production of verotoxins and adhesion molecules, which facilitate the binding of the bacteria tightly to colonocytes facilitating the transfer of the toxins. The sporadic form of the disease can be associated with pregnancy, systemic lupus erythematosus, HIV infection, and a variety of drugs, including oral contraceptives and cyclosporin or tacrolimus. The sporadic form has been linked to mutations in complement regulatory protein factor H. The form that has been given the name *thrombotic thrombocytopenic purpura* has been linked to abnormalities of the metalloproteinase that is responsible for the breakdown of large Von Willebrand factor aggregates or multimers into smaller, less active multimers (now called ADAMTS-13). There may be a deficiency or an inhibitor of this protease. The absence of the protease results in an excess of Von Willebrand factor multimers, which are prothrombotic. Familial HUS is due to a deficiency in ADAMTS-13. Mutations in other complement factors have also been described in the atypical form. The recent use of VEGF inhibition in cancer therapy has identified a unique form of TMA where endothelial activation plays a central role (Figs. 2.40, 2.41).

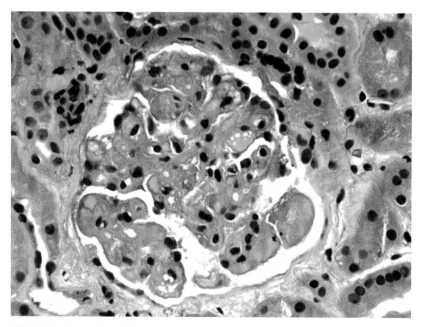

FIG. 2.40 Glomerulus of a patient treated with VEGF trap molecule with dilated denuded capillaries, swollen endothelium with focal thrombosis (hematoxylin and eosin, ×400).

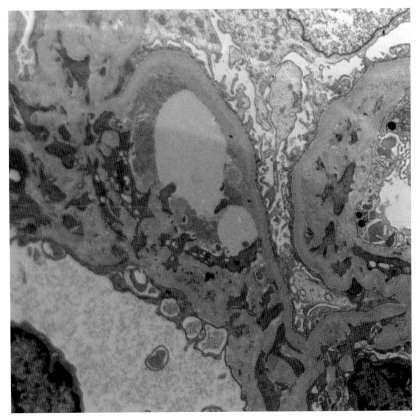

FIG. 2.41 Electron micrograph showing capillary loop where the endothelium has been denuded and the basement membrane coated with granular fibrin (transmission electron microscopy, ×8000).

Key Differential Diagnosis of Thrombotic Microangiopathy

- Fibrin may also occur associated with fibrinoid necrosis in e.g. vasculitis or crescentic glomerulonephritis.
- Karyorrhexis and tissue destruction are then evidence of the primary necrotizing process underlying the injury, rather than an intracapillary thrombotic process.

Note: Split appearance of glomerular basement membranes may also be seen because of subendothelial immune complexes (see membranoproliferative glomerulonephritis). Immunofluorescence and electron microscopy help differentiate this lesion from chronic thrombotic microangiopathy.

Selected Reading

Benz, K., Amann, K., 2010. Thrombotic microangiopathy: new insights. Current Opinion in Nephrology and Hypertension 19, 242-247.

Churg, J., Strauss, L., 1985. Renal involvement in thrombotic microangiopathies. Seminars in Nephrology 5, 46-56.

Eremina, V., Jefferson, J.A., Kowalewska, J., et al., 2008. VEGF inhibition and renal thrombotic microangiopathy. New England Journal of Medicine 358, 1129-1136.

Moake, J.L., 2002. Thrombotic microangiopathies. New England Journal of Medicine 347, 589-600.

Noris, M., Remuzzi, G., 2009. Atypical hemolytic-uremic syndrome. New England Journal of Medicine 361, 1676-1687.

Scleroderma (Progressive Systemic Sclerosis)

Progressive systemic sclerosis (PSS) is a multisystem disease that affects the skin, the gastro-intestinal tract, the lung, the heart, and the kidney. Kidney involvement occurs in approximately 60-70% of PSS patients. Age at onset of systemic sclerosis is 30-50 years and females are affected more than males, with slight predominance of African Americans versus Caucasians. Survival over 5 years in PSS ranges from 34% to 73%, with scleroderma renal crisis the most common cause of death. Scleroderma is now classified as limited or diffuse cutaneous scleroderma. In the limited form, fibrosis is mainly restricted to the hands, arms, and face with Raynaud's phenomenon preceding fibrosis, with frequent pulmonary hypertension. Most of these patients also have anticentromere antibodies. Diffuse cutaneous scleroderma is a more severe, rapidly progressing process that has adverse effects not only on large areas of skin but one or more internal organs. The kidneys, esophagus, heart, and lungs are the most frequently affected.

Scleroderma renal crisis develops in approximately 20% of patients with systemic sclerosis, but may be decreasing due to early treatment with ACEI. Patients present with malignant hypertension and acute renal failure. Grossly, petechial hemorrhages or even renal infarcts may be present in patients with scleroderma renal crisis, similar to HUS or malignant hypertension. Microscopically, there is fibrinoid necrosis of afferent arterioles. Fibrin can extend to glomeruli (Figs. 2.42, 2.43). Glomeruli may show ischemic collapse or fibrinoid necrosis (Figs. 2.42-2.45). Interlobular arteries show intimal thickening, proliferation of endothelial cells, and edema with mucoid change, whereas arterioles more often show fibrinoid necrosis (Figs. 2.46-2.48). Red blood cell (RBC) fragments are often present within the injured vessel wall, and there may be vessel wall necrosis and/or fibrin thrombi within vessels. Glomeruli may

---

Key Diagnostic Features of Scleroderma

- Fibrinoid necrosis of arterioles and interlobular arteries in acute stage
- Mucoid change of arterioles/interlobular arteries with red blood cell fragments in sub-acute stage
- Onion skinning intimal proliferation of arterioles/interlobular arteries in chronic stage

---

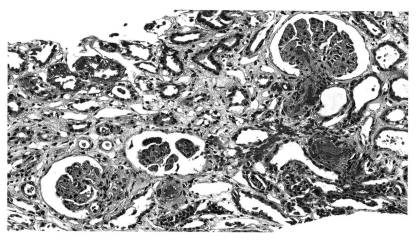

FIG. 2.42 Progressive systemic sclerosis. In scleroderma crisis, there is fibrinoid necrosis of interlobular arteries and arterioles, with fibrin thrombi sometimes extending to glomeruli. There is ischemic tubular injury, and early interstitial edema and fibrosis (hematoxylin and eosin, ×100).

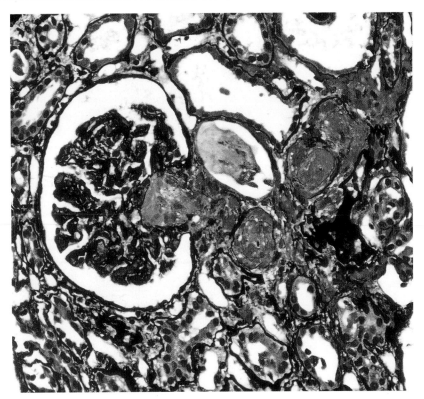

FIG. 2.43 Progressive systemic sclerosis. Fibrinoid necrosis of the arteriole is present, with fibrin thrombi occluding the lumen and extending to the hilus of the glomerulus. The glomerulus itself shows only ischemic change with corrugation of the glomerular basement membrane and retraction of the tuft (Jones silver stain, ×200).

Key Differential Diagnosis of Scleroderma

Scleroderma vs malignant hypertension:
- Malignant hypertension–associated injury typically also has underlying changes of arterionephrosclerosis and may involve smaller vessels.
- Clinical correlation is essential.

---

show ischemic collapse or fibrinoid necrosis. In chronic injury, there is reduplication of the elastic internal lamina, that is, the so-called onion-skin pattern (Figs. 2.49-2.52). Tubules may show degeneration and even necrosis, especially in scleroderma crisis (Fig. 2.46). Tubulointerstitial fibrosis develops with chronic injury. There are no immune complexes, and electron microscopy shows only increased lucency of the lamina rara interna, similar to TMA (Fig. 2.53).

The pathologic appearance overlaps with malignant hypertension and TMA. Idiopathic malignant hypertension tends to involve smaller vessels, that is, afferent arterioles, whereas scleroderma renal crisis may extend to interlobular size and larger vessels, and TMA typically involves primarily glomeruli. However, distinction of scleroderma and malignant hypertension solely on morphologic grounds is not feasible, and clinicopathologic correlation is required for specific diagnosis.

Text continued on page 336

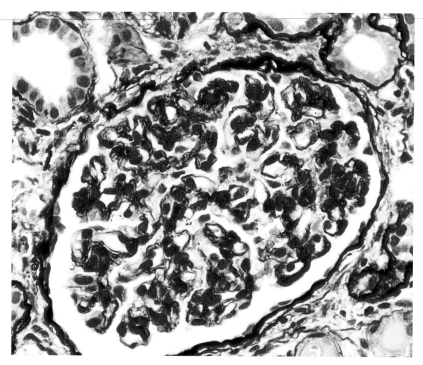

FIG. 2.44 Progressive systemic sclerosis. Even in glomeruli without demonstrable arteriolar injury or fibrin thrombi, there may be segmental corrugation and reduplication of the glomerular basement membrane, related to subacute endothelial injury (Jones silver stain, ×400).

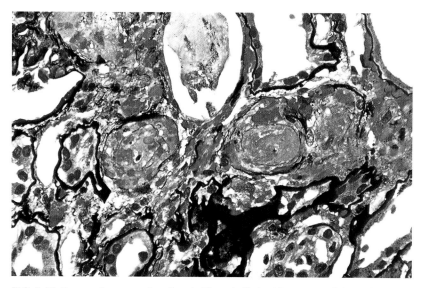

FIG. 2.45 Progressive systemic sclerosis. There is fibrinoid necrosis of the wall of this arteriole, with red blood cell fragments trapped within the wall and disruption of the internal elastic lamina (Jones silver stain, ×400).

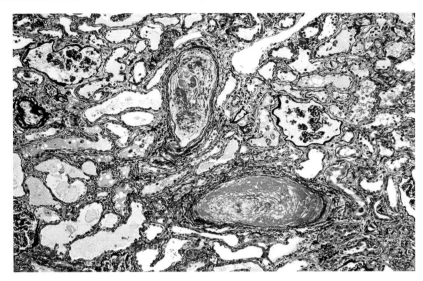

FIG. 2.46 Progressive systemic sclerosis. There is extensive injury of these medium-sized interlobular arteries, with mucoid change, necrosis, and numerous red blood cell fragments, leading to occlusion of the lumens. There is surrounding acute tubular necrosis with flattening and regeneration injury of the epithelium, and ischemic corrugation of the glomerular basement membrane (Jones silver stain, ×200).

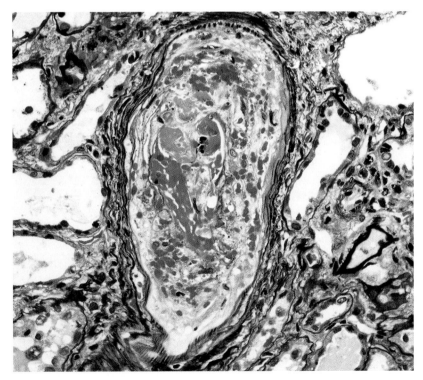

FIG. 2.47 Progressive systemic sclerosis. The mucoid expansion of the intima, with fibrin occluding the lumen, and numerous red blood cell fragments within the vessel wall are shown (Jones silver stain, ×400).

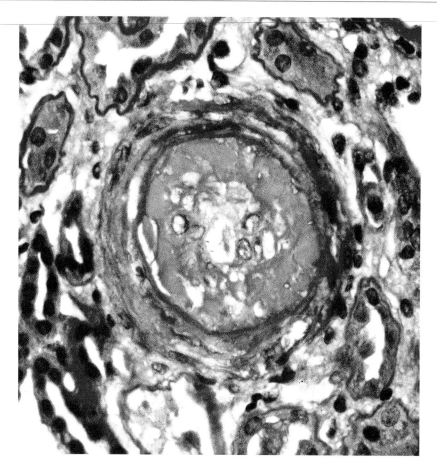

FIG. 2.48 Progressive systemic sclerosis. A less severely affected arteriole shows intimal reduplication and mucoid change of the intima, with swelling of the endothelium (periodic acid Schiff, ×200).

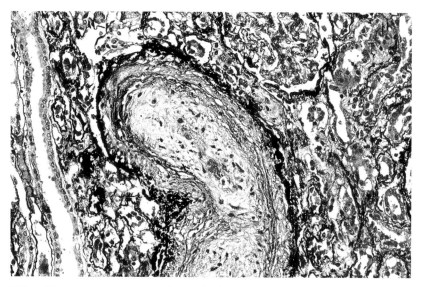

FIG. 2.49 Progressive systemic sclerosis. With more chronic injury, there is early intimal fibroplasia developing from the mucoid change, with small areas of fibrin and red blood cells. The lumen is virtually occluded (Jones silver stain, ×200).

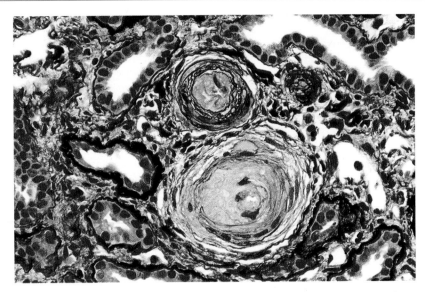

FIG. 2.50 Progressive systemic sclerosis. There is remarkable mucoid change and early concentric intimal fibroplasia of these arterioles in the more chronic phase of injury (Jones silver stain, ×200).

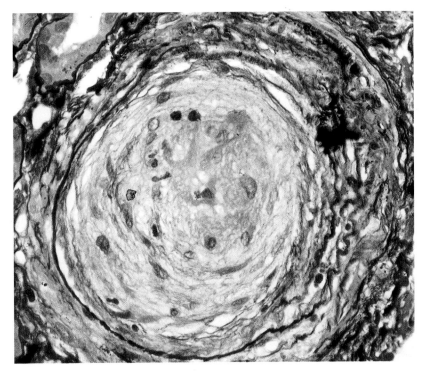

FIG. 2.51 Progressive systemic sclerosis. Intimal fibroplasia is occluding the lumen of the interlobular artery, with early so-called onion-skinning change, without any inflammation (Jones silver stain, ×400).

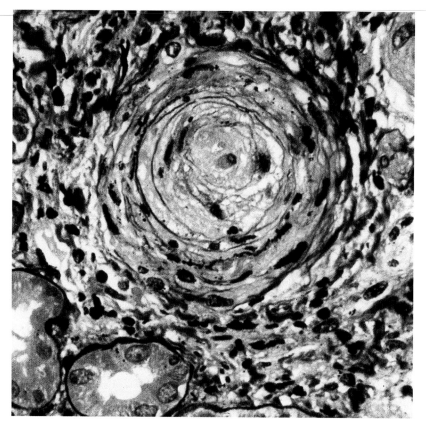

FIG. 2.52 Progressive systemic sclerosis. The well-established intimal fibroplasia following the acute injury is evident, with concentric intimal fibroplasia, the so-called onion-skinning appearance (Jones silver stain, ×400).

Etiology/Pathogenesis

The pathogenesis is unknown, but probably involves immune mechanisms, endothelial injury with unknown inciting events, associated with excess collagen accumulation. Endothelial injury is thought to play a key role in renal PSS, and occurs early in the course of the disease, but whether it is primary or initiated by immune injury has not been elucidated. Arterioles develop large gaps between endothelial cells, and the endothelium is damaged with vacuolization. Perivascular infiltrates of mononuclear immune cells, obliterative microvascular lesions, and rarefaction of capillaries develop. Scleroderma patients also have a defect in vasculogenesis and deficiency of circulating endothelial progenitor cells.

Autoantibodies are often present, including antitopoisomerase I, anticentromere, anti-RNA polymerase, each present in 25% of patients with scleroderma. Some studies have demonstrated cytotoxic antiendothelial factors in serum from scleroderma patients. Imbalance of vasodilators (e.g., nitric oxide, vasodilatory neuropeptides such as calcitonin gene-related peptide, substance P) and vasoconstrictors (e.g., endothelin-1, serotonin, thromboxane A2) has been described in PSS patients. Prolonged vasoconstriction could contribute to structural changes and fibrosis in the kidney. Increased profibrotic factors, including transforming growth factor-β and connective tissue growth factor, have been described.

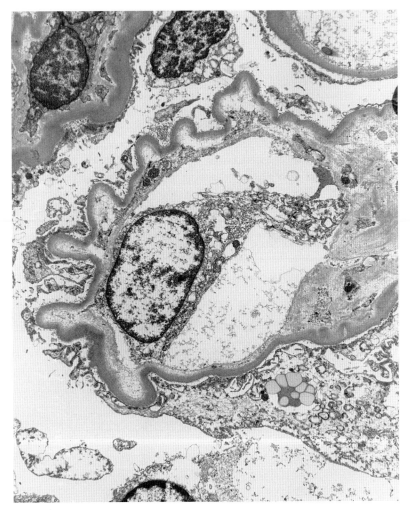

FIG. 2.53 There is corrugation of the glomerular basement membrane, with expansion of the lamina rara interna, related to chronic endothelial injury. There are no immune complexes. Overlying foot processes show extensive effacement with occasional vacuoles and lipid droplets (transmission electron microscopy, ×8000).

Selected Reading

Cannon, P.J., Hassar, M., Case, D.B., et al., 1974. The relationship of hypertension and renal failure in scleroderma (progressive systemic sclerosis) to structural and functional abnormalities of the renal cortical circulation. Medicine (Baltimore) 53, 1-46.

Donohoe, J.F., 1992. Scleroderma and the kidney. Kidney International 41, 462-477.

Gabrielli, A., Avvedimento, E.V., Krieg, T., 2009. Scleroderma. New England Journal of Medicine 360, 1989-2003.

Kuwana, M., Okazaki, Y., Yasuoka, H., et al., 2004. Defective vasculogenesis in systemic sclerosis. Lancet 364, 603-610.

Leinwand, I., Duryee, A.W., Richter, M.N., 1954. Scleroderma (based on study of over 150 cases). Annals of Internal Medicine 41, 1003-1041.

Steen, V.D., Medsger, Jr., T.A., 2000. Long-term outcomes of scleroderma renal crisis. Annals of Internal Medicine 133, 600-603.

Antiphospholipid Antibody Disease

The antiphospholipid syndrome (APS) is defined by two major components, a vascular event or pregnancy morbidity and the presence of at least one type of antiphospholipid autoantibody. Antiphospholipid antibody (APL) disease may occur in conjunction with systemic lupus erythematosus (SLE) or without other underlying systemic disease. Clinical manifestations are due to arterial and/or venous thrombosis. In women, fetal loss is common with a history of repeated miscarriages. Patients with APL antibodies may have systemic hypertension.

The kidney may be involved by TMA with acute renal failure, or symptoms may be more insidious. The involved kidney acutely shows thrombi in arterioles and interlobular arteries and also may involve glomeruli as in TMA of any cause (see detailed description of these lesions above). Chronically, the vascular lesions organize and there is fibrous intimal hyperplasia of interlobular arteries with associated focal cortical atrophy. The involvement of larger vessels occurs typically in primary APL antibody syndromes, resulting in sharply defined areas of cortical atrophy.

Etiology/Pathogenesis

APL antibodies may be lupus anticoagulants, anticardiolipin antibodies, or antibodies to beta-2 glycoprotein I. They may occur as a primary APL antibody syndrome or secondarily in association with SLE or other mixed connective tissue disease. These antibodies are prothrombotic and often result in thrombosis both systemically and occasionally in the kidney, with consequent tissue ischemia and injury, similar to that seen with TMA of any cause.

Key Morphologic Findings of Antiphospholipid Antibody Disease

- Lesions of thrombotic microangiopathy (see above)

Selected Reading

Daugas, E., Nochy, D., Huong du, L.T., et al., 2002. Antiphospholipid syndrome nephropathy in systemic lupus erythematosus. Journal of the American Society of Nephrology 13, 42-52.

Miyakis, S., Lockshin, M.D., Atsumi, T., et al., 2006. International consensus statement on an update of the classification criteria for definite antiphospholipid syndrome (APS). Journal of Thrombosis and Haemostasis 4, 295.

Nochy, D., Daugas, E., Droz, D., et al., 1999. The intrarenal vascular lesions associated with primary antiphospholipid syndrome. Journal of the American Society of Nephrology 10, 507-518.

Preeclampsia and Eclampsia

Toxemia of pregnancy includes both preeclampsia and eclampsia and can occur with or without an underlying primary renal disease. Preeclampsia is primarily a disease of nulliparas and manifests after the 20th week of gestation. It is characterized by hypertension, proteinuria, and edema. Preeclampsia occasionally progresses to a convulsive phase that is called eclampsia. This is often life threatening and clinically is manifested by a greater degree of hypertension and proteinuria. The clinical manifestations may extend to include hemolysis and red blood cell fragmentation, low platelet count, and elevated liver enzymes due to endothelial activation of the hepatic sinusoids in addition to that of the glomerular disease (HELLP syndrome).

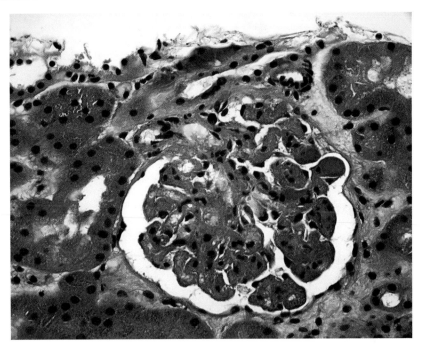

FIG. 2.54 Preeclampsia. Glomerulus demonstrates lobular accentuation with mesangial proliferation. The glomerular capillaries are collapsed. Occasional capillaries show microthrombi. The endothelial cells appear swollen (hematoxylin and eosin, ×400).

Key Diagnostic Features of Preeclampsia/Eclampsia

- Endotheliosis (swollen endothelial cells, "bloodless" appearance of glomeruli)
- Increased lucency of lamina rara interna, swollen endothelial cells by electron microscopy
- Thrombotic microangiopathy, fibrinoid necrosis in severe cases, HELLP syndrome

---

PATHOLOGY

Light microscopy shows a lesion characterized by enlarged glomeruli that appear bloodless and have swollen endothelial cells, coined the endotheliosis lesion (Figs. 2.54-2.60). More severe cases demonstrate the presence of fibrin both on light and immunofluorescence microscopy, particularly if HELLP syndrome is present. Immunofluorescence confirms the presence of fibrin. Rarely, trapped immunoglobulins are also found (Figs. 2.61, 2.62). In patients with preeclampsia and acute renal failure, the important findings are primarily ultrastructural, with evidence of endothelial cell swelling. Electron microscopy shows endothelial swelling with separation of the endothelium from the basement membrane by lucent material consistent with fibrinogen and foci of necrosis (Figs. 2.63-2.67).

Etiology/Pathogenesis

The pathology in preeclampsia/eclampsia is similar to that seen in TMAs. However, the pathogenesis is different. A range of deficiencies in placentation affects the key process of spiral artery remodeling. As pregnancy progresses to the third trimester, inadequate spiral artery

Text continued on page 347

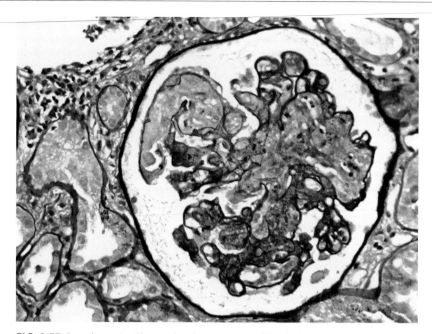

FIG. 2.55 Preeclampsia. Glomerulus demonstrates dilated glomerular capillaries, and the endothelial cells appear swollen to fill the capillary lumens (endotheliosis) (silver methenamine, ×400).

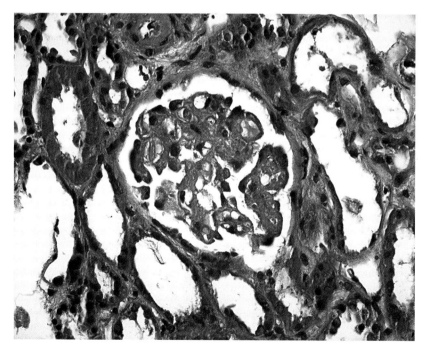

FIG. 2.56 Preeclampsia. The glomerulus demonstrates a bloodless appearance. The capillary loops are collapsed and appear to be thickened largely as a result of endothelial cell swelling (hematoxylin and eosin, ×400).

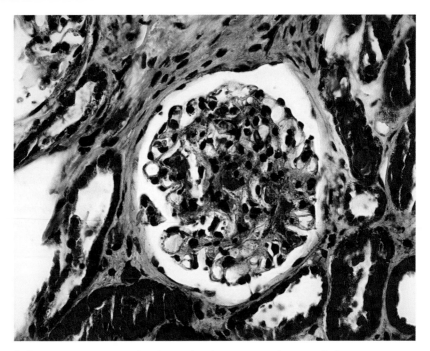

FIG. 2.57 Preeclampsia. The glomerulus demonstrates the same findings as in Fig. 2.51 with evidence of capillary thrombosis, thickening of the capillary walls and endothelial cell swelling (trichrome, ×400).

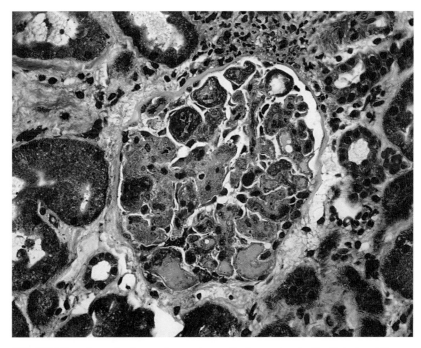

FIG. 2.58 Preeclampsia. Some glomerular capillaries are markedly dilated and there is evidence of mesangiolysis and focal necrosis (trichrome, ×400).

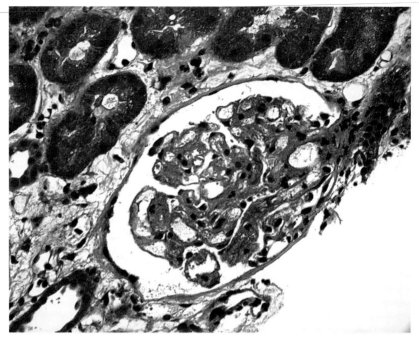

FIG. 2.59 Preeclampsia. In glomeruli not as severely involved, there is an increase in mesangial matrix and thickening of the capillary walls as a result of endothelial cell swelling (trichrome, ×400).

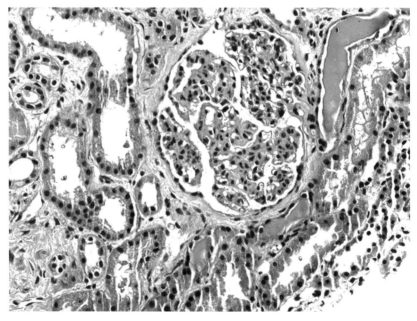

FIG. 2.60 Preeclampsia. In glomeruli not as severely involved, there is an increase in mesangial matrix and thickening of the capillary walls as a result of endothelial cell swelling (hematoxylin and eosin, ×200).

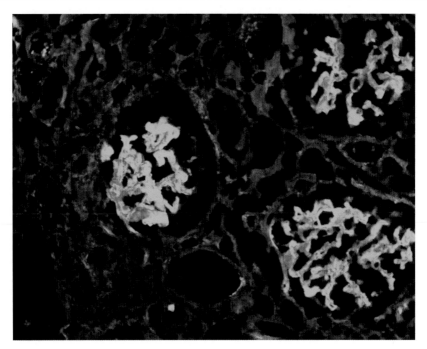

FIG. 2.61 Preeclampsia. Immunofluorescence demonstrates the presence of fibrinogen diffusely throughout the glomerulus (antifibrinogen immunofluorescence, ×200).

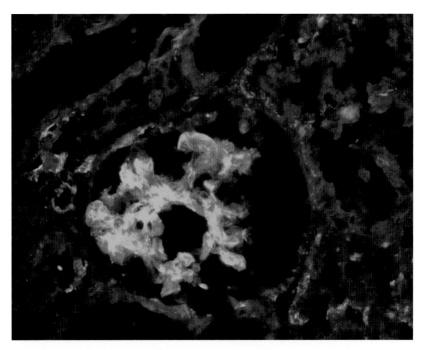

FIG. 2.62 Preeclampsia. Higher power demonstrates fibrinogen deposition in the glomerulus and surrounding peritubular capillaries (antifibrinogen immunofluorescence, ×400).

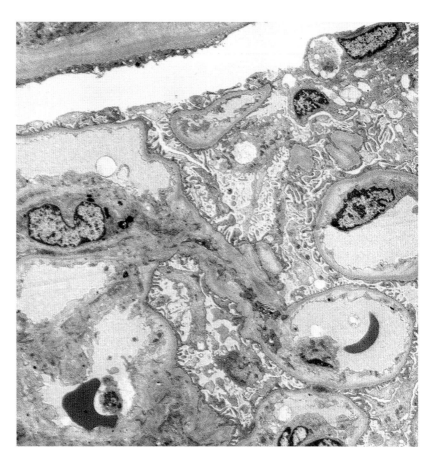

FIG. 2.63 Preeclampsia. Electron micrograph demonstrates the capillary lumina to be patent, the endothelial cells have lost fenestration and are swollen and separated from the basement membrane by electron-lucent material (transmission electron microscopy, ×2000).

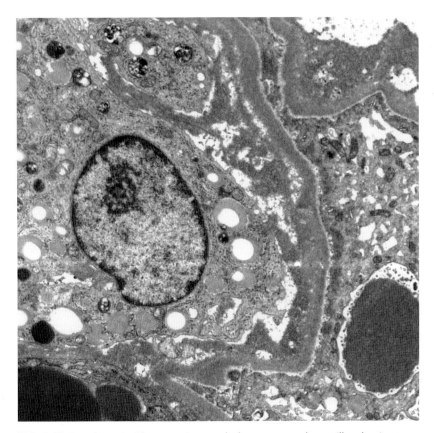

FIG. 2.64 Preeclampsia. Electron micrograph demonstrates the capillary lumina to be patent, the endothelial cells have lost fenestration and are swollen and separated from the basement membrane by granular electron-dense material (transmission electron microscopy, ×2000).

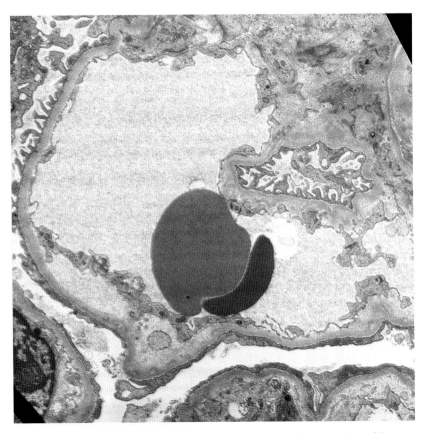

FIG. 2.65 Preeclampsia. Electron microscopy demonstrates the separation of the endothelium from the basement membrane with accumulation of lucent material. There is extensive effacement of the foot processes (transmission electron microscopy, ×3000).

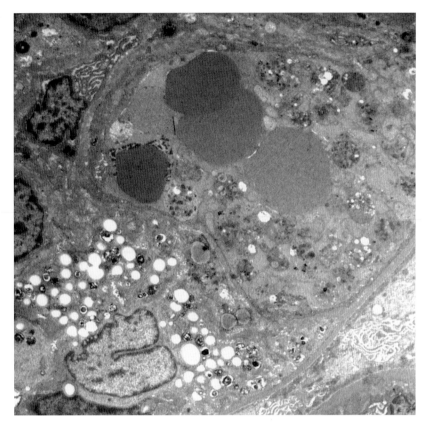

FIG. 2.66 Preeclampsia. Electron microscopy demonstrates the capillary lumen filled with platelets, fibrin, and red cells (transmission electron microscopy, ×1200).

remodeling along with multiple hemodynamic, placental, and maternal factors converge to activate the maternal immune and cardiovascular systems. Deficient uteroplacental perfusion is well recognized to be a feature in all preeclampsia syndromes as a result of preexisting vasculopathy and deficient trophoblast modeling of decidual arteries at the implantation site. Several mechanisms have been implicated in the pathogenesis of preeclampsia, including endothelial dysfunction, oxidative stress from placental hypoxia, and the renin–angiotensin system. Preeclampsia is associated with increased sensitivity to angiotensin II that may develop before the clinical manifestations of the disease. Placental vascular abnormalities often accompany the presence of preeclampsia. There is abnormal differentiation of the cytotrophoblasts and altered expression of adhesion molecules. These lesions lead to thrombosis of placental vasculature and infarction.

It has been hypothesized that the placental injuries release a factor into the systemic circulation that induces endothelial cell activation and initiation of intravascular coagulation. Genetic links have also been implicated as a result of familial aggregation of the syndrome between mother and daughters. Recent studies point to a primary importance of vascular endothelial-derived growth factor (VEGF) in preeclampsia. Increased levels of the soluble VEGF receptor, fms-like tyrosine kinase 1 (sFlt1), inhibits VEGF actions and placental growth factor (PlGF), which in turn appear to cause endothelial dysfunction and the classic endotheliosis lesion.

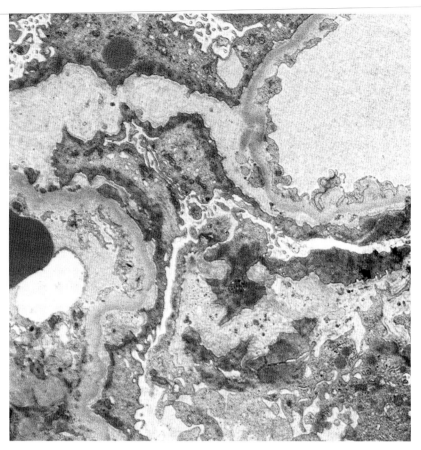

FIG. 2.67 Preeclampsia. Remodeling of the basement membrane is present with focal lamination and folding as a process of repair (transmission electron microscopy, ×5000).

Selected Reading

James, J.L., Whitley, G.S., Cartwright, J.E., 2010. Pre-eclampsia: fitting together the placental, immune and cardiovascular pieces. Journal of Pathology 221, 363-378.

Maynard, S., Epstein, F.H., Karamanchi, A.S.A., 2008. Preeclampsia and angiogenic imbalance. Annual Review of Medicine 59, 61-78.

Fibromuscular Dysplasia

A clinically important group of lesions of the renal artery are the so-called dysplastic lesions of the renal artery. These lesions may involve vessels outside of the renal artery but become clinically important when they cause obstruction initiating severe hypertension by creating a Goldblatt kidney. Fibromuscular dysplasia is a noninflammatory, nonatherosclerotic process that leads to arterial stenosis and can occur in all arterial beds. It is more common in females. The lesions can be subdivided into six separate groups, including intimal fibroplasias, medial fibroplasias, medial hyperplasia, perimedial fibroplasias, medial dissection, and periarterial fibroplasias. The term *fibromuscular dysplasia* has been used to encompass several of these separate categories but it appears useful to subclassify them because they may affect different patient populations (Table 2.2).

TABLE 2-2 Dysplastic Lesions of the Renal Artery

	Age (years) and sex incidence	Relative frequency[a] (%)	Lesion
Intimal fibroplasia	1–50 M = F	1-2	Narrowing by intimal proliferation without lipid
Medial fibroplasia with aneurysms	30–60 F > M	60-70	"String of beads"; alternating stenosis and mural thinning
Medial hyperplasia	30–60 F > M	5-15	Smooth muscle hyperplasia and thickening
Perimedial fibroplasia	30–60 F > M	15-24	Fibrosis of outer media; occasionally aneurysms
Medial dissection	30–60 F > M	5-15	Fibrosis of media with dissecting aneurysms
Periarterial fibroplasia	15–50 F > M	1	Perivascular fibrosis & inflammation

M, male; F, female.
[a]Relative to all forms of dysplastic lesions, i.e., medial fibroplasia is the most common form of renal arterial dysplasia.

Etiology/Pathogenesis

Little is known relative to the pathogenesis, but it is thought to be related to a potential defect in matrix synthesis and regulation. A genetic predisposition with a reported autosomal mode of inheritance has been reported in some families. Hormonal influence, ischemic damage, and mechanical stretch have all been postulated.

PATHOLOGY

The most common of the dysplastic lesions is medial fibroplasia. This usually results in a multifocal stenotic lesion alternating with microaneurysms. This pattern of disease leads to the characteristic string-of-beads appearance seen on arteriography (Figs. 2.68, 2.69). Histopathologically, there is atrophy of the muscle and fibrosis of the wall in the region of the small aneurysms alternating with the stenotic lesions where there is medial muscular hypertrophy with an increase of interstitial collagen (Fig. 2.70). The second most frequently encountered variation of fibromuscular hyperplasia is perimedial fibroplasias. In contrast to medial fibroplasias, segmental aneurysmal dilatation is not present but focal aneurysms occasionally occur (Fig. 2.71). The lesions consist of thickening of the outer half of the media with an increase in fibrous tissue (Fig. 2.72). The muscle is disoriented and there is generalized thickening of the wall although the elastic and intima as well as the inner portion of the media retain a normal architecture. Far less common is medial hyperplasia. Here there is hyperplasia of the muscle that results in uniform thickening of the vessel wall and results in generalized narrowing of the lumen (Fig. 2.73). Periarterial fibroplasias is a rare lesion in which fibrosis of the adventia extends into the surrounding adipose and connective tissue, resulting in constriction of the vessel from without rather than from within the vessel wall. In intimal fibroplasias, the fibrotic lesion involves only the intima of the vessel, with the elastica and media maintaining a normal structure (Fig. 2.74). There is hyperplasia of the intima, which is essentially indistinguishable from the proliferative stage of arteriosclerosis but is not associated with an increased deposition of lipid. The lesion has been reported in an individual as young as 1 year of age but is most commonly seen in the third and fourth decades.

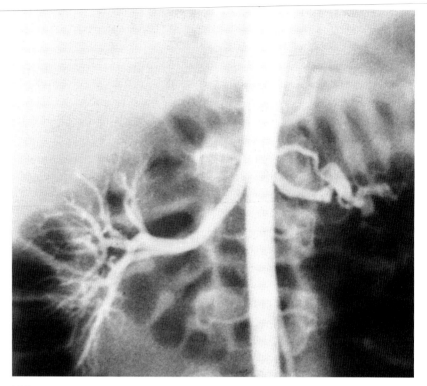

FIG. 2.68 Medial fibroplasias. Radiograph from a patient with fibromuscular dysplasia demonstrating the "string of beads" appearance of the renal arteries.

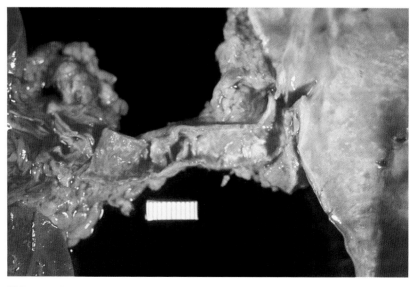

FIG. 2.69 Medial fibroplasias. Fibromuscular dysplasia. The artery shows irregular saccular dilatations with bands of narrowing between the aneurysmal dilatations. These correspond to the "string of beads" findings on the radiograph.

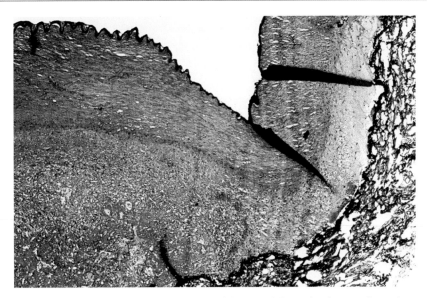

FIG. 2.70 Medial fibroplasias. Elastic stain of the vessel shows focal areas of atrophy of the smooth muscle and fibrosis in the region of the aneurysmal dilatations (elastic stain, ×200).

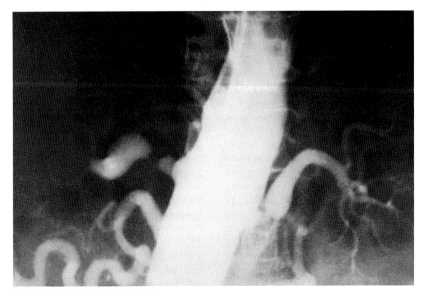

FIG. 2.71 Perimedial fibroplasia. Radiograph showing area of constriction and a focal aneurysmal dilatation distal to the constriction.

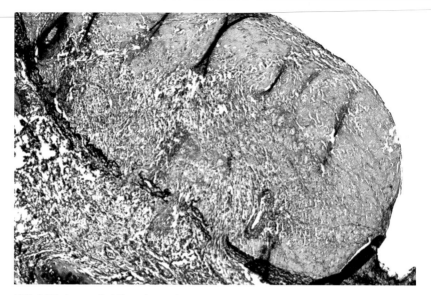

FIG. 2.72 Perimedial fibroplasia. Elastic stain demonstrates thickening of the outer half of the media and an increase in fibrous tissue (elastic stain, ×200).

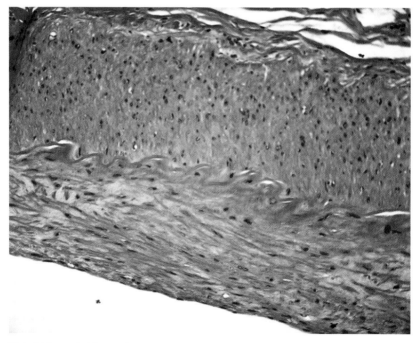

FIG. 2.73 Medial hyperplasia. Hyperplasia of the muscular layers of the wall results in uniform thickening of the vessel wall with generalized narrowing of lumen without aneurysmal dilation (hematoxylin and eosin, ×400).

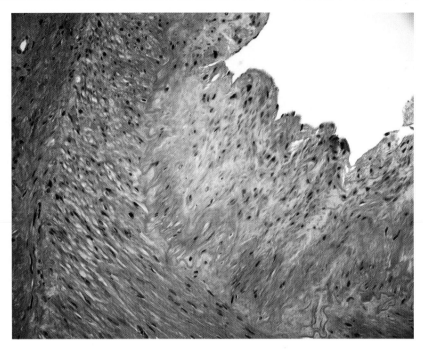

FIG. 2.74 Periarterial fibroplasias. Fibrosis is predominantly present in the adventitia with irregular changes within the muscular media (hematoxylin and eosin, ×400).

Selected Reading

Kashgarian, M., 1995. Hypertensive disease and kidney structure. In: Laragh, J.H., Brenner, B.M., (Eds.), "Hypertension". Raven Press, New York, pp. 433-444.

Perdu, J., Boutouyrie, P., Bourgai, C., et al., 2007. Inheritance of arterial lesions in renal fibromuscular dysplasia. Journal of Human Hypertension 21, 393-400.

Arterionephrosclerosis

Patients usually have a history of hypertension and may have renal insufficiency and varying proteinuria. Proteinuria can be nephrotic range, particularly if hypertension is severe. Arterionephrosclerosis is associated with renal insufficiency in African Americans more commonly than in Caucasians.

"Benign" nephrosclerosis results in small kidneys with finely granular surface and thinned cortex in late stages (Fig. 2.75). Microscopically, there is vascular wall medial thickening with frequent afferent arteriolar hyaline deposits (Figs. 2.76, 2.77). The hyalinization is due to endothelial injury and increased pressure, leading to an insudate of plasma macromolecules. With accelerated hypertension, endothelial cells are swollen and RBC fragments can be trapped within the vessel wall (Fig. 2.78). Interlobular and larger arteries show varying medial hypertrophy and intimal fibrosis with reduplication of the internal elastic lamina (Figs. 2.79-2.81). There are associated focal glomerular ischemic changes with variable thickening and wrinkling of the basement membrane, and/or global sclerosis, tubular atrophy and interstitial fibrosis. Global sclerosis can be either of the obsolescent type (i.e., glomerular tuft sclerosed and Bowman's space filled with collagenous material) or of the solidified type (global solidification of the tuft without collagenous material within Bowman's space) (Figs. 2.82-2.86). Globally sclerosed glomeruli can even become continuous with the surrounding interstitial fibrosis as Bowman's capsule is resorbed. The globally sclerosed glomerulus may then be difficult to discern and may even disappear as a recognizable structure (Fig. 2.84). Secondary

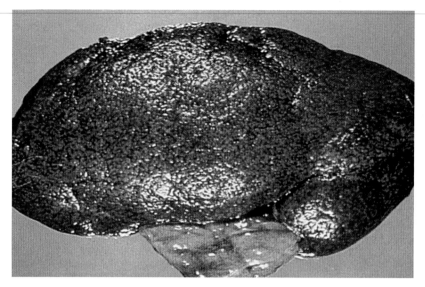

FIG. 2.75 The kidney shows a finely granular surface, related to arteriolar sclerosis with associated glomerular obsolescence and tubulointerstitial fibrosis. The broad-based scars are due to disease in slightly larger, interlobular arteries with depressed cortical areas of scarring.

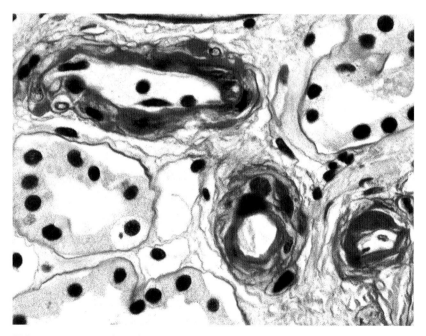

FIG. 2.76 Arterionephrosclerosis. Endothelial injury is frequently accompanied by hyalinosis, a lesion due to an insudation of plasma proteins. The material is glassy smooth and periodic acid Schiff (PAS)–positive (PAS, ×200).

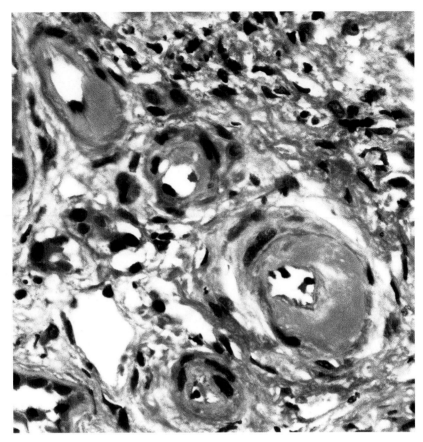

FIG. 2.77 Arterionephrosclerosis. Moderate to severe hyalinosis is present in this arteriole. It is cut multiple times in this section, because of its tortuosity. The hyalinosis is eccentric (hematoxylin and eosin, ×200).

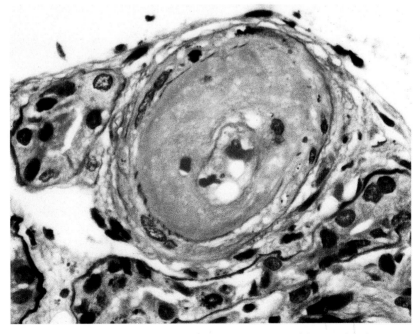

FIG. 2.78 Arterionephrosclerosis. There is severe hyalinosis of this interlobular artery, with swollen endothelial cells and a few red blood cell fragments, indicative of early, accelerated endothelial injury (Jones silver stain, ×200).

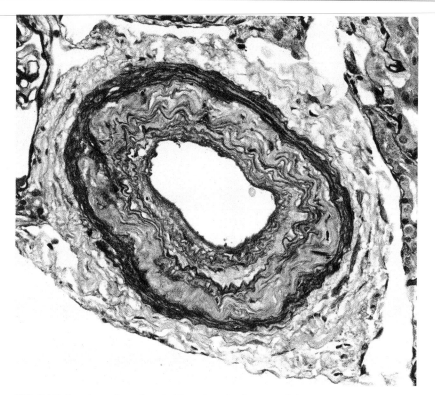

FIG. 2.79 Arterionephrosclerosis. There is reduplication of the intima, with intimal fibroplasia, resulting in a thicker, less compliant wall of this interlobular artery (periodic acid Schiff, ×200).

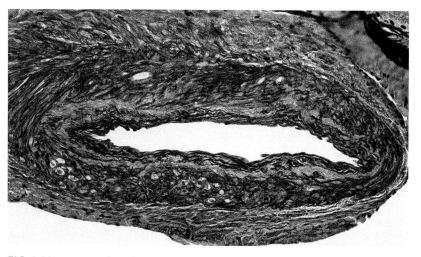

FIG. 2.80 Arterionephrosclerosis. There is intimal fibrosis, thickening of the media, and increased thickness of the adventitia (periodic acid Schiff, ×100).

FSGS may also occur, often with associated GBM corrugation and periglomerular fibrosis and subtotal foot process effacement (Figs. 2.87-2.89). In addition, the associated vascular lesions and the clinical history, with hypertension preceding other manifestations of renal disease, are useful in favoring a secondary etiology of the segmental sclerosis rather than primary FSGS. Immunofluorescence may show trapping of IgM and C3 in glomeruli. Electron microscopy confirms the corrugated, wrinkled GBM and ischemic changes with increased

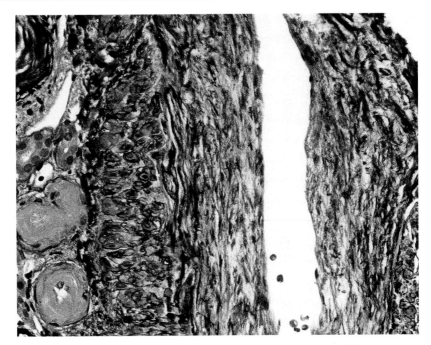

FIG. 2.81 Arterionephrosclerosis. A large artery shows marked intimal fibroplasia. Adjacent arterioles show severe hyalinosis (Jones silver stain, ×200).

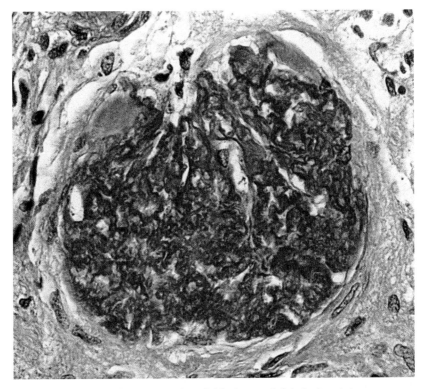

FIG. 2.82 Arterionephrosclerosis. The solidified type of global sclerosis is characterized by solidification of the entire glomerular tuft (periodic acid Schiff, ×200).

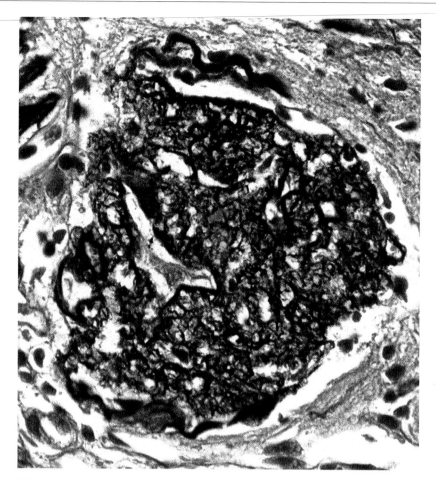

FIG. 2.83 Arterionephrosclerosis. The solidified glomerulus is completely solidified, with wrinkled glomerular basement membrane clearly discernible on silver stain (Jones silver stain, ×200).

Key Diagnostic Features of Arterionephrosclerosis

- Vascular sclerosis and hyalinosis, out of proportion to glomerular/tubulointerstitial lesions
- Extensive global glomerulosclerosis
- +/− segmental glomerulosclerosis
- Lamina rara interna expansion and variable foot process effacement by electron microscopy

---

lucency of the lamina rara interna without immune deposits (Fig. 2.90). Some foot process effacement may also be present, but it is usually not as extensive as in primary FSGS. Hyaline deposits are often present in arterioles as well as in sclerosed segments of glomeruli (Fig. 2.91).

Although none of these lesions is pathognomonic, the constellation of these changes in the absence of other lesions of primary glomerular disease is indicative of arterionephrosclerosis (ANS).

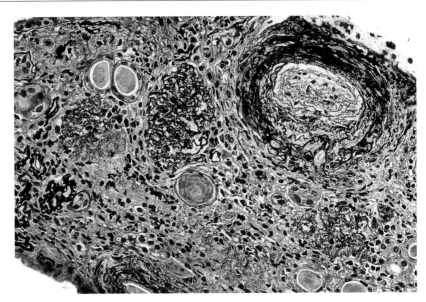

FIG. 2.84 Arterionephrosclerosis. Two solidified glomeruli are shown, along with an artery with intimal fibroplasia. The glomerulus on the far right is becoming resorbed, with dissolution of Bowman's capsule, becoming continuous with the surrounding interstitial fibrosis. The adjacent glomerulus is still easily recognizable by silver stain, but Bowman's capsule is no longer intact. The remnant of another glomerulus is evident on the left, with small area of contours of GBM still visible on silver stain. There is severe associated tubular atrophy, so-called thyroidization with interstitial fibrosis (Jones silver stain, ×200).

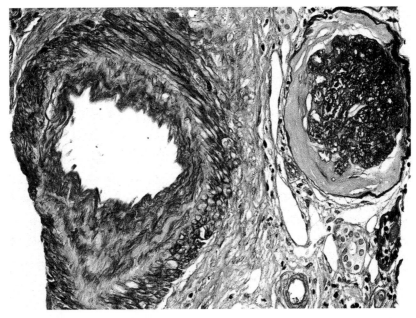

FIG. 2.85 Arterionephrosclerosis. Glomeruli may also become globally sclerosed by becoming obsolescent. The obsolescent glomerulus has a totally sclerosed glomerular tuft with fibrous material filling in and obliterating Bowman's capsule. The adjacent artery shows intimal reduplication, and there is surrounding tubulointerstitial fibrosis (periodic acid Schiff, ×200).

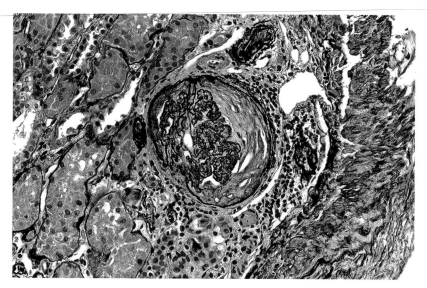

FIG. 2.86 Arterionephrosclerosis. The obsolescent glomerulus is easily differentiated from the solidified type by silver stain, highlighting the retracted, globally sclerosed glomerular tuft and the collagenous material filling in Bowman's space. There is surrounding tubulointerstitial fibrosis (Jones silver stain, ×200).

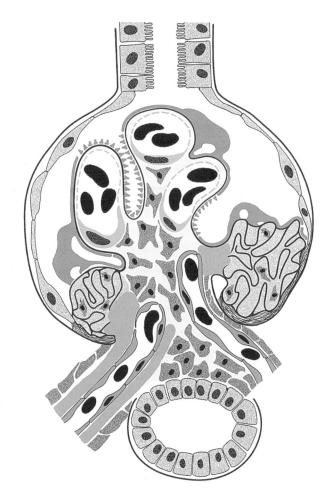

FIG. 2.87 Arterionephrosclerosis may also show glomerular lesions, with secondary segmental glomerulosclerosis, often characterized by hilar location of segmental sclerosis with associated hyalin, vascular sclerosis, and periglomerular fibrosis.

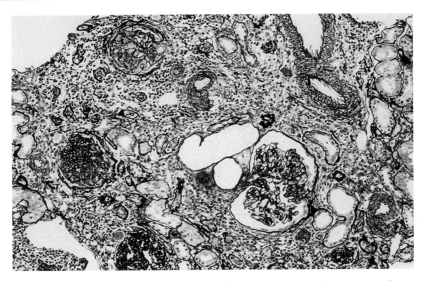

FIG. 2.88 Arterionephrosclerosis. There may be associated secondary segmental glomerulosclerosis, as shown on the left, associated with globally sclerotic glomeruli, arteriolo- and arteriosclerosis. There is proportional tubulointerstitial fibrosis (Jones silver stain, ×100).

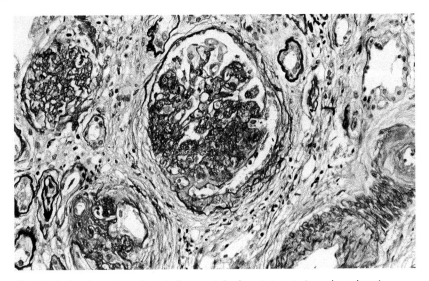

FIG. 2.89 Arterionephrosclerosis. Segmental sclerosis in arterionephrosclerosis typically has associated periglomerular fibrosis, obsolescent glomeruli, vascular disease out of proportion to segmental sclerosis, and subtotal foot process effacement (periodic acid Schiff, ×200).

Etiology/Pathogenesis

Hypertension has been presumed to cause end-organ damage in the kidney. In a large series of renal biopsies in patients with essential hypertension, arteriolar nephrosclerosis was present in 81.2%, and the severity of arteriolar sclerosis correlated significantly with level of diastolic blood pressure. However, in several large autopsy series of patients with presumed benign hypertension, significant renal lesions were rare. Further, the level of blood pressure does not directly predict degree of end-organ damage: African Americans have higher risk for more

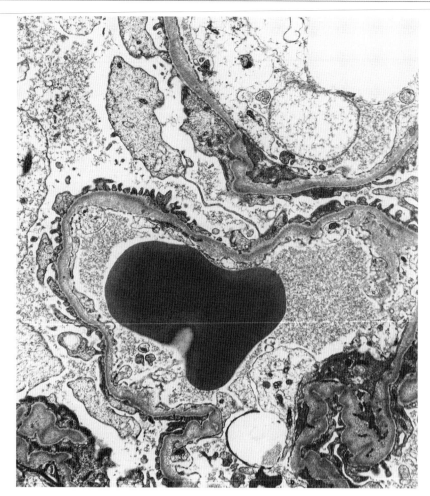

FIG. 2.90 Arterionephrosclerosis. Although segmental sclerosis was present in this patient with arterionephrosclerosis, there is only minimal foot process effacement, and there is segmental increase in lamina rara interna lucent material, and segmental corrugation of the GBM (transmission electron microscopy, ×11,250).

severe end-organ damage at any level of blood pressure. It is possible that underlying microvascular disease causes the hypertension and the renal disease in susceptible patients. Underlying causes include possible genetic and structural components, such as low-term birth weight, linked to increased risk of cardiovascular disease and hypertension in adulthood. Low birth weight is also associated with fewer nephrons at birth, and enlarged glomeruli. Low birth weight occurs more commonly in African Americans than in Caucasians, and healthy African Americans have larger glomeruli than age- and body mass–matched Caucasians. The fewer nephrons are postulated to be exposed to greater hemodynamic stress. In addition, genetic polymorphisms contributing to retarded intrauterine development might also play a role in augmented fibrotic responses to injuries later in life.

Our biopsy data suggest a different phenotype of scarring in ANS in African Americans versus Caucasians. The solidified type of global glomerulosclerosis was more frequent in African Americans, contrasting the predominance of the obsolescent type of global sclerosis in Caucasians. The solidified type was also associated with more severe disease clinically, echoing its original description as "decompensated benign nephrosclerosis."

Whether hypertension causes the ANS, or a subtle primary microvascular renal injury causes the hypertension, which in turn accelerates the sclerosis, has not been proven.

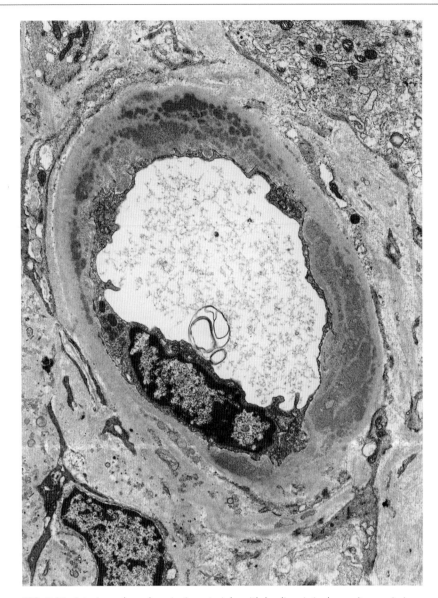

FIG. 2.91 Arterionephrosclerosis. An arteriole with hyalinosis is shown (transmission electron microscopy, ×11,250).

Mutations in apolipoprotein L1 are tightly linked to the excess ANS observed in African Americans and also to other nondiabetic chronic kidney disease in this population. This mutation confers protection against some trypanosomal disease, and thus its relatively high prevalence in African Americans may have been influenced by natural selection because of a survival advantage. The mechanisms of increased risk of kidney disease are unknown.

Selected Reading

Barker, D.J., Osmond, C., Golding, J., et al., 1989. Growth in utero, blood pressure in childhood and adult life, and mortality from cardiovascular disease. British Medical Journal 298 (6673), 564-567.

Böhle, A., Ratschek, M., 1982. The compensated and decompensated form of benign nephrosclerosis. Pathology, Research and Practice 174, 357-367.

Brenner, B.M., Garcia, D.L., Anderson, S., 1988. Glomeruli and blood pressure. Less of one, more the other? American Journal of Hypertension 1, 335-347.

Fogo, A., Breyer, J.A., Smith, M.C., et al., 1997. Accuracy of the diagnosis of hypertensive nephrosclerosis in African Americans: a report from the African American Study of Kidney Disease (AASK) Trial. AASK Pilot Study Investigators. Kidney International 51, 244-252.

Freedman, B.I., Iskandar, S.S. Buckalew, V.M., et al., 1994. Renal biopsy findings in presumed hypertensive nephrosclerosis. American Journal of Nephrology 14, 90-94.

Genovese, G., Friedman, D.J., Ross, M.D., et al., 2010. Association of trypanolytic ApoL1 variants with kidney disease in African Americans. Science 329, 841-845.

Innes, A., Johnston, P.A., Morgan, A.G., et al., 1993. Clinical features of benign hypertensive nephrosclerosis at time of renal biopsy. Quarterly Journal of Medicine 86, 271-275.

Katz, S.M., Lavin, L., Swartz, C., 1979. Glomerular lesions in benign essential hypertension. Archives of Pathology Laboratory Medicine 103, 199-203.

Keller, G., Zimmer, G., Mall, G., et al., 2003. Nephron number in patients with primary hypertension. New England Journal of Medicine 348 (2), 101-108.

Marcantoni, C., Ma, L.J., Federspiel, C., et al., 2002. Hypertensive nephrosclerosis in African-Americans vs. Caucasians. Kidney International 62, 172-180.

McManus, J.F.A., Lupton, Jr., C.H., 1960. Ischemic obsolescence of renal glomeruli: the natural history of the lesions and their relation to hypertension. Laboratory Investigations 9, 413-434.

Sommers, S.C., Relman, A.S., Smithwick, R.H., 1958. Histologic studies of kidney biopsy specimens from patients with hypertension. American Journal of Pathology 34, 685-713.

Accelerated/Malignant Hypertension

Malignant or accelerated hypertension is rarer than previously in the United States. However, in other developing countries, malignant hypertension at initial presentation is still not uncommon. The average age is 40 years and men are affected more commonly than women. Patients may have a history of "benign" hypertension, or present de novo with malignant hypertension, defined as blood pressure usually higher than 200/130 mmHg. Less than 1% of patients with hypertension, either primary or secondary, develop the malignant phase. Patients usually present with severe headaches, vomiting, visual disturbances, stupor, coma, convulsions, congestive heart failure, oliguria, or renal failure. Any one or all of the above may be present. Patients may have proteinuria, even nephrotic range, which decreases with control of blood pressure. Hematuria may also be present in some patients. Severe retinopathy is present with hemorrhage and exudates, with papilledema being present only in malignant, but not accelerated, hypertension. If left untreated, survival is poor, whereas long-term survival is >90% if blood pressure is controlled.

Malignant (accelerated) nephrosclerosis grossly shows petechial hemorrhage of the subcapsular surface, with mottling and occasional areas of infarct (Fig. 2.92). Microscopically, arterioles show mucoid change and endothelial cell swelling with RBC fragments in accelerated hypertensive injury (Fig. 2.93). In malignant hypertension, there is fibrinoid necrosis of arterioles, and interlobular arteries have a concentric onion-skin pattern of intimal fibrosis (hyperplastic arteriolopathy), overlapping with the appearance of PSS and TMA (Figs. 2.94-2.96). Larger arteries do not usually show specific lesions in primary malignant hypertension. In secondary hypertension, there may be underlying intimal fibrosis and reduplication of the elastica. Glomeruli may be normal, or show focal segmental necrosis or severe congestion. With more chronic, ongoing injury, there is corrugation of the GBM with occasional reduplication (Figs. 2.97, 2.98). These changes typically are superimposed on lesions of benign ANS, such as medial hypertrophy, arteriolar hyaline, intimal fibrosis, and global glomerulosclerosis with proportional tubulointerstitial fibrosis. By immunofluorescence, there may be

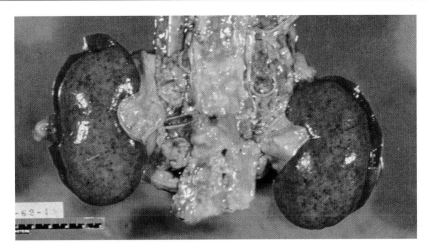

FIG. 2.92 Malignant hypertension. Grossly, there are petechial hemorrhages, secondary to the arteriolar necrosis, giving rise to a "flea-bitten" appearance.

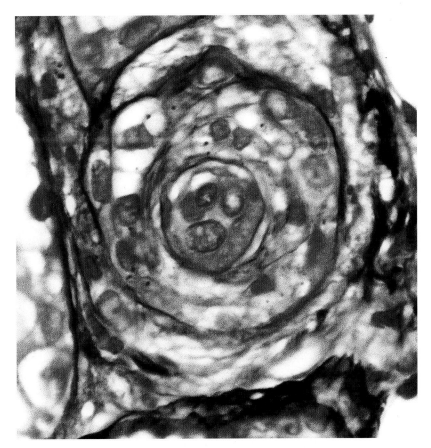

FIG. 2.93 Accelerated hypertension. There is endothelial swelling and mucoid change with red blood cell fragments within the wall, but without frank fibrinoid necrosis, associated with accelerated hypertension (Jones silver stain, ×200).

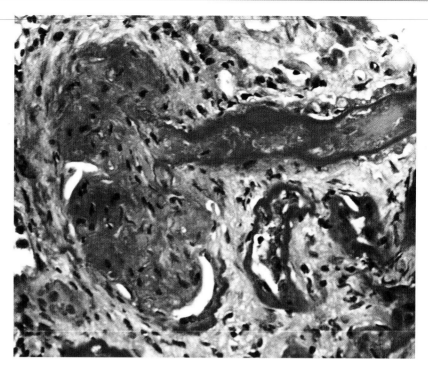

FIG. 2.94 Malignant hypertension. There is frank fibrinoid necrosis of the arteriole, which has led to obliteration of the glomerulus. There is surrounding tubulointerstitial fibrosis. This appearance cannot be distinguished morphologically from the acute injury in progressive systemic sclerosis, and clinicopathologic correlation is needed (hematoxylin and eosin, ×200).

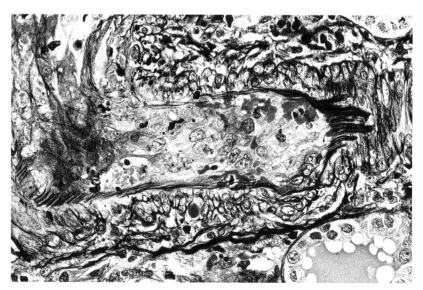

FIG. 2.95 Malignant hypertension. An interlobular artery is occluded by swollen endothelial cells with karyorrhectic debris, occasional polymorphonuclear leukocytes, and chunks of fibrin within the swollen endothelium. The media is still intact (Jones silver stain, ×200).

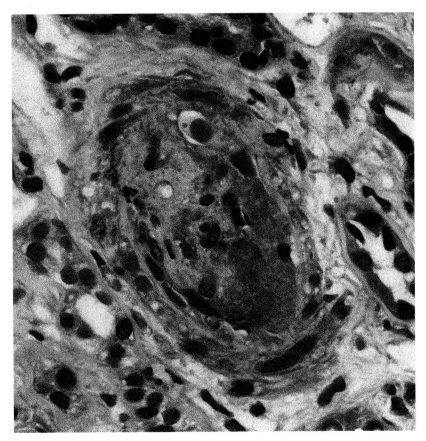

FIG. 2.96 Malignant hypertension. There is extensive injury of the interlobular artery, with occlusion by endothelial swelling with mucoid change and fibrin thrombi, with fibrinoid necrosis extending into the media (Masson trichrome stain, ×400).

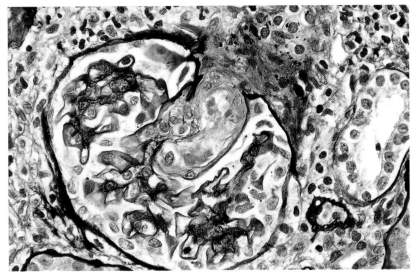

FIG. 2.97 Malignant hypertension. There is endothelial swelling and fibrin occluding the arteriole at the glomerular hilus, with ischemic retraction of the glomerular tuft (Jones silver stain, ×400).

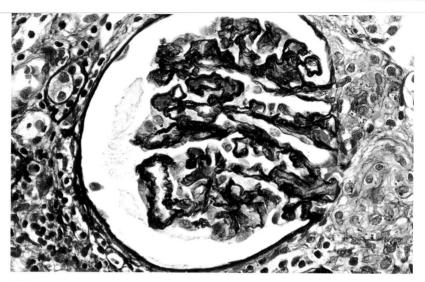

FIG. 2.98 Malignant hypertension. Even glomeruli without thrombotic occlusion may show ischemic injury with corrugation of the glomerular basement membrane and segmental reduplication (Jones silver stain, ×400).

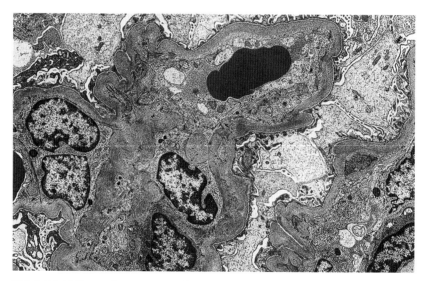

FIG. 2.99 Malignant hypertension. There is expansion of the lamina rara interna and corrugation of the glomerular basement membrane, with segmental effacement of the overlying foot processes (transmission electron microscopy, ×9750).

trapping of IgM and C3 in sclerotic areas. Necrotic vessels and glomeruli may stain for fibrinogen. Electron microscopy shows corrugation of the GBM and expansion of the lamina rara interna (Fig. 2.99). Foot processes may show segmental effacement. Fibrin tactoids may be visualized by electron microscopy. There are no immune complexes.

Etiology/Pathogenesis

Hyperplastic arteriolar lesions and fibrinoid necrosis of the arterioles plays a key role in development of the signs and symptoms. However, the etiology is unknown. Abnormalities in the renin–angiotensin system have been postulated to play a role. An animal model with rats transgenic for renin mirrors many aspects of malignant hypertension.

Key Diagnostic Features of Accelerated/Malignant Hypertension

- Fibrinoid necrosis of arterioles in acute stage
- Mucoid change, red blood cell fragments in vessel wall in subacute stage
- Onion-skinning of arterioles in chronic stage

Selected Reading

Bohle, A., Helmchen, U., Grund, K.E., et al., 1977. Malignant nephrosclerosis in patients with hemolytic uremic syndrome (primary malignant nephrosclerosis). Current Topics in Pathology 65, 81-113.

Caetano, E.R., Zatz, R., Saldanha, L.B., et al., 2001. Hypertensive nephrosclerosis as a relevant cause of chronic renal failure. Hypertension 38 (2), 171-176.

Hsu, H., Churg, J., 1980. The ultrastructure of mucoid "onionskin" intimal lesions in malignant nephrosclerosis. American Journal of Pathology 99 (1), 67-80.

Lip, G.Y., Beevers, M., Beevers, G., 1994. The failure of malignant hypertension to decline: a survey of 24 years' experience in a multiracial population in England. Journal of Hypertension 12 (11), 1297-1305.

Murphy, C., 1995. Hypertensive emergencies. Emergency Medicine Clinics of North America 13, 973-1001.

Atheroemboli

Atheroembolic disease occurs in older patients who have underlying atherosclerosis. Men are more frequently affected than women, reflecting higher incidence of atherosclerotic disease. Cholesterol emboli most often involve multiple organs, and have been reported in virtually all tissues. The kidney is the most commonly involved organ at autopsy (75%), followed by spleen (55%), pancreas (52%), gastrointestinal tract (31%), and the adrenals (20%).

The histologic diagnosis of cholesterol emboli is based on the finding of the characteristic needle-shaped slits of dissolved cholesterol crystals in the lumina of blood vessels (Figs. 2.100-2.104). The crystals are dissolved by routine tissue processing, but are birefringent and stain positive for fat on frozen section. The cholesterol emboli usually lodge in vessels of 150-300 μm diameter. In the kidney, therefore, the lesions are most common in arcuate and interlobular arteries, although glomeruli may also be involved (Fig. 2.105). When there is massive showering of cholesterol emboli, there may be patchy cortical necrosis and tubular necrosis and injury secondary to ischemia. If the process is more gradual, there may be a mixture of necrosis due to acute local ischemia from occluded vessels and more chronic ischemic changes such as glomerular scarring, tubular atrophy, and interstitial fibrosis. The early response, based on animal models, consists of mononuclear cell infiltration in the vessel and foreign body giant cell reaction surrounding the crystals (Fig. 2.101). Polymorphonuclear leukocytes and eosinophils may also be seen transiently in the vessel lumen in the first 24 hours after embolization (Fig. 2.102). The vessel may then become thrombosed in the subacute stage from 24 to 72 hours. After the initial acute phase of injury, there is endothelial cell proliferation and intravascular fibrosis (Fig. 2.103). Cholesterol crystals may remain detectable for as long as 9 months after the acute event.

Immunofluorescence and electron microscopy show no specific changes, but occasionally the tissue submitted for these studies may contain the only cholesterol emboli in the biopsy (Figs. 2.106, 2.107). Diagnostic cholesterol emboli are very localized, and multiple step sections and examination of all tissue is necessary to ensure optimal detection. Cholesterol emboli are typically present superimposed on changes of ANS, that is, sclerosis of arterioles and arteries and global glomerulosclerosis (Fig. 2.104). Rarely, there may be associated focal segmental glomerulosclerosis, likely secondary, and significant proteinuria.

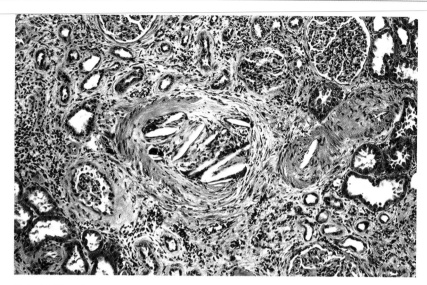

FIG. 2.100 Atheroemboli. Atheroemboli typically lodge in arterioles and interlobular arteries. Multiple cleft-shaped spaces, reflecting the empty space left after dissolution of the cholesterol by standard processing, are present in the artery in the middle, with surrounding inflammatory cell reaction. In the early weeks, this infiltrate consists primarily of mononuclear cells. An older lesion, more organized and with more subtle cholesterol emboli, is seen in the arteriole on the right, with a single cleft-like space and surrounding hyperplasia and fibrosis of the arteriole (hematoxylin and eosin, ×100).

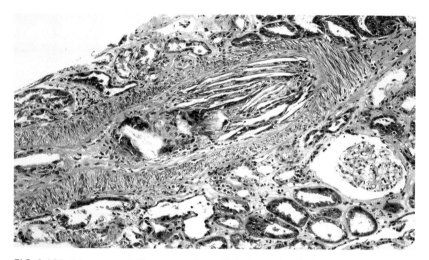

FIG. 2.101 Atheroemboli. The acute phase of cholesterol emboli is shown, with multiple stacks of varying shapes of cleft-like spaces in an artery with surrounding giant cell and mononuclear cell reaction. There is minimal fibrosis (Masson trichrome stain, ×200).

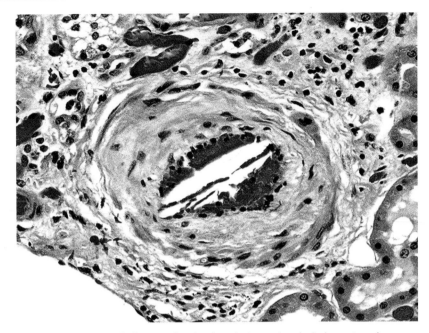

FIG. 2.102 Atheroemboli. Immediately after cholesterol emboli showering, there are only rare inflammatory cells with a mix of polymorphonuclear leukocytes and monocytes, with red blood cell fragments, fibrin, and platelets surrounding the cleft-like spaces occluding this interlobular artery (hematoxylin and eosin, ×200).

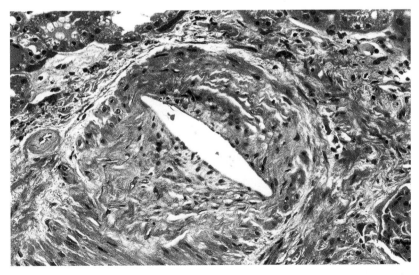

FIG. 2.103 Atheroemboli. Intimal fibrosis and mild cell proliferation with occasional mononuclear cells are seen in this artery with a single cleft-like space, representing a dissolved cholesterol embolus. When these cleft-like spaces are oriented at an angle parallel to the lumen of the artery, they may easily be overlooked (hematoxylin and eosin, ×200).

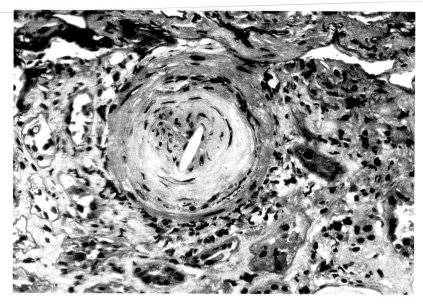

FIG. 2.104 Atheroemboli. A single, small inconspicuous cholesterol embolus was present in this patient, who presented with acute worsening of hypertension and acute decline in renal function. There is surrounding mononuclear cell reaction and underlying arteriosclerosis (Jones silver stain, ×200).

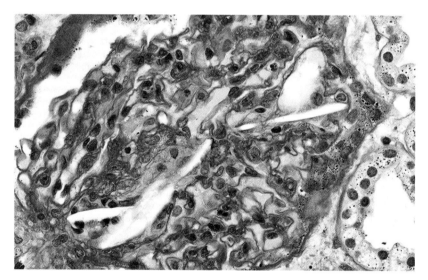

FIG. 2.105 Atheroemboli. Cholesterol emboli may rarely enter the glomerulus. Here there is focal surrounding mononuclear cell reaction. Numerous cholesterol emboli were found in other arterioles and arteries in this patient (periodic acid Schiff, ×400).

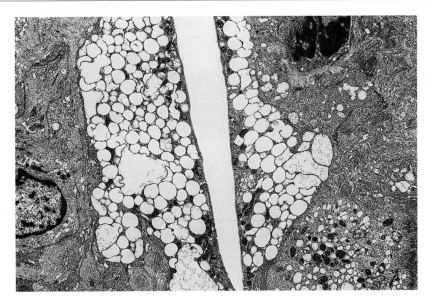

FIG. 2.106 Atheroemboli. Occasionally the only cholesterol embolus in the sample may be present in the sample dedicated for electron microscopy. The clear needle-shaped space left by the cholesterol crystal is illustrated, with surrounding foamy macrophage reaction (transmission electron microscopy, ×6000).

Etiology/Pathogenesis

Atherosclerosis is the requisite underlying condition for occurrence of atheroemboli. Cholesterol emboli may happen spontaneously, or more commonly following invasive procedures or vascular surgery. In autopsies of patients with mild atherosclerosis of the aorta, cholesterol emboli were rare (1.7%-4%), rising to 7%-30% in patients with severe disease or abdominal aortic aneurysms. Some 25% of patients who had undergone aortography had cholesterol emboli, and in patients who had undergone resection of an abdominal aneurysm, cholesterol emboli were present in 77%.

The surface of the atheromatous plaque is covered by endothelial cells with an underlying fibrous cap, consisting of smooth muscle cells, macrophages, and extracellular matrix proteins. The center of the plaque contains necrotic cellular debris, cholesterol bound to proteins and cholesteryl esters, macrophages, and foam cells. When the plaque ruptures, grumous fluid extrudes (athere, Greek for gruel), including the cholesterol crystals, which shower the organs below the site of plaque rupture. Atherosclerotic plaques are much more common in the abdominal aorta than in the thoracic aorta and have a particular propensity for the areas adjacent to or surrounding the ostia of branch vessels. Thus, the distribution of cholesterol emboli is largely to organs below the diaphragm.

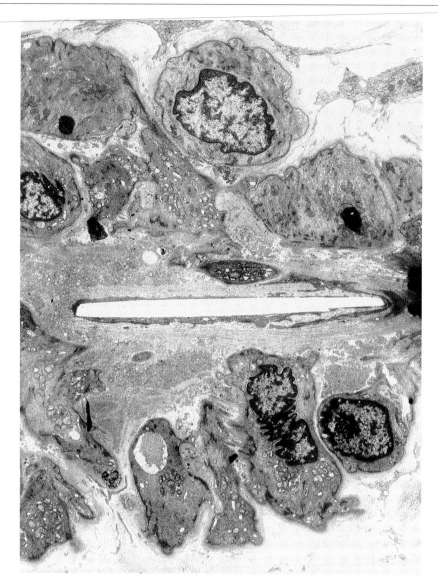

FIG. 2.107 Atheroemboli. The needle-shaped space left by the cholesterol crystal is seen distorting and pushing the endothelium in this small arteriole (transmission electron microscopy, ×3000).

Selected Reading

Fine, M.J., Kapoor, W., Falanga, V., 1987. Cholesterol crystal embolization: a review of 221 cases in the English literature. Angiology 38 (10), 769-784.

Flory, C.M., 1945. Arterial occlusions produced by emboli from eroded aortic atheromatous plaques. American Journal of Pathology 21, 549-565.

Fogo, A., Stone, W.J., 1992. Atheroembolic renal disease. In: Martinez-Maldonado, M., (Ed.), Hypertension and Renal Disease in the Elderly. Blackwell Scientific, Cambridge, MA, 261-271.

Gore, I., McCombs, H.L., Lindquist, R.L., 1964. Observations on the fate of cholesterol emboli. Journal of Atherosclerosis Research 4, 527-535.

Greenberg, A., Bastacky, S.I., Iqbal, A., et al., 1997. Focal segmental glomerulosclerosis associated with nephrotic syndrome in cholesterol atheroembolism: clinicopathological correlations. American Journal of Kidney Disease 29 (3), 334-344.

Ramirez, G., O'Neill, W.M., Lambert, R., et al., 1978. Cholesterol embolization. A complication of angiography. Archives of Internal Medicine 138, 1430-1432.

Tubulointerstitial Diseases

Introduction

The tubulointerstitial compartment is affected in all forms of renal disease with changes that include tubular epithelial injury, atrophy, hypertrophy/hyperplasia, and fibrosis. These changes can be primary with the tubule and interstitium as the target of damage but are often secondary to primary glomerular or vascular disease where tubular atrophy and interstitial scarring accompany primary glomerular or vascular disease. This chapter will focus on those tubular and interstitial diseases where the tubules and interstitium are the primary target of the pathogenic process and which results in structural and functional alterations.

Primary tubular and interstitial diseases are a group of diverse renal diseases with involvement of the renal tubules and interstitium resulting from a variety of different etiologies and pathogenic mechanisms. The various etiologies and mechanisms include infection, obstruction, immune mediated, ischemic, and toxic tubular and interstitial injury (Table 3.1). Despite the diverse etiology, the clinical presentations usually have great similarities. In acute

TABLE 3-1 Etiologies of Tubular and Interstitial Diseases

Infections
  Bacterial
  Viral
  Parasitic
Toxins
  Drug-induced
    Direct toxic-mediated
    Hypersensitivity mediated
  Environmental toxins
    Heavy metals
    Hydrocarbons
    Fungal toxins
Metabolic diseases
  Diabetes
  Hypercalcemia
  Urate nephropathy
  Oxalate nephropathy
Physical
  Obstruction
  Radiation
Vascular disease
  Acute tubular injury
  Arterionephrosclerosis
Neoplasms
  Lymphoma
  Multiple myeloma

cases, the clinical presentation may be so severe as to result in acute renal failure. In less severe and chronic cases, the functional manifestations usually include impaired urinary concentrating ability, impaired ability to secrete acid into the urine, diminished reabsorption of sodium, hyperkalemia, and azotemia. In advanced cases, the presentation may be that of chronic renal failure or end-stage kidney. In cases of moderate renal failure, a sudden worsening of renal failure may herald an activation of a new tubulointerstitial nephritis. It is under circumstances such as these that renal biopsy is often performed to identify the underlying process.

The World Health Organization Collaborating Center for Histologic Classification of Renal Diseases proposed a new classification that takes into account the etiologic pathogenetic and clinical features in addition to the histology (Table 3.2). In this chapter, we will focus on morphology as applied to renal biopsy diagnosis.

Infection is a major cause of tubulointerstitial nephritis. In the WHO classification, four different forms of renal involvement are described:

1. Acute infectious tubulointerstitial nephritis, which is the result of the direct invasion of the renal parenchyma by microorganisms and subsequent proliferation of bacteria, fungi, or viruses. Classical acute bacterial pyelonephritis is the paradigm of this form.
2. Acute tubulointerstitial nephritis associated with systemic infection but not caused by direct renal infection, which may be due to a hypersensitivity reaction. The histologic picture is often similar to that of drug-induced tubulointerstitial nephritis. The interstitial nephritis associated with Legionnaires disease is an example of this type of involvement.

TABLE 3-2 WHO Classification of Tubulointerstitial Diseases

Infection
  Acute infectious tubulointerstitial nephritis
  Acute tubulointerstitial nephritis associated with systemic infection
  Chronic infectious tubulointerstitial nephritis (chronic pyelonephritis)
  Specific renal infection
Drug-induced tubulointerstitial nephritis
  Acute drug-induced tubulotoxic injury
  Drug-induced hypersensitivity tubulointerstitial nephritis
  Chronic drug-induced tubulointerstitial nephritis
Tubulointerstitial nephritis associated with immune disorders
  Induced by antibodies reacting with tubular antigens
  Induced by autologous or exogenous antigen–antibody complexes
  Induced by, or associated with, cell-mediated hypersensitivity
  Induced by immediate (IgE-type) hypersensitivity
Obstructive uropathy
Vesicoureteral reflux-associated nephropathy (reflux nephropathy)
Tubulointerstitial nephritis associated with papillary necrosis
Heavy metal–induced tubular and tubulointerstitial lesions
Acute tubular injury/necrosis
  Toxic
  Ischemic
Tubular and tubulointerstitial nephropathy caused by metabolic disturbances
Hereditary renal tubulointerstitial disorders
Tubulointerstitial nephritis associated with neoplastic disorders
Tubulointerstitial lesions in glomerular and vascular diseases
Miscellaneous disorders
  Balkan endemic nephropathy

---

3. Chronic infectious tubulointerstitial nephritis in which bacteria have an important role but renal injury may persist and occur in the absence of continued bacterial infection. Xanthogranulomatous pyelonephritis and malakoplakia are examples.
4. Specific renal infections such as tuberculosis and leprosy, which have distinctive histologic manifestations that are similar to involvement by these organisms in other organ systems.

Acute Pyelonephritis

In acute bacterial pyelonephritis associated with ascending infection, the inflammatory infiltrate is predominately polymorphonuclear, involving both medullary and cortical portions of the kidney. Polymorphonuclear leukocytes are present within the tubular lumina as well as invading the tubular epithelium and being abundantly present in the interstitium (Fig. 3.1). Areas of necrosis and abscess formation may be seen as well. Hematogenous infection of the kidney results in the presence of numerous small cortical abscesses without significant medullary involvement (Fig. 3.2). The abscesses are frequently glomerulocentric, and tubular involvement may not be prominent (Fig. 3.3). While the presence of a neutrophilic invasion of the tubular lumina or of abscesses is characteristic of acute bacterial tubulointerstitial nephritis (Figs. 3.4-3.6), it should be remembered that the cellular infiltrate frequently includes some lymphocytes, plasma cells, macrophages, and occasionally eosinophils, and the differential diagnosis should include consideration of the possibility of idiopathic or drug-induced tubulointerstitial nephritis that is not infectious. In addition, in viral renal infections

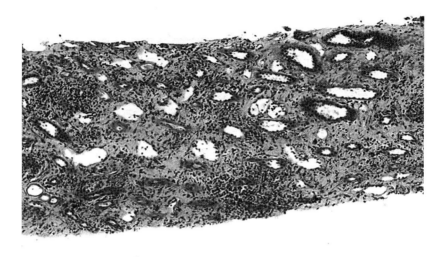

FIG. 3.1 Acute pyelonephritis. Low-power image of a renal biopsy showing diffuse interstitial infiltrate that is predominately polymorphonuclear leukocytic. There is interstitial edema; some tubular atrophy and leukocytes can be seen in the lumen of the tubules (hematoxylin and eosin, ×100).

Key Diagnostic Feature of Acute Pyelonephritis

- Intratubular plugs of polymorphonuclear leukocytes.

Differential Diagnosis of Acute Pyelonephritis

- Polymorphonuclear leukocytes may be associated with degenerated cells or may be a reaction to crystals such as in light chain cast nephropathy (LCCN). These can be distinguished by examination of the tissue for such crystals and by immunofluorescent staining to detect monoclonal staining in LCCN.

---

such as with adenovirus and hanta virus, the infiltrate is often hemorrhagic and mononuclear cells tend to predominate (Figs. 3.7, 3.8).

Etiology/Pathogenesis

Acute uncomplicated pyelonephritis typically occurs in healthy, young women and must be distinguished from acute complicated pyelonephritis (i.e., in the presence of obstruction or reflux) and from chronic pyelonephritis. Acute infectious tubulointerstitial nephritis is generally designated as pyelonephritis, implying that there is involvement of the collecting system as well as the renal parenchyma by the inflammatory process. Both acute and chronic pyelonephritis are frequently associated with congenital or acquired obstructive lesions of the lower urinary tract or are associated with conditions resulting in retention of residual urine in the bladder. A variety of pathogens can be identified using staining techniques for microorganism identification, which include Brown–Brenn, periodic acid Schiff (PAS), and Grocott silver stains. *Escherichia coli* is the major causative pathogen in both uncomplicated upper and lower urinary tract infection in young women, being present in approximately 70-95% of cases. In

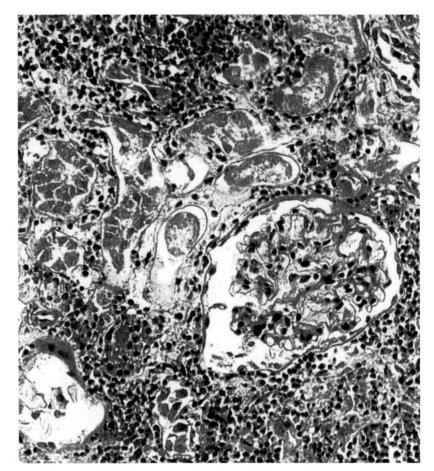

FIG. 3.2 Acute pyelonephritis. There is a diffuse interstitial infiltrate with polymorphonuclear leukocytes (hematoxylin and eosin, ×200).

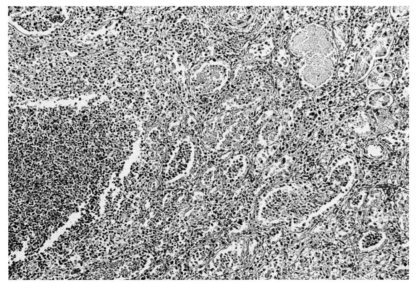

FIG. 3.3 Acute pyelonephritis with abscess formation. The abscesses are frequently glomerulocentric and are destructive of the renal parenchyma (hematoxylin and eosin, ×200).

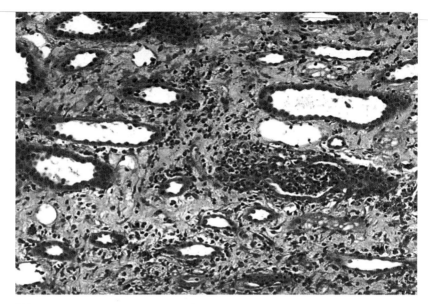

FIG. 3.4 Acute pyelonephritis. The infectious nature of an active interstitial nephritis is best identified by the presence of polymorphonuclear leukocytes within the lumen of the tubules (hematoxylin and eosin, ×400).

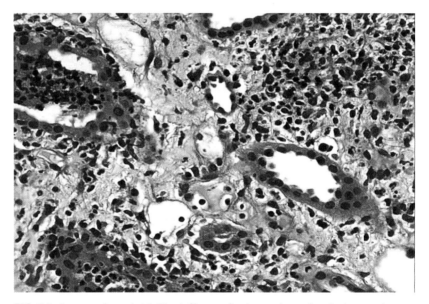

FIG. 3.5 Acute pyelonephritis. The infiltrate of polymorphonuclear leukocytes is not only present within the interstitium and in the tubular lumens but evidence of tubulitis also is seen (hematoxylin and eosin, ×400).

older age groups, there is an increase in infections due to *Klebsiella* spp. (6% in women and 11% in men) and *Enterococcus* spp. (3% in women and 7% in men). Hematogenous infections are most frequently caused by *Staphylococcus aureus* or atypical bacteria (mycobacterium avium-intracellulare or Ehrlichia) (Figs 3.9, 3.10) or fungal organisms including Candida and Aspergillus. These are especially important in immunosuppressed individuals. Although renal biopsy rarely gives a sampling of the renal papilla and pelvis, it is important to remember that these structures are involved in infection. Genetic factors may be associated with risk of acquiring acute pyelonephritis in children and adults. A case–control study of women

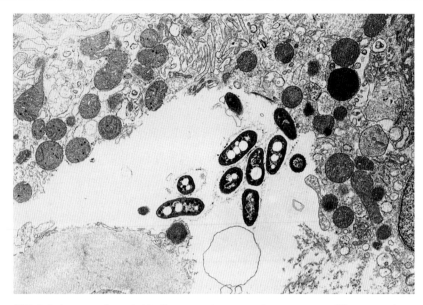

FIG. 3.6 Acute pyelonephritis. Electron microscopy demonstrates coliform organisms within the lumen of a tubule (transmission electron microscopy, ×10,000).

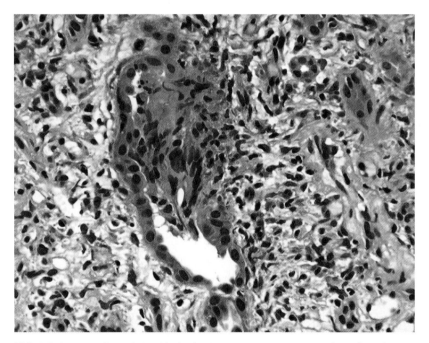

FIG. 3.7 Acute pyelonephritis. Viral infections may mimic acute pyelonephritis but can be often distinguished by the presence of atypical tubular epithelial cells. Viral infection is described separately later (hematoxylin and eosin, ×400).

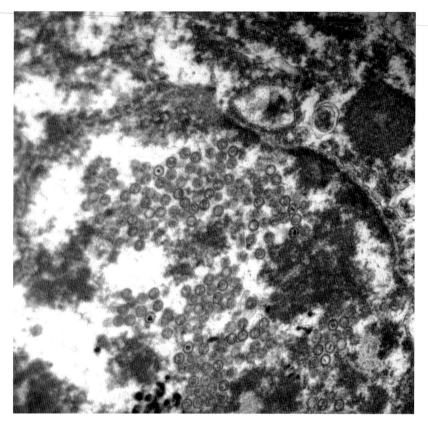

FIG. 3.8 Acute pyelonephritis. Viral infections may mimic acute pyelonephritis but can be often distinguished by the presence of atypical tubular epithelial cells. Here Herpes virus is detected in the nucleus.

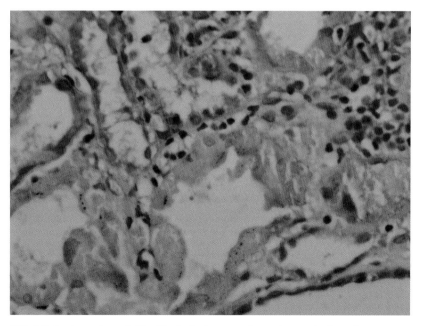

FIG. 3.9 Acute pyelonephritis. Atypical microorganisms also can be found. *Mycobacterium avium-intracellulare* is seen in this example.

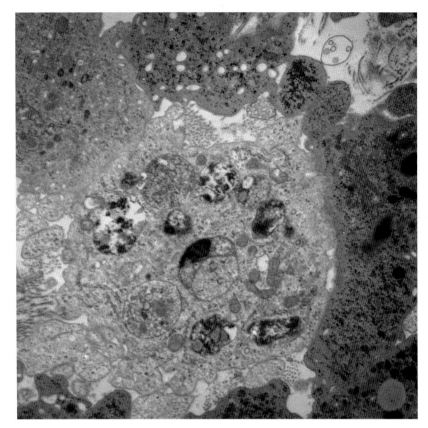

FIG. 3.10 Acute pyelonephritis. Atypical microorganisms also can be found. Intracellular *Ehrlichia* was found in this biopsy.

suggested that polymorphisms in Toll-like receptor pathway genes are associated with altered risk of acute pyelonephritis.

Selected Reading

Hawn, T.R., Scholes, D., Li, S.S., et al., 2009. Toll-like receptor polymorphisms and susceptibility to urinary tract infections in adult women. PLoS One 4, e5990.

Ki, M., Park, T., Choi, B., et al., 2004. The epidemiology of acute pyelonephritis in South Korea, 1997-1999. American Journal of Epidemiology 160, 985-993.

Scholes, D., Hooton, T.M., Roberts, P.L., et al., 2005. Risk factors associated with acute pyelonephritis in healthy women. Annals of Internal Medicine 142, 20.

Chronic Pyelonephritis and Reflux Nephropathy

Chronic pyelonephritis is a controversial term. It is often difficult to separate chronic infectious tubulointerstitial nephritis or true chronic pyelonephritis from many other chronic interstitial diseases as the histologic changes are relatively nonspecific. Chronic interstitial scarring, tubular atrophy, and the presence of an infiltrate of lymphocytes and plasma cells are lesions common to many disorders. Similar changes can be seen in arterionephrosclerosis, chronic urinary tract obstruction, chronic glomerular diseases, diabetic nephropathy, and numerous other causes. For this reason, chronic infectious tubular interstitial nephritis cannot be diagnosed with any degree of certainty on the limited sampling usually achieved by renal biopsy. A better diagnosis can be made when information concerning the renal papilla, calyces, and pelvis is available from radiologic examination as well as the gross morphology of the kidney obtained with sophisticated imaging techniques such as ultrasonography or magnetic resonance imaging.

Chronic pyelonephritis results in a coarse renal scarring that is characteristically focal in its distribution. Microscopically, the findings consist of tubular atrophy, interstitial scarring, and a chronic inflammatory infiltrate (Figs. 3.11-3.13). The tubules are either collapsed or dilated and lined by a flattened epithelium and sometimes filled with colloid casts (Fig. 3.14).

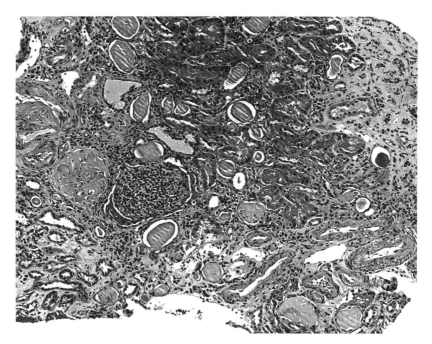

FIG. 3.11 Chronic pyelonephritis manifests a nonspecific interstitial infiltrate predominately with lymphocytes. There is evidence of destruction of the renal parenchyma with atrophy of tubules (hematoxylin and eosin, ×200).

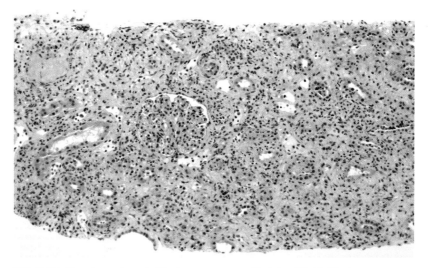

FIG. 3.12 Chronic pyelonephritis shows a nonspecific interstitial infiltrate predominately with lymphocytes. The parenchyma is diffusely infiltrated (hematoxylin and eosin, ×200).

Key Diagnostic Features of Chronic Pyelonephritis/Reflux Nephritis

- Jigsaw pattern/geographic pattern of scarring
- Thyroidization of tubules (suggestive, not pathognomonic)

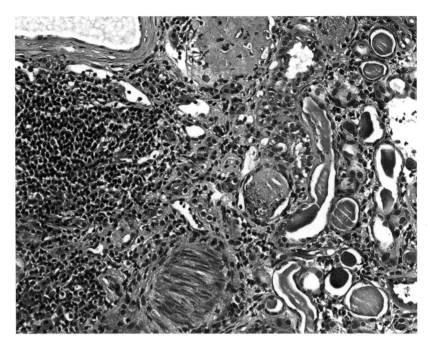

FIG. 3.13 Chronic pyelonephritis. Tubules are filled with proteinaceous casts associated with a diffuse interstitial infiltrate of lymphocytes and interstitial scarring (hematoxylin and eosin, ×200).

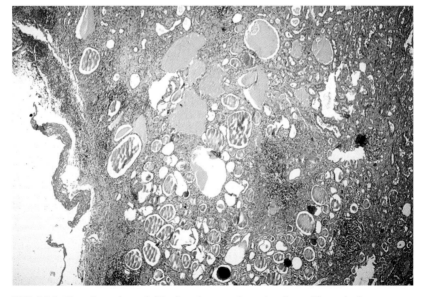

FIG. 3.14 Chronic pyelonephritis. Scarring may be extensive, with marked destruction of the normal architecture leading to end-stage renal disease. The dilatation of the tubules filled with proteinaceous material has often been termed thyroidization (hematoxylin and eosin, ×200).

> ## Differential Diagnosis of Reflux Nephropathy/Chronic Pyelonephritis
>
> - This must be distinguished from scarring due to vascular disease, based on the more extensive vascular sclerosis seen in that entity, and from primary focal segmental glomerulosclerosis (FSGS) (see FSGS).
> - Other specific causes of chronic tubulointerstitial scarring, such as viral infection, crystals, or drugs, must be excluded by examining for viral change, crystals (including polarization of tissue), and features of hypersensitivity reaction such as eosinophils and/or nonnecrotizing granulomas.

This latter pattern has been termed "thyroidization." The inflammatory infiltrate is quite variable but consists predominately of lymphocytes as well as plasma cells and, to a lesser extent, mononuclear cells but may contain neutrophils.

In chronic pyelonephritis associated with reflux or obstruction, Tamm–Horsfall protein can be identified in the interstitium by the presence of strongly PAS-positive amorphous or finely fibrillar material. In instances where reflux has contributed to the development of chronic pyelonephritis, focal and segmental glomerulosclerosis may be extremely prominent and may suggest the possibility of a primary glomerular lesion. The histopathologic changes of chronic pyelonephritis have also been described with so-called reflux nephropathy associated with vesicoureteral reflux.

Etiology/Pathogenesis

Chronic pyelonephritis is the consequence of persistence of untreated and incompletely resolved acute pyelonephritis, and thus has many of the same risk factors and pathogeneses. In addition, structural abnormalities promoting reflux contribute to the lesions of chronic pyelonephritis and reflux nephropathy.

Selected Reading

Tolkoff-Rubin, N.E.R.R., 1983. Urinary tract infection. Tubulo-interstitial nephropathies. Contemporary issues in nephrology, vol. 10. Churchill Livingstone, New York, pp. 49-82.

Xanthogranulomatous Pyelonephritis

Xanthogranulomatous pyelonephritis is a distinct type of infectious pyelonephritis. It occurs most often in middle-aged women with a history of recurrent urinary tract infections. Microscopically, there is a diffuse granulomatous inflammatory infiltrate, which includes large numbers of foamy histiocytes and occasional multinucleated giant cells in addition to lymphocytes, plasma cells, and neutrophils (Figs. 3.15, 3.16,). The lesion is destructive, and renal parenchyma may not be easily identified within affected areas.

Etiology/Pathogenesis

Escherichia coli is the most frequently associated etiologic agent but *Proteus mirabilis* and *Staphylococcus aureus* have also been reported as causative agents. It is due to a defect in macrophage processing of bacteria. Occasionally, microabscesses containing basophilic bacterial colonies surrounded by eosinophilic homogenous material (Botryomycosis) can be identified.

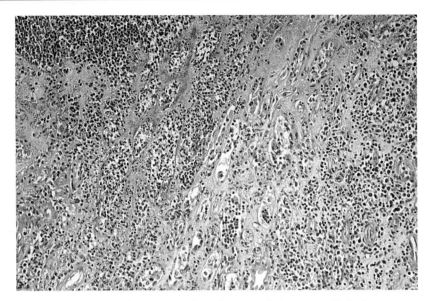

FIG. 3.15 Xanthogranulomatous pyelonephritis is a distinct type of infectious pyelonephritis. There is a diffuse granulomatous infiltrate, which includes macrophages as well as polymorphonuclear leukocytes (hematoxylin and eosin, ×200).

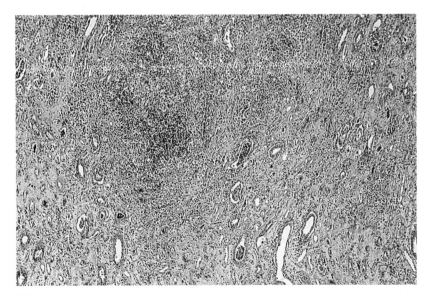

FIG. 3.16 Xanthogranulomatory pyelonephritis. Granulomatous structures can involve both cortex and medulla as seen here. Microabscesses containing eosinophilic homogenous material are also present (hematoxylin and eosin, ×100).

Selected Reading

Hill, G.S., Droz, D., Nochy, D., 2001. The woman who loved well but not too wisely, or the vicissitudes of immunosuppression. American Journal of Kidney Disease 37, 1324-1329.

Zorzos, I., Moutzouris, V., Korakianitis, G., et al., 2003. Analysis of 39 cases of xanthogranulomatous pyelonephritis with emphasis on CT findings. Scandinavian Journal of Urology and Nephrology 37, 342-347.

Malakoplakia

Malakoplakia has a similar gross and microscopic appearance to xanthogranulomatous pyelo-nephritis. Confluent nodules of the homogenous yellow-tan tissue are seen to replace large areas of renal parenchyma grossly. Microscopically, there is an inflammatory infiltrate, which consists of histiocytes with relatively few lymphocytes and plasma cells (Fig. 3.17). Charac-teristic Michaelis–Gutmann bodies are found both within cells and extracellularly in the stroma (Fig. 3.18). These calcospherites stain positively with Von Kossa (calcium) and PAS and are thought to represent an aggregation of calcium-containing crystals induced by a central nidus of bacterial breakdown products, and fibroblastic proliferation and scarring are extremely prominent.

Etiology/Pathogenesis

Malakoplakia is an unusual consequence of an inflammatory reaction most frequently second-ary to infection by *E. coli*, and is thought to be initiated by inadequate clearance of bacteria, perhaps related to immune deficiency or leukocyte abnormalities. It is similar to xanthogranu-lomatous pyelonephritis and may represent a chronic sequelae of this process.

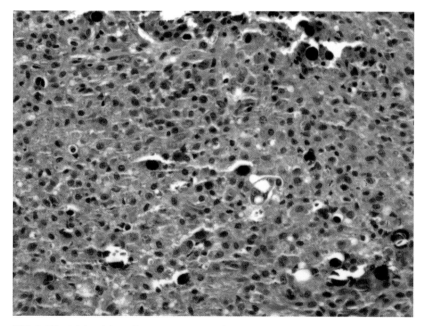

FIG. 3.17 Malakoplakia. There is prominent fibroblastic proliferation and inflammatory infiltrate, with numerous histiocytes and only scattered lymphocytes and plasma cells (hematoxylin and eosin, ×200).

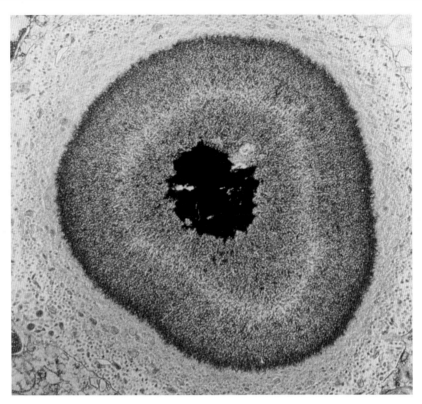

FIG. 3.18 Malakoplakia. Characteristic Michaelis–Gutmann body with central core, by electron microscopy (transmission electron microscopy, ×8000).

Selected Reading

Hill, G.S., Droz, D., Nochy, D., 2001. The woman who loved well but not too wisely, or the vicissitudes of immunosuppression. American Journal of Kidney Disease 37, 1324-1329.

Mignon, F., Mery, J.P., Mougenot, B., et al., 1984. Granulomatous interstitial nephritis. Advances in Nephrology from the Necker Hospital 13, 219-245.

Acute Tubulointerstitial Nephritis—Drug-Related

Acute interstitial nephritis is most often induced by drug therapy. Although the clinical manifestations may be variable, they are usually heralded by fever and hematuria as well as azotemia. Eosinophilia occurs in a majority of cases. Urinalysis reveals hematuria, sterile pyuria, and moderate proteinuria. Eosinophils may be detected in the urinary sediment. A skin rash is seen in some patients lending support to the concept that the disease is immunologically mediated. The azotemia may be severe and patients may present with acute renal failure, leading to the use of the renal biopsy as a diagnostic procedure.

One of the most distinguishing features of acute drug-induced tubulointerstitial nephritis is the nature of the interstitial infiltrate. The interstitium is edematous with tubules separated by a pale staining interstitium (in contrast to the dense staining of fibrosis) and infiltrated with a significant number of eosinophils and mononuclear cells (Figs. 3.19-3.21). The infiltrate is characteristically focal and most prominent at the cortical medullary junction and often surrounds individual tubules. The mononuclear portion of the infiltrate is predominately lymphocytes with some macrophages and plasma cells that sometime form granulomas (Figs. 3.22, 3.23). The eosinophils tend to concentrate in small foci and may form eosinophilic microabscesses (Figs. 3.24, 3.25). Neutrophils can be present but are uncommon (Fig. 3.26).

Text continued on page 396

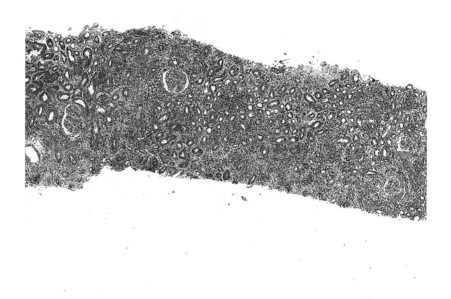

FIG. 3.19 Acute interstitial nephritis. There is a diffuse interstitial infiltrate with evidence of interstitial edema. Glomeruli are relatively well preserved (hematoxylin and eosin, ×100).

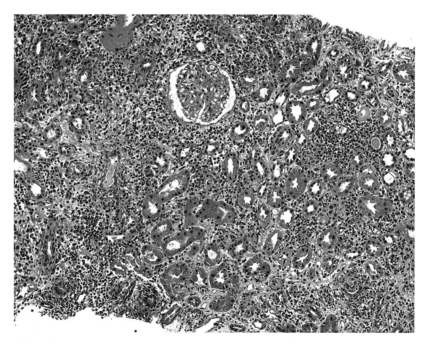

FIG. 3.20 Acute interstitial nephritis. Higher power demonstrates the presence of mononuclear cells throughout the interstitium; the tubule lumina are relatively free of leukocytic infiltrate (hematoxylin and eosin, ×200).

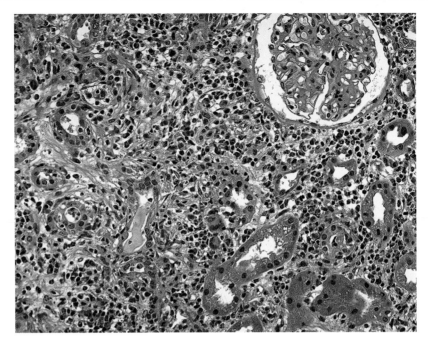

FIG. 3.21 Acute interstitial nephritis. There is infiltration of the tubules by the interstitial infiltrate, which is distinctive of tubulitis (hematoxylin and eosin, ×400).

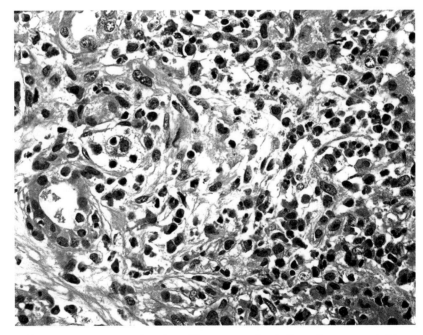

FIG. 3.22 Acute interstitial nephritis. The mononuclear infiltrate is accompanied by abundant eosinophils and may have a granulomatous appearance (hematoxylin and eosin, ×400).

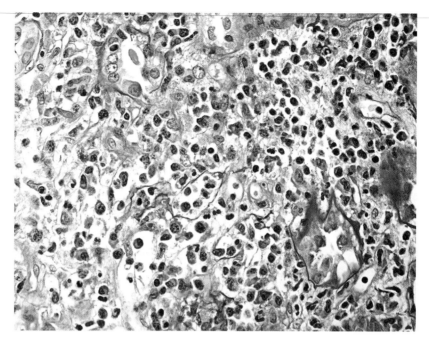

FIG. 3.23 Acute interstitial nephritis. The granulomata often involve the tubules in a destructive fashion (hematoxylin and eosin, ×400).

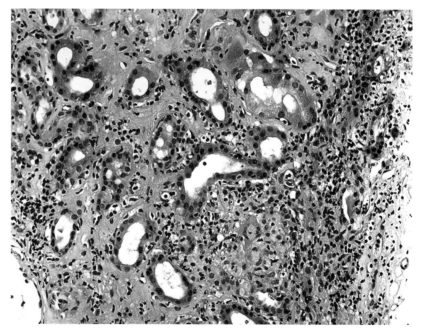

FIG. 3.24 Acute interstitial nephritis. The eosinophilic infiltrate can sometimes be dense and form small eosinophilic abscesses (hematoxylin and eosin, ×200).

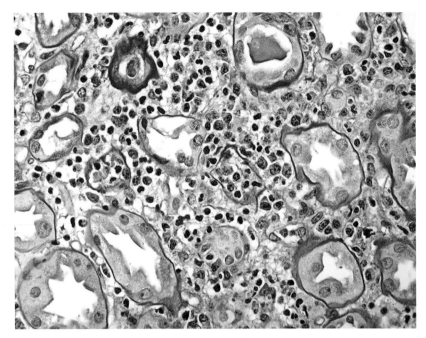

FIG. 3.25 Acute interstitial nephritis. There is destruction of the tubular epithelium with relative preservation of the basement membrane (periodic acid Schiff, ×400).

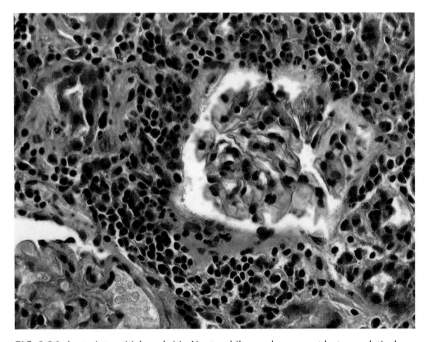

FIG. 3.26 Acute interstitial nephritis. Neutrophils may be present but are relatively uncommon (hematoxylin and eosin, ×400).

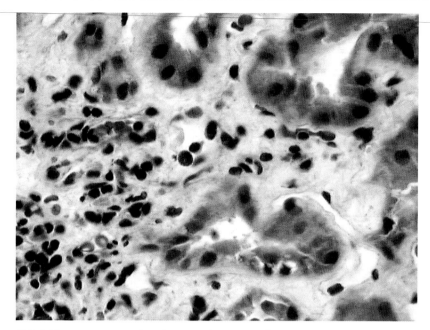

FIG. 3.27 Acute interstitial nephritis. Higher power of tubulitis demonstrating interstitial edema and invasion of the tubular epithelium by lymphocytes (hematoxylin and eosin, ×400).

A second distinguishing characteristic is the presence of tubulitis (Figs. 3.27, 3.28). Particularly with PAS stains, lymphocytes can be seen invading the tubules beneath the tubular basement membrane (TBM). Variable degrees of tubular epithelial cell damage (Figs. 3.29-3.31) with evidence of regeneration as identified by the presence of mitotic figures and pleomorphic nuclei are almost always found, but extensive necrosis of the epithelium is rare.

Etiology/Pathogenesis

It is now widely recognized that a large variety of drugs including β-lactam antibiotics, nonsteroidal anti-inflammatory drugs, diuretics, anticonvulsants, proton pump inhibitors, and an increasingly diverse group of other drugs can be associated with an allergic acute tubular interstitial nephritis. Although drugs have been implicated in most cases of allergic interstitial nephritis, additional causes include autoimmune disorders. A similar picture can be found in patients with lupus nephritis and rarely in association with anti-TBM antibodies. Biopsy-proven instances of acute oliguric tubular interstitial nephritis with a similar histologic picture but without any known drug exposure have also been reported. One special group includes the association of acute tubulointerstitial nephritis with uveitis (i.e., TINU syndrome) and bone marrow and lymph node granulomas. This syndrome occurs predominately in adolescent girls and young women and is presumed to have an autoimmune etiology. This entity must be distinguished from renal sarcoid involvement, which also characteristically has numerous, even at times confluent, granulomas.

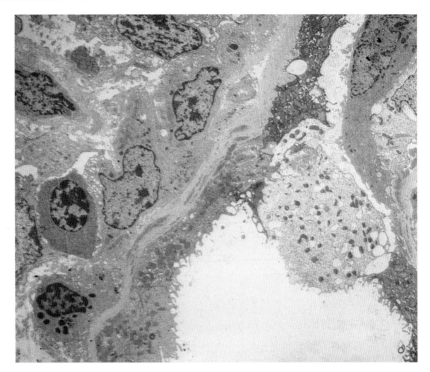

FIG. 3.28 Acute interstitial nephritis. Electron micrograph demonstrates the mononuclear infiltrate with the eosinophils, plasma cells, and activated lymphocytes (transmission electron microscopy, ×2000).

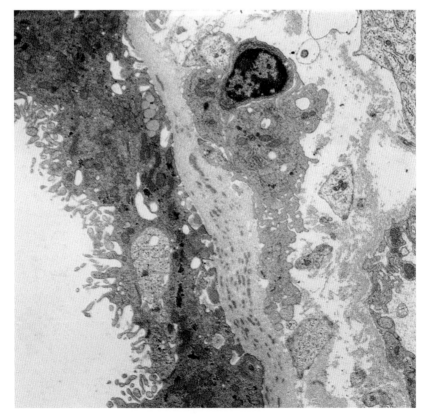

FIG. 3.29 Acute interstitial nephritis. Mononuclear cells traversing the endothelium of a peritubular capillary are shown (transmission electron microscopy, ×3000).

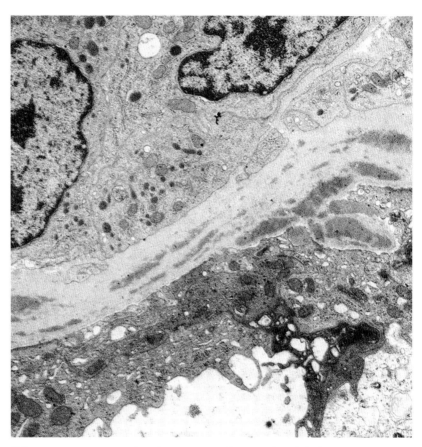

FIG. 3.30 Acute interstitial nephritis. Varying degrees of epithelial damage are present, demonstrated here by loss of the apical membrane and swelling of the cells (transmission electron microscopy, ×3000).

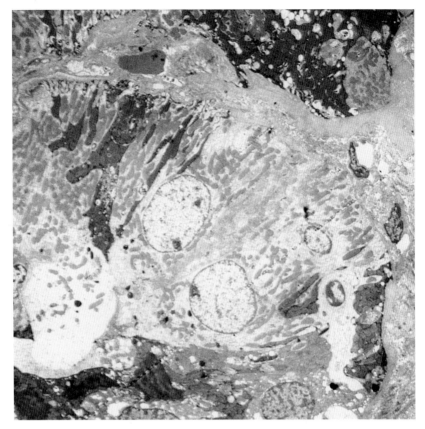

FIG. 3.31 Acute interstitial nephritis. More severe damage with evidence of cellular necrosis is also seen (transmission electron microscopy, ×4000).

Selected Reading

Haas, M., Spargo, B.H., Wit, E.J., et al., 2000. Etiologies and outcome of acute renal insufficiency in older adults: a renal biopsy study of 259 cases. American Journal of Kidney Disease 35, 544-546.

Rastegar, A., Kashgarian, M., 1998. The clinical spectrum of tubulointerstitial nephritis. Kidney International 54, 313-327.

Acute Tubulointerstitial Nephritis—Viral Infection

Bacterial infections result in predominantly intratubular polymorphonuclear leukocytes, characteristic of acute pyelonephritis (see Acute Pyelonephritis). Viral infections may give rise to a more predominantly chronic interstitial infiltrate, with admixed mononuclear cells and more scarce polymorphonuclear leukocytes. In viral renal infections such as with adenovirus and hanta virus, the interstitium is often hemorrhagic and mononuclear cells tend to predominate (see Fig. 3.7). Other viruses may also infect the kidney, notably HIV, BK virus, and cytomegalovirus, and are discussed under the Transplantation section and under HIV-associated nephropathy.

Etiology/Pathogenesis

Viruses may cause renal injury by direct parenchymal infection (e.g., cytomegalovirus) and/or by cytokine injury secondary to systemic and/or infiltrating cell/dendritic cell infection. Direct evidence of parenchymal infection may be seen by viral inclusions, or cytopathic changes, with enlarged, smudgy nuclei. Adenovirus infection occurs in immunocompromised hosts. In contrast, Hanta virus infection may occur in immunocompetent patients. The varying clinical syndromes due to Hanta virus in Europe versus the United States appear to reflect differences in the carrier rodent population. Subclinical Hanta virus infection has been postulated to result in hypertension consequent to parenchymal scarring, based on serological studies, but the causality has not been proven.

Selected Reading

Peters, C.J., Simpson, G.L., Levy, H., 1999. Spectrum of hantavirus infection: hemorrhagic fever with renal syndrome and hantavirus pulmonary syndrome. Annual Review of Medicine 50, 531-545.

Settergren, B., Ahlm, C., Alexeyev, O., et al., 1997. Pathogenetic and clinical aspects of the renal involvement in hemorrhagic fever with renal syndrome. Renal Failure 19, 1-14.

Teague, M.W., Glick, A.D., Fogo, A.B., 1991. Adenovirus infection of the kidney: mass formation in a patient with Hodgkin's disease. American Journal of Kidney Disease 18, 499-502.

Anti-TBM Antibody Nephritis

Anti-TBM antibody nephritis is very rare and presents with acute kidney injury with increased serum creatinine. By light microscopy, there is lymphoplasmacytic interstitial infiltrate with occasional neutrophils, with tubulitis and associated acute tubular injury with vacuolation, sloughing of tubular epithelial cells, and edema (Figs. 3.32, 3.33). There are no specific changes in glomeruli or arteries, except when anti-TBM staining is associated with anti-GBM antibody glomerulonephritis. In such cases, glomeruli show destructive, crescentic lesions. By immunofluorescence microscopy, there is intense linear staining along TBMs with IgG (Figs. 3.34, 3.35), most often associated with complement that may be discontinuous or continuous linear. Deposits are not visualized by electron microscopy.

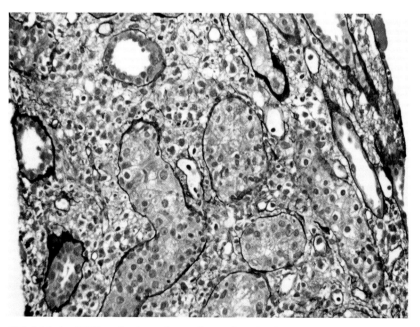

FIG. 3.32 Anti-TBM antibody nephritis. There is lymphoplasmacytic interstitial infiltrate with tubulitis and associated acute tubular injury (periodic acid Schiff, ×200). *TBM,* tubular basement membrane.

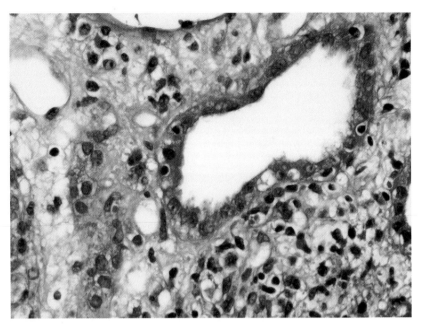

FIG. 3.33 Anti-TBM antibody nephritis. There is lymphoplasmacytic interstitial infiltrate with tubulitis and occasional eosinophils and associated acute tubular injury, changes that are not distinguishable from hypersensitivity drug reaction by light microscopy (hematoxylin and eosin, ×200). *TBM*, tubular basement membrane.

Key Diagnostic Features of Anti-TBM Antibody Nephritis

- Intense interstitial nephritis with lymphoplasmacytic infiltrate with occasional neutrophils
- Linear deposition of IgG and C3 along TBMs

TBM, tubular basement membrane.

Differential Diagnosis of Anti-TBM Antibody Nephritis

- Primary anti-TBM antibody nephritis does not show specific findings in glomeruli or vessels. Circulating anti-TBM antibodies may be detected in the serum of these patients, and show reactivity with normal TBMs.
- In some patients with anti-GBM antibody glomerulonephritis, anti-TBM linear staining is present, usually weaker and not typically associated with intense injury. In these patients, glomeruli show typical changes of anti-GBM antibody glomerulonephritis.

TBM, tubular basement membrane.

Etiology/Pathogenesis

Primary anti-TBM antibodies are exceedingly rare, but have been described in some patients to a 58-kilodalton protein called tubulointerstitial nephritis antigen. This antibody reaction may occasionally be triggered by drug exposure, and is also rarely seen in the transplant. Anti-TBM antibodies have been detected in 50-70% of patients with anti-GBM antibody glomerulonephritis, but typically with only focal and less intense TBM linear IgG staining. Patients with membranous nephropathy may rarely have anti-TBM antibodies, in most cases

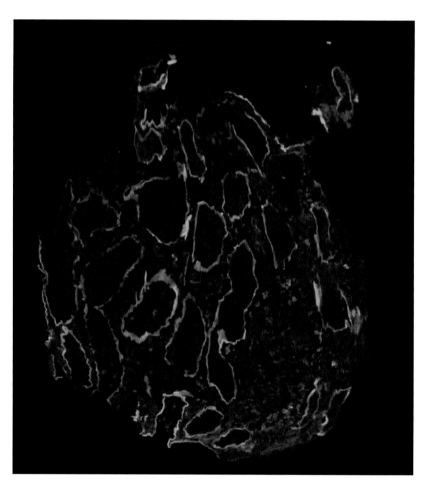

FIG. 3.34 Anti-TBM antibody nephritis. In anti-TBM antibody nephritis, there is linear staining with IgG along TBMs (anti-IgG immunofluorescence, ×200). *TBM,* tubular basement membrane.

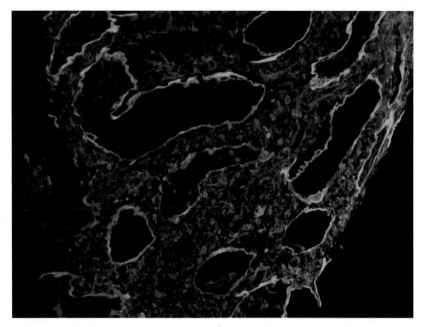

FIG. 3.35 Anti-TBM antibody nephritis. The linear staining with IgG along tubular basement membranes is evident (anti-IgG immunofluorescence, ×200). *TBM,* tubular basement membrane.

directed against the tubulointerstitial nephritis antigen. In the transplant setting, the occasional appearance of anti-TBM linear staining is thought to be related to antigenic polymorphism and does not affect prognosis or outcome.

Selected Reading

Andres, G., Brentjens, J., Kohli, R., et al., 1978. Histology of human tubulo-interstitial nephritis associated with antibodies to renal basement membranes. Kidney International 13, 480-491.

Brentjens, J.R., Matsuo, S., Fukatsu, A., et al., 1989. Immunologic studies in two patients with antitubular basement membrane nephritis. American Journal of Medicine 86, 603-608.

Clayman, M.D., Martinez-Hernandez, A., Michaud, L., et al., 1985. Isolation and characterization of the nephritogenic antigen producing anti-tubular basement membrane disease. Journal of Experimental Medicine 161, 290-305.

IgG4-Related Tubulointerstitial Nephritis

Tubulointerstitial nephritis may have many causes. Recently, a group of multiorgan diseases called IgG4-related disease, with high levels of serum IgG4 and IgG4-positive plasma cell parenchymal infiltration, has been recognized. The term *auto-immune pancreatitis* has frequently been used, but the widespread systemic involvement has led to the adaptation of the term IgG4-related systemic disease. Frequently involved organs include the gall bladder, inducing sclerosing cholangitis; the salivary glands, inducing sialadenitis; the peritoneum, with resulting retroperitoneal fibrosis; interstitial pneumonitis, periaortitis, and tubulointerstitial nephritis; and more rarely the breast, prostate, lymph nodes, and pituitary gland. In a recent large series of patients with this entity, about 20% had evidence of renal involvement, predominantly evident as tubulointerstitial nephritis. Even though slightly more than half of the patients with renal involvement did not show the characteristic pancreatic lesions, all showed similar features in the kidney. Patients were dominantly middle-aged elderly men, and by definition had high levels of serum IgG and IgG4, with frequent hypocomplementemia. Imaging studies may show enlarged kidneys or even a renal mass. This entity generally responds well to corticosteroids.

The light microscopic appearance is that of tubulointerstitial nephritis, with a plasma cell–rich infiltrate (Fig. 3.36). The interstitial fibrosis is patchy, expansile, and destructive, with a vague whorling pattern (Fig. 3.37-3.39), and may have accompanying eosinophils. In a minority of lesions, the infiltrate may just be plasma cell rich without the distinctive whorling pattern of interstitial fibrosis. There is accompanying tubular atrophy. IgG4 subclass staining shows dominance of IgG4-positive plasma cells, with >10 cells per high-power field in the most dense area of infiltrate (Fig. 3.40).

In one small series, granular TBM-dominant IgG4 deposits were detected in four of five cases with corresponding deposits by electron microscopy (Figs. 3.41-3.44). However, in a larger series, TBM deposits were only detected in one patient with concomitant membranous glomerulopathy.

Key Diagnostic Features of IgG4-Related Tubulointerstitial Nephritis

- Plasma cell–rich tubulointerstitial nephritis
- Whorling, destructive interstitial fibrosis
- IgG4-positive plasma cells, >10/hpf in densest area

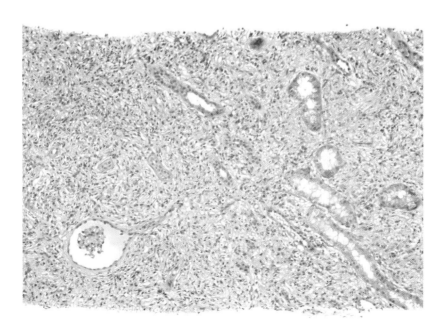

FIG. 3.36 IgG4-related tubulointerstitial nephritis. There is an expansile tubulointerstitial nephritis with lymphoplasmacytic infiltrate and tubular atrophy. Glomeruli are well-preserved in this case (hematoxylin and eosin, ×100). (Case kindly shared by Lynn D. Cornell, M.D., Consultant, Anatomic Pathology, Assistant Professor of Laboratory Medicine and Pathology, College of Medicine, Mayo Medical School).

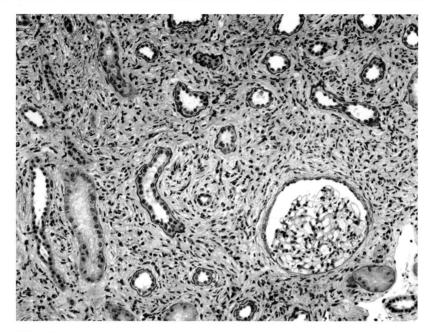

FIG. 3.37 IgG4-related tubulointerstitial nephritis. The expansile interstitial nephritis with frequent plasma cells and whorling pattern of fibrosis are evident, with sparing of glomeruli (Jones silver stain, ×200). (Case kindly shared by Lynn D. Cornell, M.D., Consultant, Anatomic Pathology, Assistant Professor of Laboratory Medicine and Pathology, College of Medicine, Mayo Medical School).

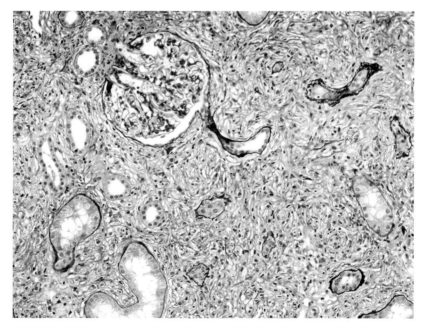

FIG. 3.38 IgG4-related tubulointerstitial nephritis. There is advanced fibrosis with a whorling expansile fibrotic process and scattered plasma cells, with sparing of glomeruli (Jones silver stain, ×200). (Case kindly shared by Lynn D. Cornell, M.D., Consultant, Anatomic Pathology, Assistant Professor of Laboratory Medicine and Pathology, College of Medicine, Mayo Medical School).

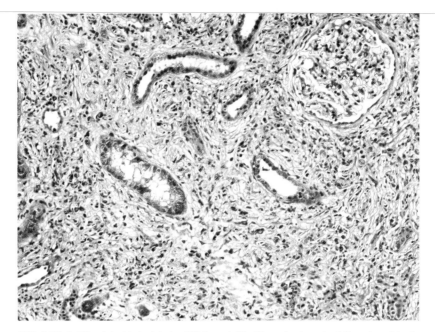

FIG. 3.39 IgG4-related tubulointerstitial nephritis. There is abundant fibrosis evident by blue staining on Masson Trichrome stain, with frequent interstitial plasma cells and fibroblasts (Masson Trichrome stain). (Case kindly shared by Lynn D. Cornell, M.D., Consultant, Anatomic Pathology, Assistant Professor of Laboratory Medicine and Pathology, College of Medicine, Mayo Medical School).

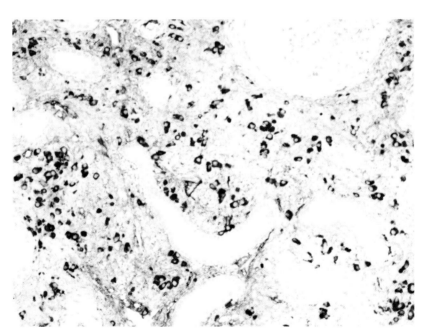

FIG. 3.40 IgG4-related tubulointerstitial nephritis. The plasma cell infiltrate is composed predominantly of IgG4-positive plasma cells (anti-IgG4 immunohistochemistry, ×400). (Case kindly shared by Lynn D. Cornell, M.D., Consultant, Anatomic Pathology, Assistant Professor of Laboratory Medicine and Pathology, College of Medicine, Mayo Medical School).

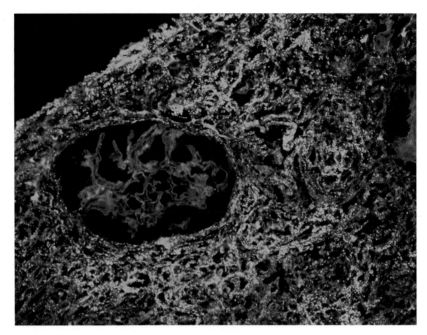

FIG. 3.41 IgG4-related tubulointerstitial nephritis. In some cases of this disease, there may be granular tubular basement membrane deposits, without corresponding glomerular deposits (anti-IgG immunofluorescence, ×100). (Case kindly shared by Lynn D. Cornell, M.D., Consultant, Anatomic Pathology, Assistant Professor of Laboratory Medicine and Pathology, College of Medicine, Mayo Medical School).

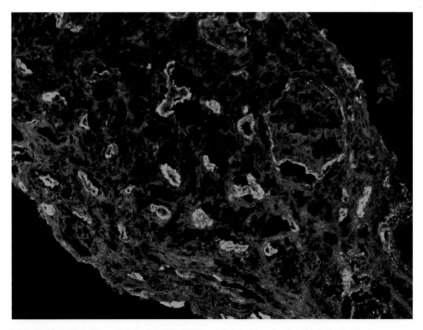

FIG. 3.42 IgG4-related tubulointerstitial nephritis. Focal granular tubular basement membrane deposits with anti-IgG are evident (anti-IgG immunofluorescence, ×200). (Case kindly shared by Lynn D. Cornell, M.D., Consultant, Anatomic Pathology, Assistant Professor of Laboratory Medicine and Pathology, College of Medicine, Mayo Medical School).

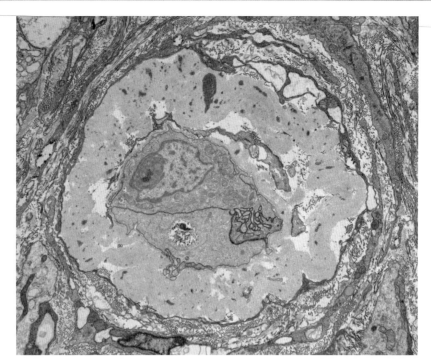

FIG. 3.43 IgG4-related tubulointerstitial nephritis. The tubular basement membrane is thickened and fibrotic with scattered small and occasional medium deposits with surrounding collagen (transmission electron microscopy, ×8000). (Case kindly shared by Lynn D. Cornell, M.D., Consultant, Anatomic Pathology, Assistant Professor of Laboratory Medicine and Pathology, College of Medicine, Mayo Medical School).

Differential Diagnosis of IgG4-Related Tubulointerstitial Nephritis

- Other causes of tubulointerstitial nephritis should be excluded (see Tubulointerstitial Nephritis). These include virus or other infections, heavy metal, light chain casts, crystals, or other autoimmune tubulointerstitial nephritis. In patients with pancreatitis or increased serum IgG4 or accumulation of plasma cells with whorling pattern fibrosis, IgG4 staining should be done to specifically make the diagnosis.

Etiology/Pathogenesis

The pathogenesis remains poorly understood. IgG4 is the rarest circulating IgG subclass in normal subjects, and is elevated after chronic antigen exposure, such as has been observed in beekeepers after repeated exposure to bee venom or patients undergoing immunotherapy with allergen exposure. IgG4 may easily dissociate into two immunoglobulin half molecules because of its weak disulfide bridges, and these portions of IgG4 may then associate with other moieties. IgG4 does not fix complement, and may thus function as an anti-inflammatory agent by forming complexes that can block antigen binding by the more pathogenic IgG1. Clearly, the heightened IgG4 levels do not directly explain hypocomplementemia or inflammatory injury. Investigators have hypothesized that anti-inflammatory cytokines produced in response to an initial injury result in increased interleukin-10 and tumor necrosis factor alpha, both anti-inflammatory. Further induction of fibrogenic interleukin-13 is then postulated to induce fibrosis and release of IgG4 in response to this injury. IgG4 from some patients with autoimmune pancreatitis showed immunoreactivity against epithelium in pancreatic ducts, bile ducts, and salivary gland ducts.

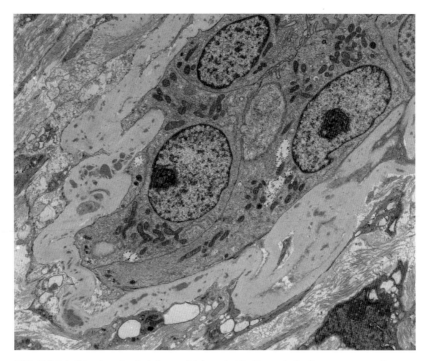

FIG. 3.44 IgG4-related tubulointerstitial nephritis. The tubular basement membrane is corrugated and thickened with scattered deposits (transmission electron microscopy, ×8000) and cell remnants. (Case kindly shared by Lynn D. Cornell, M.D., Consultant, Anatomic Pathology, Assistant Professor of Laboratory Medicine and Pathology, College of Medicine, Mayo Medical School).

Selected Reading

Cornell, L.D., 2010. IgG4-related tubulointerstitial nephritis. Kidney International 78, 951-953.

Cornell, L.D., Chicano, S.L., Deshpande, V., et al., 2007. Pseudotumors due to IgG4 immune-complex tubulointerstitial nephritis associated with autoimmune pancreatocentric disease. American Journal of Surgical Pathology 31, 1586-1597.

Saeki, T., Nishi, S., Imai, N., et al., 2010. Clinicopathological characteristics of patients with IgG4-related tubulointerstitial nephritis. Kidney International 78, 1016-1023.

Sarcoidosis

Considering the potential differential diagnoses, it must be noted that if the interstitial infiltrate is not prominent, it may be difficult to distinguish acute drug-induced tubular interstitial nephritis from nephrotoxic tubular injury or ischemic acute tubular necrosis since a minimal infiltrate with occasional eosinophils has been described in each of these entities. When the interstitial infiltrate is so intense that it forms granulomas, the differential diagnosis must include sarcoidosis (Figs. 3.45-3.47). In a large series of 46 biopsies from a single institution, drug-induced granulomatous interstitial nephritis was diagnosed in nearly a third of cases. About 10% of cases remained idiopathic after investigation and follow-up. Remaining causes included granulomatosis with polyangiitis (GPA, also called Wegener granulomatosis), foreign body giant cell reaction, reaction to Calmette-Guerin instillation in the urinary bladder for cancer treatment, and xanthogranulomatous pyelonephritis. In general, however, sarcoid involvement of the kidney is characterized by the presence of randomly distributed distinct granulomas with or without areas of central necrosis (Figs. 3.48, 3.49). When the granulomas

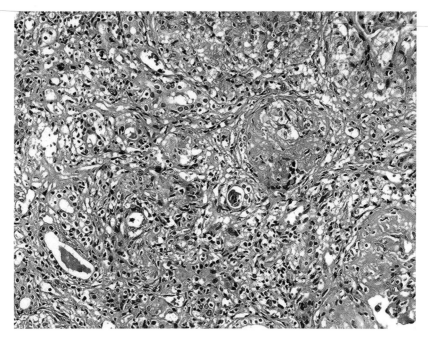

FIG. 3.45 Sarcoidosis may present as a granulomatous interstitial nephritis with well-defined sarcoid granulomata as seen here (hematoxylin and eosin, ×200).

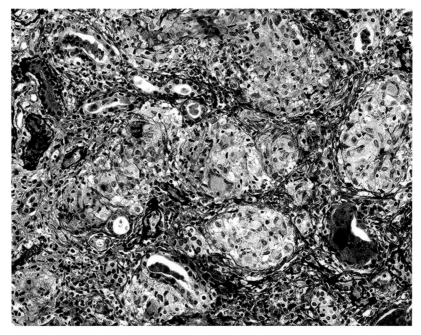

FIG. 3.46 Sarcoidosis. Silver stains demonstrate the architecture of the granulomata with evidence of interstitial fibrosis (Jones, ×200).

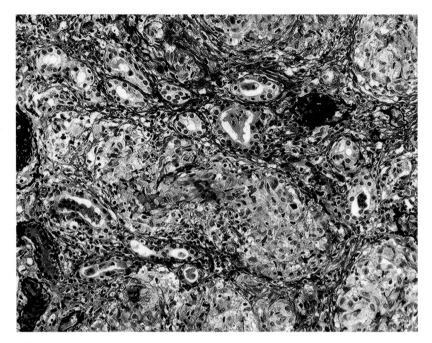

FIG. 3.47 Sarcoidosis. The granulomata consists predominately of mononuclear cells and epithelioid macrophages, and occasional foci of necrosis are seen (Jones, ×200).

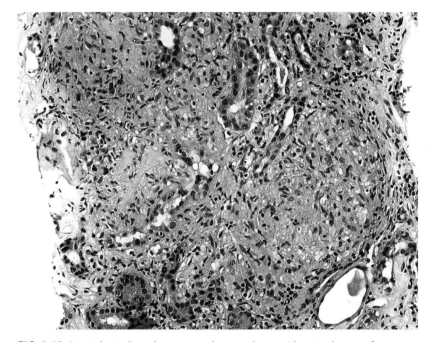

FIG. 3.48 Sarcoidosis. Granulomata may become large with central areas of necrosis. Examination for fungi and tuberculosis is essential when necrosis is present (hematoxylin and eosin, ×200).

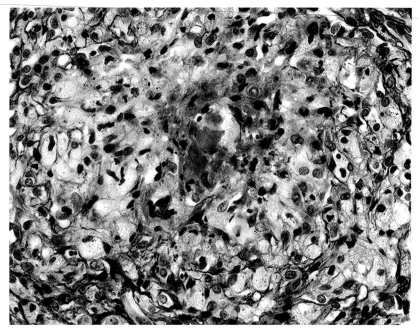

FIG. 3.49 Sarcoidosis. Central areas of necrosis may be present in granulomas (Jones, ×400).

Key Diagnostic Feature of Sarcoid

- Nonnecrotizing granulomas

Key Differential Diagnoses of Sarcoid

- Nonnecrotizing granulomas may be present in drug reactions also, but are usually less abundant, and often have accompanying eosinophils.
- Necrotizing lesions of glomeruli should invoke consideration of pauciimmune necrotizing crescentic glomerulonephritis, or even anti–glomerular basement membrane glomerulonephritis. Crescents are typical of those entities, and are not part of sarcoid.
- Necrotizing granulomas due to tuberculous or fungal infection can be diagnosed by appropriate special stains.

---

are confluent (Figs. 3.50, 3.51), involving the glomeruli or with prominent necrosis, consideration in the differential diagnosis must include granulomatosis with polyangiitis (GPA, also called Wegener granulomatosis). Glomerular involvement is rare in sarcoidosis.

The presence of necrotizing granulomas should bring up the possibility of tuberculosis or fungal infection of the kidney, and investigated as appropriate by special stains.

Etiology/Pathogenesis

Sarcoidosis is a multisystem granulomatous disorder of unknown etiology that is characterized pathologically by the presence of noncaseating granulomas in involved organs, and in the kidney is a diagnosis of exclusion. Sarcoid is presumed to have autoimmune etiology, but the pathogenesis remains unknown.

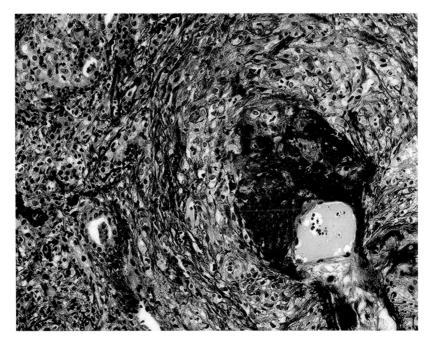

FIG. 3.50 Sarcoidosis. When granulomata are confluent and areas of necrosis are present, the differential diagnosis must include granulomatosis with polyangiitis (GPA, also called Wegener granulomatosis) (Jones, ×200).

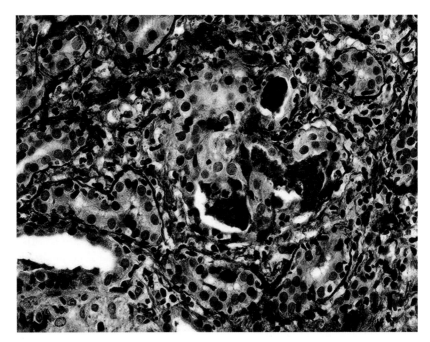

FIG. 3.51 Sarcoidosis. Glomeruli may also be involved in the granulomatous process (Jones, ×400).

Selected Reading

Bijol, V., Mendez, G.P., Nose, V., et al., 2006. Granulomatous interstitial nephritis: A clinicopathologic study of 46 cases from a single institution. International Journal of Surgical Pathology 14, 57-63.

Joss, N., Morris, S., Young, B., et al., 2007. Granulomatous interstitial nephritis. Clinical Journal of the American Society of Nephrology 2, 222-230.

Mahevas, M., Lescure, F.X., Boffa, J.J., et al., 2009. Renal sarcoidosis: clinical, laboratory, and histologic presentation and outcome in 47 patients. Medicine (Baltimore) 2009 88, 9-106.

Acute Kidney Injury/Acute Tubular Necrosis

A common indication for renal biopsy is the development of the syndrome of acute kidney injury, formerly called acute renal failure. Acute kidney injury is the clinical situation in which there is a sudden loss of renal function. It is usually characterized by oliguria and the rapid development of azotemia. Some forms of acute kidney injury, however, may not exhibit oliguria and may even be polyuric. A rapid cessation in renal function can occur as a result of extrarenal events as well as intrinsic renal disease.

Acute kidney injury/acute tubular necrosis (the latter also called acute tubular injury) is an acute process in which the clinical course has several phases, including initiation, extension, maintenance, and repair. Acute kidney injury/acute tubular necrosis is most commonly initiated by hypovolemia and/or hypotension and the injury is extended by induction of an inflammatory response. Acute kidney injury/acute tubular necrosis is not completely reversible in up to 25% of patients. The duration of each of these phases and especially the maintenance and recovery phases is highly variable depending on the presence of previously existing renal disease, on the volume and electrolyte status of the individual, the length and severity of the initiation, drug therapy and whether there are other contributory factors that can alter renal perfusion, such as treatment with angiotensin blockade and diuretics. This sequence of events can vary in time from several weeks to months from initiation to recovery. Hypotension and hypovolemia are the most common causes of acute kidney injury/acute tubular necrosis, both in the community and in hospitalized patients with multi organ failure. The kidneys are most vulnerable to moderate hypoperfusion when autoregulation is impaired. This is seen in elderly patients or in patients with atherosclerosis, hypertension, diabetes, or early chronic kidney disease, where arterial and arteriolar nephrosclerosis is present, and in patients who are receiving angiotensin-receptor blockers or angiotensin-converting enzyme inhibitors.

ISCHEMIC ACUTE TUBULAR INJURY

The histologic picture varies with the evolution of the lesion in relationship to the onset of the acute kidney injury. Individual cell necrosis with denudation of the basement membrane and shedding of epithelial cells and necrotic debris into the tubular lumen is characteristic (Figs. 3.52-3.58). Hyaline, granular, and pigmented casts are seen in the distal portions of the nephron. These casts consist of Tamm–Horsfall protein, which stains positively with PAS stains. In the specific instances of acute tubular necrosis following hemolysis or following muscle damage, deeply pigmented hemoglobin and myoglobin casts are also present. In segments of the tubules that do not show significant necrosis, the tubules are often dilated and lined by flattened epithelial cells, often called tubular simplification (Figs. 3.59-3.61). In PAS stains, the brush border of proximal tubules is often thinned or absent (Fig. 3.62). Further, the interstitium is markedly edematous. As the lesion progresses following the initial injury, evidence of tubular regeneration with mitotic figures can be seen. There may be a mild interstitial inflammatory infiltrate with small numbers of lymphocytes, macrophages, neutrophils, or occasionally eosinophils present. In these late stages, the distinction between ischemic acute

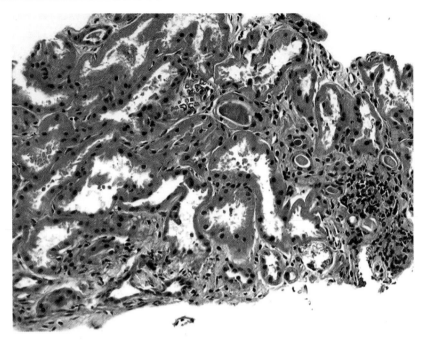

FIG. 3.52 Acute tubular injury. In acute tubular injury, there is dilation of the tubules and interstitial edema. In addition, the proximal tubules show evidence of loss of the brush border with blebbing of the apical membrane into the tubular lumen (hematoxylin and eosin, ×100).

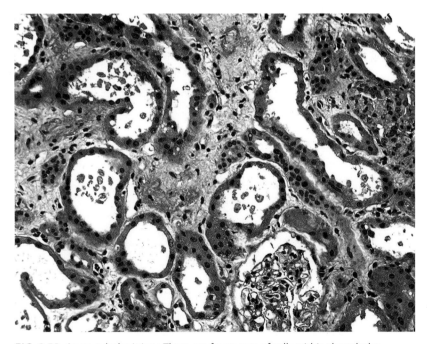

FIG. 3.53 Acute tubular injury. There are fragments of cells within the tubular lumina. Flattening of the tubular epithelium, loss of nuclei, and a marked interstitial infiltrate with occasional inflammatory cells are also present (hematoxylin and eosin, ×200).

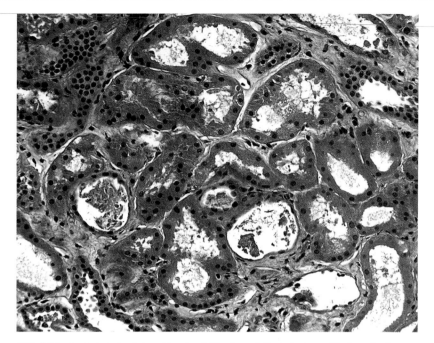

FIG. 3.54 Acute tubular injury. Focal calcification of the tubular epithelium is also seen with evidence of denudation of the basement membrane (hematoxylin and eosin, ×200).

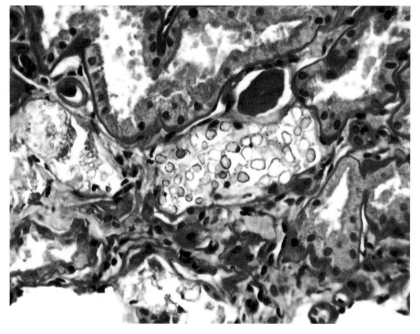

FIG. 3.55 Acute tubular injury. Foci of calcified epithelial cells can sometimes be present with flattened regenerating epithelium along the basement membrane (hematoxylin and eosin, ×400).

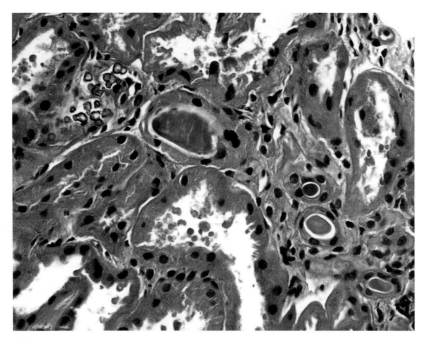

FIG. 3.56 Acute tubular injury. Proteinaceous casts are present in the distal tubules made up of Tamm–Horsfall protein (hematoxylin and eosin, ×400).

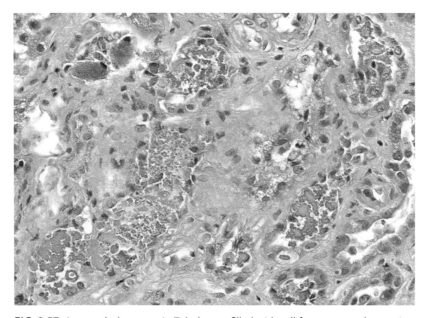

FIG. 3.57 Acute tubular necrosis. Tubules are filled with cell fragments and necrotic epithelium. These can form the nidus for dystrophic calcification.

tubular injury and acute tubulointerstitial nephritis may be challenging. However, generally the infiltrate is much less prominent in cases of acute tubular injury.

One caveat that must always be remembered in evaluating the biopsy of a patient with acute kidney injury is not to quickly assign the cause to acute tubular injury. Because of the paucity of findings in acute tubular injury, one must search carefully for other potential causes, including glomerular diseases such as minimal change disease causing nephrotic syndrome,

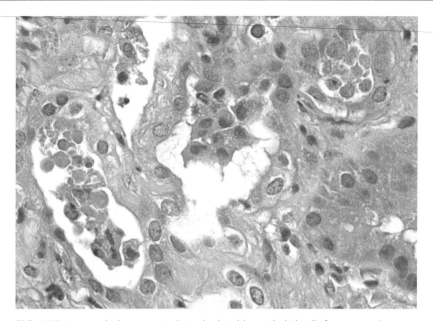

FIG. 3.58 Acute tubular necrosis. Detached viable epithelial cells form casts that can be shed into the urine.

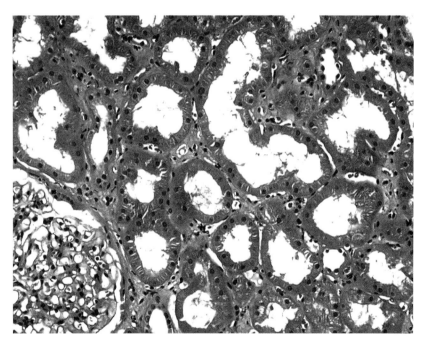

FIG. 3.59 Acute tubular injury. In cases where there is no evident necrosis, the most prominent finding is loss of the architecture of the proximal tubules with dilatation and flattening of the epithelium (hematoxylin and eosin, ×200).

where a patient can present with oliguria due to hypovolemia secondary to shifts in extracellular fluid as a result of the massive proteinuria.

Whereas electron microscopy generally does not add significantly to the evaluation of most tubular interstitial diseases, it is helpful in evaluating the tubular epithelial changes in both ischemic and toxic types of acute tubular injury (Figs. 3.63-3.65). In ischemic acute tubular injury, scattered epithelial cell changes show a variety of different cytopathic alterations. There

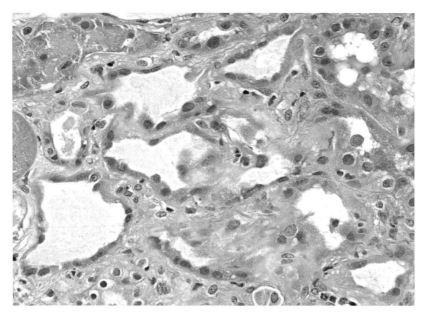

FIG. 3.60 Acute tubular injury. Injured tubules are lined with an admixture of attenuated, apoptotic, and regenerating epithelium.

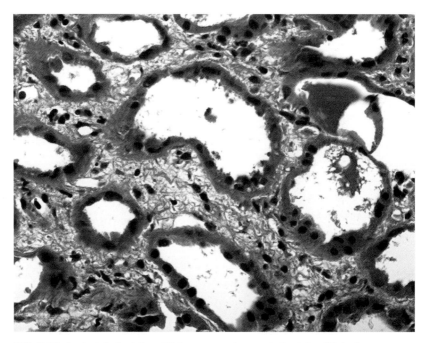

FIG. 3.61 Acute tubular injury. Higher power demonstrates interstitial edema, flattening of the epithelium, and loss of occasional nuclei (hematoxylin and eosin, ×400).

is loss of the brush border, blebbing of the apical membrane with shedding of apical membrane blebs into the tubular lumina, high-amplitude swelling with condensation of the cristae of the mitochondria, individual cell apoptosis as seen as cell shrinkage with nuclear fragmentation, and a variety of other degenerative changes, including necrosis. Electron microscopy may therefore be useful in evaluating those instances where the diagnosis is questionable or where other causes are suspected.

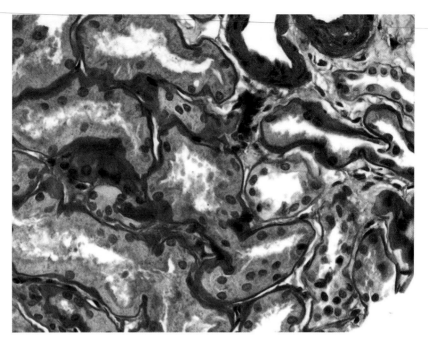

FIG. 3.62 Acute tubular injury. PAS stains demonstrate loss of the brush border with evidence of apical blebbing (periodic acid Schiff, ×400).

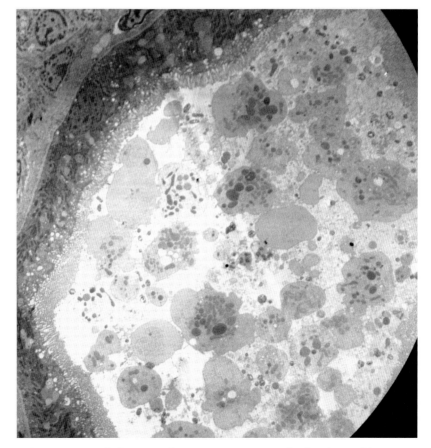

FIG. 3.63 Acute tubular injury. Electron microscopy reveals of evidence of fragments of epithelial cells filling the tubular lumen (transmission electron microscopy, ×2000).

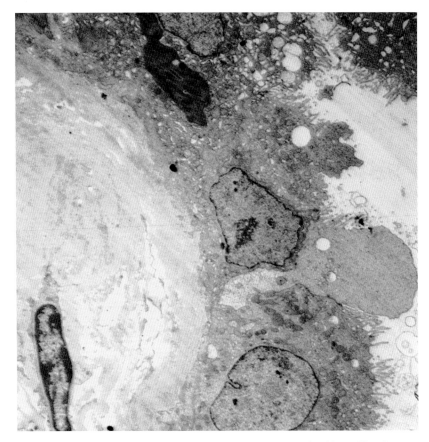

FIG. 3.64 Acute tubular injury. Higher power demonstrating focal loss of brush border of the proximal tubules with the development of apical blebs (transmission electron microscopy, ×4000).

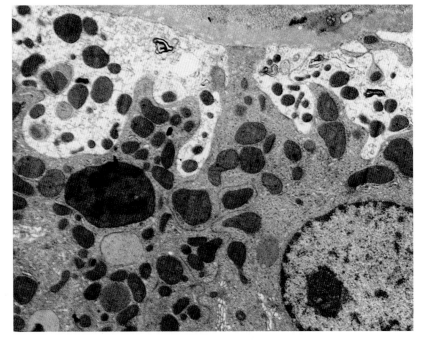

FIG. 3.65 Toxic acute tubular injury. Sublethal injury is seen with marked intracellular edema and condensation of adjacent cells (transmission electron microscopy, ×8000).

ACUTE PHOSPHATE NEPHROPATHY

A clinically distinct subset of ischemic acute kidney injury has recently been observed in older patients following colonoscopy. "Acute phosphate nephropathy" is a clinical pathologic entity where acute kidney injury occurs following administration of an oral sodium phosphate purgative in preparation for colonoscopy or bowel surgery. The abrupt onset of acute kidney injury typically occurs in a female patient with advanced age who usually has preexisting kidney disease, including hypertension and/or diabetes. Prior use of drugs that alter renal perfusion including angiotensin-converting enzyme inhibitors, angiotensin receptor blockers, nonsteroidal anti-inflammatory drugs, and diuretics predispose the potential of acute kidney injury, particularly when patients are volume depleted by the bowel preparation or have an episode of hypotension during the procedure. Additional risk factors for developing acute phosphate nephropathy as an adverse event of oral sodium phosphate purgative use are bowel obstruction, or active colitis.

Biopsies performed in the acute phase have tubular epithelial changes typical of ischemic acute kidney injury as described previously with the distinctive feature of extensive deposition of calcium phosphate in necrotic tubules (Figs. 3.66, 3.67). In biopsies with 10 or more glomeruli, more than 30 calcifications can be identified. This contrasts with the occasional dystrophic tubular calcification that can be observed in ischemic acute kidney injury and in some cases of acute tubular interstitial nephritis. The calcifications appear both as calcified necrotic tubular epithelium and as desquamated epithelial cells with surface calcification appearing as rounded concretions in the tubular lumen. (Figs. 3.68, 3.69) These crystals are nonpolarizable, and stain purplish on hematoxylin and eosin stains, and positive for phosphate by von Kossa stains (Fig. 3.70). Tubules without calcification demonstrate varying degrees of epithelial injury in the early stages of acute renal failure and tubular atrophy later in the course of the disease (Fig 3.71). Since the acute kidney injury occurs in the presence of the transient elevation of serum phosphate that results from ingestion of a large dose of sodium phosphate, the protective effect of urinary macromolecules is abrogated and dystrophic calcification of necrotic, apoptotic, and sublethally injured tubular epithelium is facilitated. While dystrophic calcification occurs in ischemic and toxic acute kidney injury of other causes and is commonly seen in allografts, the extent of calcification is generally not as extensive as seen with this clinical entity. Biopsies performed later in patients who develop chronic kidney disease following the colonoscopy have nonspecific findings of interstitial fibrosis and tubular atrophy associated with the tubular calcifications.

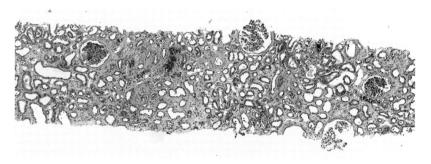

FIG. 3.66 Acute phosphate nephropathy. Biopsy showing extensive tubular calcifications involving approximately 25% of the nonatrophic tubules (hematoxylin and eosin, ×100).

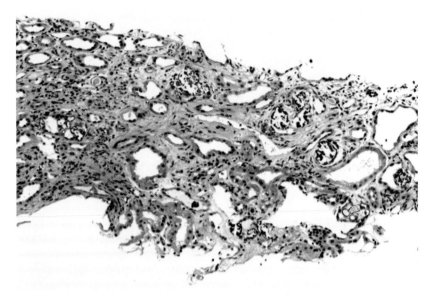

FIG. 3.67 Acute phosphate nephropathy. Higher power demonstrating the density of tubules involved with epithelial calcification (hematoxylin and eosin, ×200).

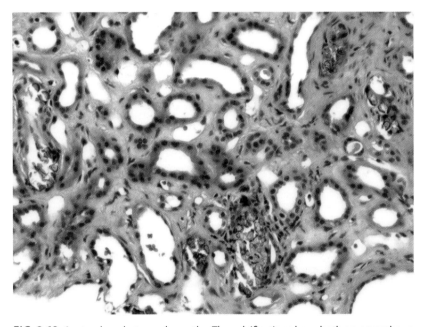

FIG. 3.68 Acute phosphate nephropathy. The calcifications have both an amorphous and bubble-like structure (hematoxylin and eosin, ×400).

Etiology/Pathogenesis

The use of a purgative results in loss of fluid and electrolytes, resulting in hypovolemia and electrolyte disturbances that predispose the individual to acute kidney injury. The use of a phosphate purgative results in hypovolemia and renal hypoperfusion in the presence of a transient elevation of serum phosphate, thus resulting in excess phosphate in the filtrate, and precipitation of calcium phosphate.

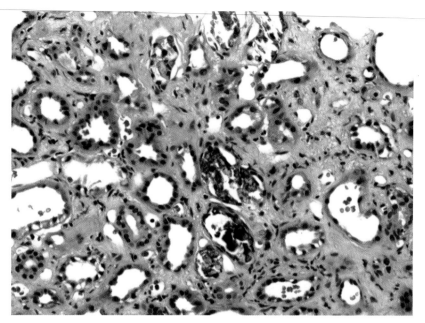

FIG. 3.69 Acute phosphate nephropathy. The calcifications begin as dystrophic calcification of necrotic epithelium (hematoxylin and eosin, ×400).

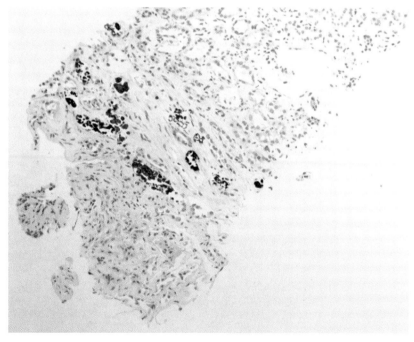

FIG. 3.70 Acute phosphate nephropathy. The calcifications are composed of calcium phosphate as determined by Von Kossa staining, ×200.

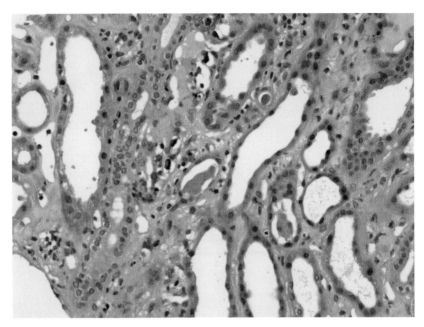

FIG. 3.71 Acute phosphate nephropathy. Extensive tubular injury is present in noncalcified tubules in the acute phase (hematoxylin and eosin, ×400).

Selected Reading

Markowitz, G.S., Perazella, M.A., 2009. Acute phosphate nephropathy. Kidney International 76, 1027-1034.

NEPHROTOXIC ACUTE TUBULAR NECROSIS

The clinical picture may be similar to that of ischemic acute tubular injury with a sudden onset of acute kidney injury. In many instances, however, particularly in industrial exposures, the onset may be insidious, and the patient may not have oliguria but present with polyuric renal insufficiency.

Histologically, severe acute toxic tubular injury is associated with extensive epithelial necrosis, which tends to involve all nephrons more uniformly than that seen in the ischemic form (Fig. 3.72). The proximal tubule is most severely involved and necrotic cells are dislodged from the basement membrane, and the tubular lumens are filled with cellular debris. Focal calcification of the necrotic material occurs very rapidly and can be seen within 1 to 2 days. As the lesion develops, regeneration of the tubular epithelium can be identified initially by flattened epithelial cells, which over several days become cuboidal and then columnar and then finally develop a normal proximal tubule architecture. In addition, specific renal epithelial changes can be seen with different toxins. In acute lead nephropathy, for example, dark intranuclear inclusions can be identified (Fig. 3.73) and oxalate crystals, polarizable and sheaf-shaped, are associated with glycol nephrotoxicity. In aminoglycoside nephrotoxicity, lysosomal myeloid bodies can be identified by electron microscopy (Fig. 3.74). Amiodarone toxicity is characterized by the presence of atypical mitochondria (Fig 3.75). In patients with rhabdomyolysis, acute tubular injury can be caused by direct toxicity of intratubular casts of myoglobin (Figs. 3.76, 3.77). Immunohistochemistry allows specific diagnosis (Fig. 3.78). In patients with severe liver failure and bilirubin levels >10 mg/dL, acute kidney injury may be contributed to by so-called bile nephrosis, characterized by greenish-tinged brown casts of bilirubin in tubules (Figs. 3.79, 3.80). These specific casts, or the casts of hemoglobin seen

Text continued on page 430

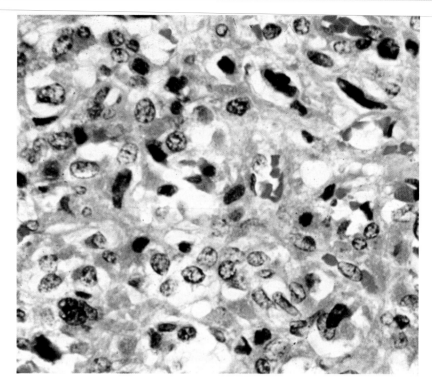

FIG. 3.72 Toxic acute tubular necrosis. There is evidence of cellular necrosis, with atypical nuclei representing regenerating epithelium (hematoxylin and eosin, ×400).

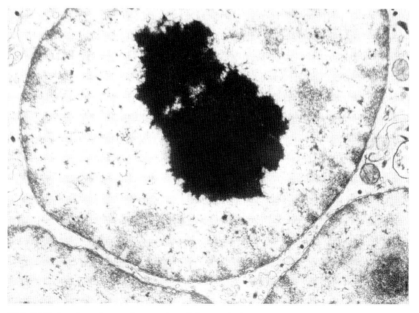

FIG. 3.73 Lead nephropathy. Nuclei of the epithelial cells contain dense bodies consisting of lead–metallothyanide complexes (transmission electron microscopy, ×12,000).

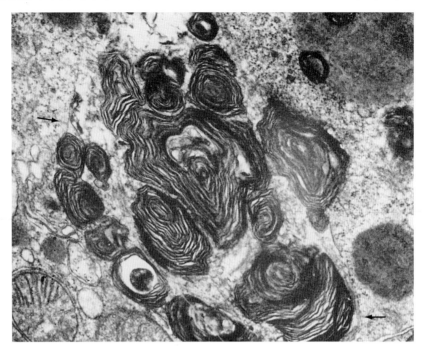

FIG. 3.74 Aminoglycoside nephrotoxicity. Myeloid bodies (arrows) are present in an intracellular localization (transmission electron microscopy, ×12,000).

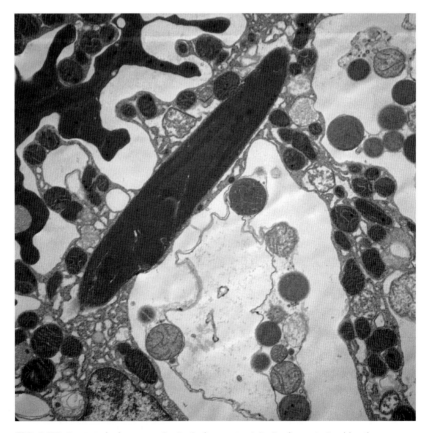

FIG. 3.75 Acute tubular necrosis. Amiodarone toxicity is characterized by the presence of atypical mitochondria (transmission electron microscopy, ×8000).

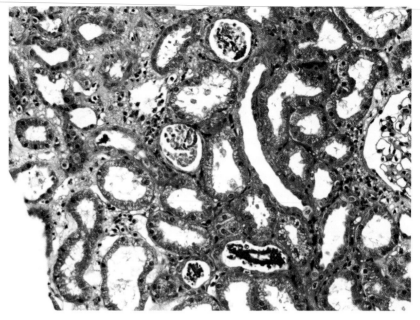

FIG. 3.76 Myoglobin casts. In rhabdomyolysis-induced acute tubular injury, myoglobin casts are seen within tubular lumina with associated acute tubular injury. These are coarsely granular with a reddish-brown tinge (hematoxylin and eosin, ×100).

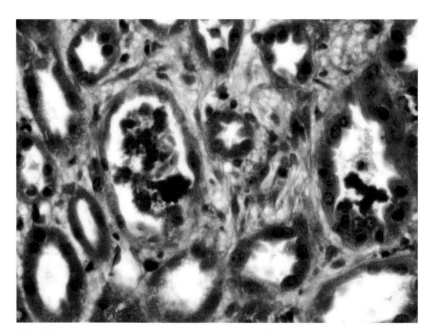

FIG. 3.77 Myoglobin casts. There is granular reddish-brown cast material within tubules with associated tubular injury with flattening of tubular epithelium and surrounding mild edema and early interstitial fibrosis (hematoxylin and eosin, ×400).

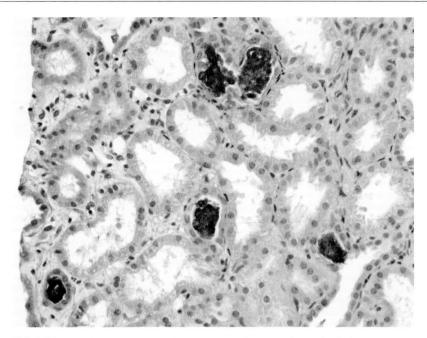

FIG. 3.78 Myoglobin casts. Myoglobin casts can be stained specifically by immunohistochemistry, revealing that these reddish-brown casts specifically consist of myoglobin (antimyoglobin, ×200).

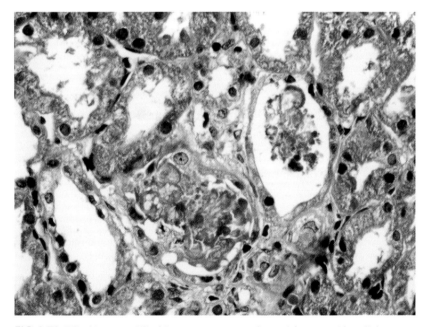

FIG. 3.79 Bilirubin casts. Bilirubin casts are seen as brownish casts with a slight green tinge with associated tubular injury with flattened tubular epithelium (hematoxylin and eosin, ×200).

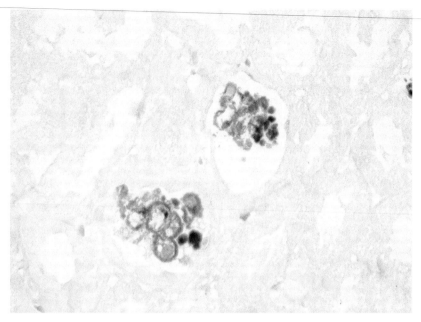

FIG. 3.80 Bilirubin casts. Bilirubin casts are seen as distinctly green with a special stain for bilirubin (Hall stain, ×200).

Key Diagnostic Features of Acute Tubular Injury

- Ischemic: Flattening, regeneration of tubules, mostly proximal
- Toxic: Frank necrosis, more widespread injury, specific findings according to etiology

---

Key Differential Diagnosis of Acute Tubular Injury

- Obstruction may also give rise to dilated, flattened appearance of tubules, but with preserved brush border and with concomitant dilatation of Bowman's spaces. Specific inciting causes, such as crystals, should be sought.

---

with acute hemolytic injury, should not be confused with Tamm–Horsfall proteinaceous casts or so-called lymph vessel casts that are seen with lymphatic obstruction (Fig. 3.81).

Osmotic nephrosis is a distinct form of toxic tubular injury (Fig 3.82). There is prominent vacuolization and swelling of the proximal tubules. It can be induced by many different compounds including intravenous contrast media, sugars including glucose, mannitol, and sucrose, and plasma expanders such as hydroxyethyl starch and dextrans. Recently, maltose-based IV Ig (intravenous immune globulin) has been added to the list of offending agents (Fig 3.83).

Both hereditary and acquired causes of hemolysis including transfusion reactions can lead to hemoglobinuric acute renal failure. It is the result of a combination of the tubular toxic effects of hemoglobin and tubular obstruction with hemoglobin casts. The tubular epithelium appears flattened and the lumen is obstructed by hemoglobin casts and fragments of hemolyzed red blood cells (Figs. 3.84-3.86).

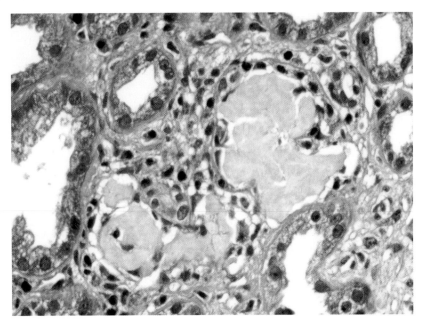

FIG. 3.81 Lymph vessel casts. In cases of obstruction to lymphatic outflow, lymphatic fluid may back-leak and dissect into tubular lumina. These so-called lymph vessel casts appear as pale material with lymphatic endothelium overlying the globular cast material (hematoxylin and eosin, ×400).

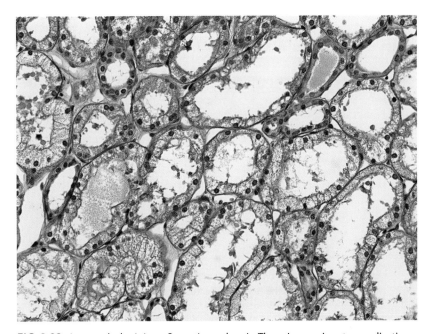

FIG. 3.82 Acute tubular injury. Osmotic nephrosis. There is prominent vacuolization and swelling of the proximal tubules (hematoxylin and eosin, ×400).

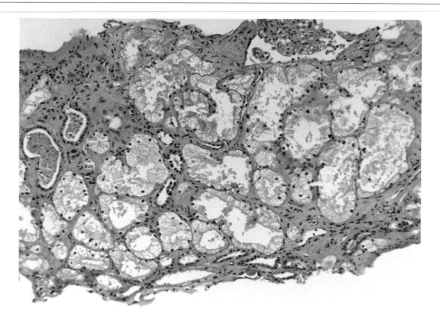

FIG. 3.83 Acute tubular injury. Intravenous Ig was the etiology in this example (hematoxylin and eosin, ×200).

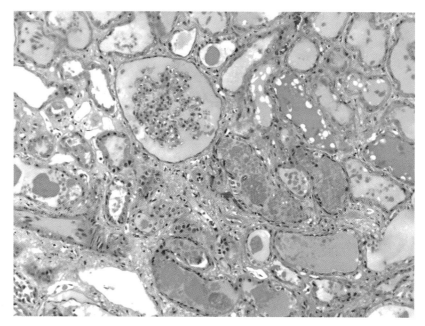

FIG. 3.84 Hemoglobinuric acute renal failure. The tubular epithelium appears flattened and the lumen is obstructed by hemoglobin casts and fragments of hemolyzed red blood cells (hematoxylin and eosin, ×200).

Etiology/Pathogenesis

Intrinsic renal causes of acute kidney injury include severe acute glomerulonephritis, vasculitis, thrombotic microangiopathies, malignant hypertension, as well as acute tubulointerstitial nephritis and the entity classically called acute tubular necrosis. Although "necrosis" is included in the term to distinguish it from other intrinsic causes of renal disease, tubular

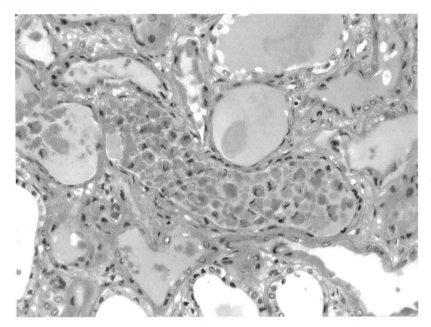

FIG. 3.85 Hemoglobinuric acute renal failure. Higher power shows lysed reticulocytes forming an obstructing cast (hematoxylin and eosin, ×400).

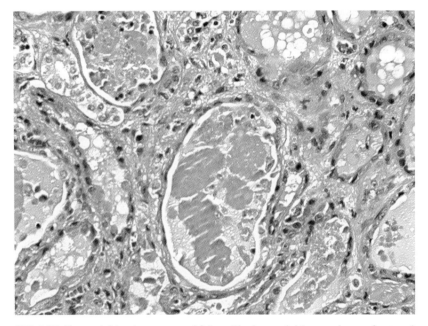

FIG. 3.86 Hemoglobinuric acute renal failure. The hemoglobin casts have a fractured appearance (hematoxylin and eosin, ×400).

epithelial damage is not always readily evident by light microscopy, and the term *acute tubular injury* is now commonly used. Acute tubular injury is generally divided into two subcategories, postischemic acute tubular injury and nephrotoxic acute tubular injury. Morphologic changes of cellular injury are usually more subtle in the ischemic form and with more obvious cytopathologic changes in the toxic form. In addition, the patterns of tubular damage differ between the two forms. In the ischemic form tubular damage is patchy, affecting the relatively short length of the straight segments of the proximal tubule and focal areas of the ascending limbs of the loops of Henle. Ischemia plays a major role in its pathogenesis. In the toxic form, the tubular epithelial damage is more extensive along segments of the proximal tubule, and the segments involved may vary with the specific toxin. Although distal tubular damage does occur, it is less extensive and more inconsistent than in ischemic acute tubular necrosis. Although most instances of severe nephrotoxic acute tubular injury are the result of industrial accidents or accidental or intentional ingestion of toxins, it must be recognized that numerous therapeutic agents such as aminoglycoside antibiotics, antineoplastic agents such as cisplatin, and plant toxins found in herbal remedies all may be associated with renal epithelial damage and are the most frequently encountered forms of nephrotoxicity in a renal biopsy practice.

Heavy Metal Nephropathy (Lead and Cadmium Nephropathy)

It has long been recognized that heavy metals can lead to a dose-dependent toxic necrosis of renal epithelial cells. Because the kidney is the principal excretory organ of the body and a major route for excretion of toxins absorbed by any route, the kidney and urinary tract are particularly vulnerable to toxic damage. Acute toxicity clinically presents similarly to ischemic tubular necrosis. Chronic nephrotoxicity is more insidious in its onset and in its clinical manifestations. It can mimic other primary renal diseases and may manifest itself by minor functional abnormalities or by the systemic effects of renal damage, including hypertension and gradually progressive renal failure. Chronic exposure to lead, mercury, cadmium, platinum, gold, lithium, silver, copper, and iron have all been associated with the development of a chronic nonspecific interstitial nephritis. The histologic findings in heavy metal nephropathy show proximal tubular injury with intranuclear inclusion bodies of metal–metallothionein complexes (see Fig. 3.73).

Etiology/Pathogenesis

The pathogenesis of the renal disease is related to the proximal tubule reabsorption of filtered lead or cadmium, with subsequent accumulation with metallothioneins in the proximal tubule cells. The renal tubular cells have a considerable capacity to synthesize metallothionein, thereby binding and detoxifying heavy metal ions. When the detoxifying capacity is surpassed, tubular damage results in interstitial inflammation and fibrosis.

Selected Reading

Abuelo, J., 2007. Normotensive ischemic acute renal failure. New England Journal of Medicine 357, 797-805.

Bennett, W.M., 1985. Lead nephropathy. Kidney International 28, 212-220.

Bohle, A.J.J., Meyer, D., Schubert, G.E., 1976. Morphology of acute renal failure. Comparative data from biopsy and autopsy. Kidney International 10, S9-16.

Dickenmann, M., Oettl, T., Mihatsch, M., 2008. Osmotic nephrosis: acute kidney injury with accumulation of proximal tubular lysosomes due to administration of exogenous solutes. American Journal of Kidney Disease 51, 491-503.

Humes, H., 1988. Aminoglycoside nephrotoxicity. Kidney International 33, 900-911.

Racusen, L., Kashgarian, M., 2007. Ischemic and Toxic Acute Tubular Injury. In: Jennette, J.C., et al., (Eds.), Heptinstall's Pathology of the Kidney, Sixth ed. Lippincott Williams and Wilkins, pp. 1139-1198.

Analgesic Nephropathy and Papillary Necrosis

Because the lesion is a chronic progressive one, the clinical presentation is extremely variable, but a common feature is nocturia and polyuria. This is due to the extensive medullary damage frequently associated with renal papillary necrosis resulting in a loss of the concentrating ability (Fig. 3.87). Because renal biopsies rarely give a significant sample of the inner medulla, it is often difficult to assign the relatively nonspecific cortical changes of interstitial fibrosis and tubular atrophy seen to this entity. Nonetheless, analgesic nephropathy has extensive interstitial scarring, which is usually bland with relatively few inflammatory cells that, if present, are generally small lymphocytes (Figs. 3.88-3.92). Extensive tubular atrophy is also seen. Glomerulosclerosis is also present as a secondary change, but more commonly the glomeruli are not damaged and become crowded because of the tubular atrophy. These cortical changes are relatively nonspecific but in the presence of radiologic evidence of papillary necrosis are consistent with the diagnosis of analgesic nephropathy. It should be remembered in the differential diagnosis that sickle cell disease and diabetes may also be associated with papillary necrosis.

Etiology/Pathogenesis

A particular form of chronic nephrotoxicity that is of special interest is the lesion associated with analgesic abuse. It has been long recognized that chronic excessive use of analgesic drugs is associated with the development of chronic renal failure due to a chronic tubulointerstitial nephritis. Although phenacetin combined with caffeine and codeine is the compound most frequently implicated in the earliest reports, abuse of a number of common

---

Key Diagnostic Feature of Chronic Tubulointerstitial Nephritis

- Inflammation and interstitial fibrosis and tubular atrophy out of proportion to glomerular and/or vascular injury

Note: Specific etiologies must be sought – see below.

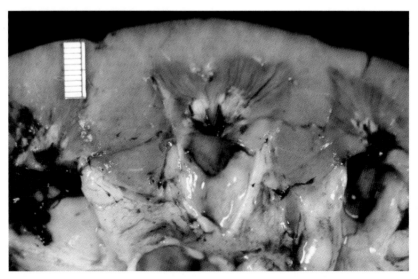

FIG. 3.87 Analgesic nephropathy. There is extensive interstitial fibrosis associated with papillary necrosis.

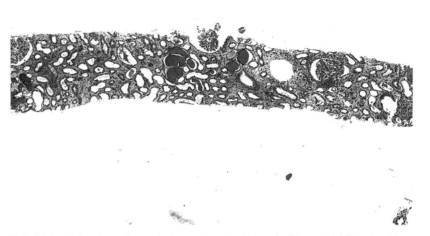

FIG. 3.88 Analgesic nephropathy is associated with marked interstitial fibrosis with a relative paucity of interstitial infiltrate. Tubular atrophy with numerous casts are present. Glomeruli are generally not involved or demonstrate sclerosis (hematoxylin and eosin, ×50).

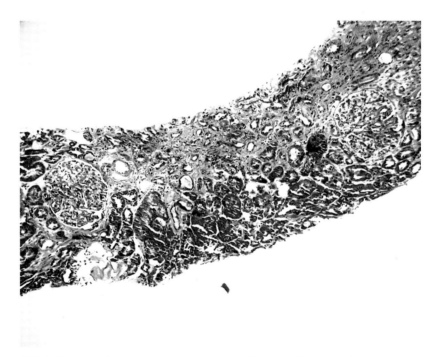

FIG. 3.89 Analgesic nephropathy. The extensive interstitial fibrosis is demonstrated here on trichrome stain associated with marked tubular atrophy (trichrome, ×100).

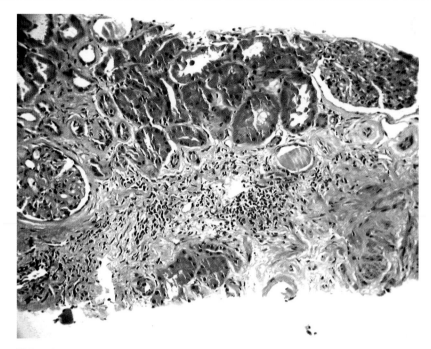

FIG. 3.90 Analgesic nephropathy. Higher power demonstrates a nonspecific lymphocytic infiltrate (hematoxylin, phloxine, and saffron, ×200).

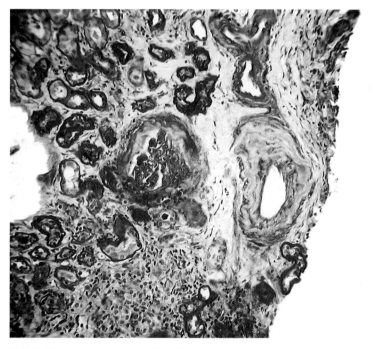

FIG. 3.91 Analgesic nephropathy. There are vascular changes accompanying the chronic interstitial nephritis (periodic acid Schiff, ×200).

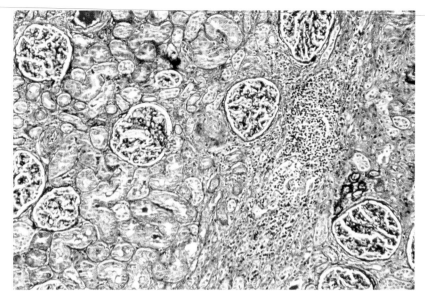

FIG. 3.92 Analgesic nephropathy. There is diffuse fibrosis and trichrome stain with relative preservation of glomeruli (trichrome, ×100).

analgesics including acetaminophen and nonsteroidal anti-inflammatory drugs have more recently also been implicated in the development of this lesion.

Selected Reading

De Broe, M.E., Elseviers, M.M., 1998. Analgesic nephropathy. New England Journal of Medicine 338, 446-452.

Mihatsch, M.J., Khanlari, B., Brunner, F.P., 2006. Obituary to analgesic nephropathy – an autopsy study. Nephrology Dialysis Transplantation 21, 3139-3145.

Light Chain Cast Nephropathy and Tubulopathy

Proteinaceous casts are common in all forms of chronic interstitial nephritis. The cast nephropathy associated with multiple myeloma deserves special mention because it has a distinctive histologic appearance, and the cast material is involved in the direct pathogenesis of the lesion. Light chain, or so-called myeloma, cast nephropathy is seen in approximately half of patients with multiple myeloma who have renal disease. The remainder of patients with multiple myeloma who have related renal disease have either light chain deposition or amyloid deposition, or rarely combined lesions, as discussed elsewhere. The casts in myeloma cast nephropathy consist of Bence Jones or light chain proteins combined with Tamm–Horsfall protein. Casts can be diffuse or focal involving distal convoluted and collecting tubules and often have a fractured or crystalline appearance (Figs. 3.93-3.95). They frequently are surrounded by multinucleated giant cells formed from infiltrating macrophages (Figs. 3.96-3.98). Disruption of the tubules can be seen focally and acute polymorphonuclear or granuloma-like inflammation may extend into the adjoining interstitium (Fig. 3.99). The cytoplasm of the proximal tubules frequently contains large hyaline protein droplets or needle-like inclusion bodies (Figs. 3.100, 3.101). There is interstitial fibrosis and a lymphocytic infiltration associated with tubular atrophy. Thus, except for the distinctive nature of the casts and the granulomatous reaction to them, the lesion may mimic other forms of chronic interstitial nephritis. Immunofluorescence microscopy is helpful in cases of suspected light chain cast nephropathy.

Text continued on page 443

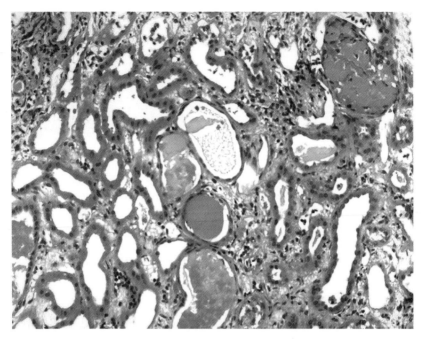

FIG. 3.93 Cast nephropathy. Tubules are dilated and filled with proteinaceous casts completely occluding some tubular lumina (hematoxylin and eosin, ×200).

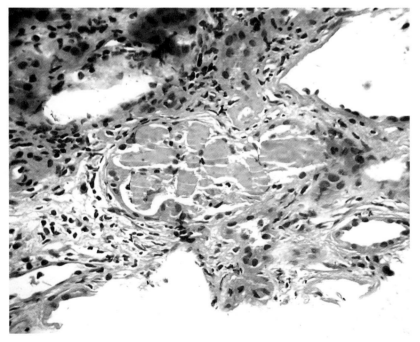

FIG. 3.94 Cast nephropathy. The casts have a fractured appearance and also demonstrate a cellular reaction (hematoxylin and eosin, ×400).

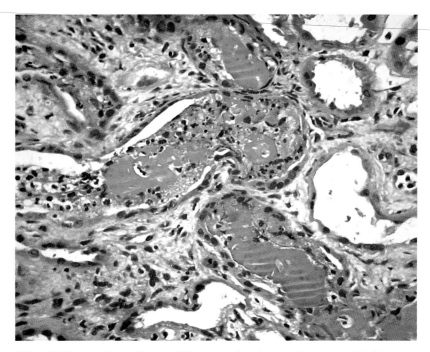

FIG. 3.95 Cast nephropathy. In addition, there is evidence of tubular epithelial damage and interstitial edema (hematoxylin, phloxine, and saffron, ×400).

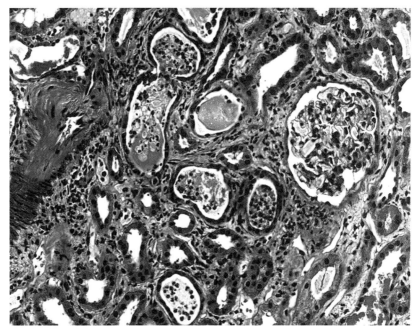

FIG. 3.96 Cast nephropathy. The casts are surrounded by multinucleated giant cells formed from infiltrating macrophages (trichrome, ×200).

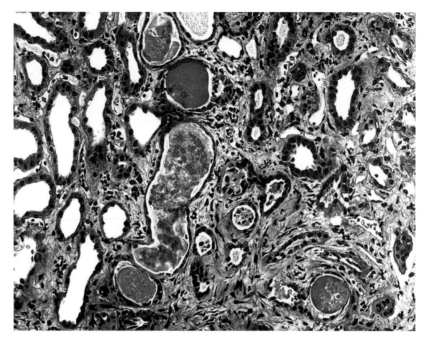

FIG. 3.97 Cast nephropathy. There is evidence of tubular necrosis and an inflammatory response is seen involving the interstitium (trichrome, ×200).

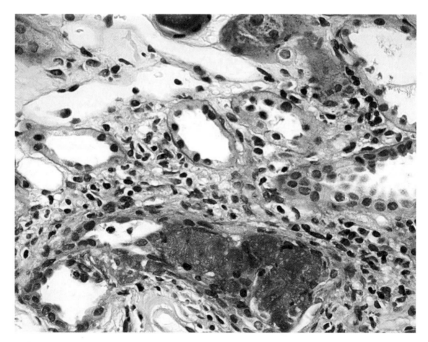

FIG. 3.98 Cast nephropathy. There is Tamm–Horsfall protein intermingled with the light chains (periodic acid Schiff, ×400).

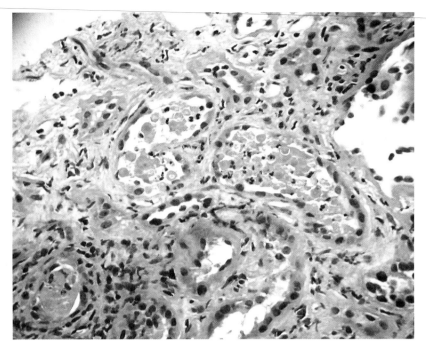

FIG. 3.99 Cast nephropathy. The fractured casts are surrounded by hyaline material within the epithelial cells (hematoxylin and eosin, ×400).

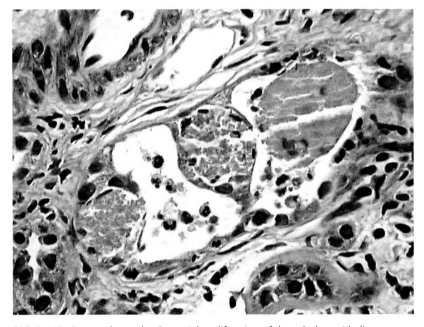

FIG. 3.100 Cast nephropathy. Syncytial proliferation of the tubular epithelium surrounding cast material (trichrome, ×400).

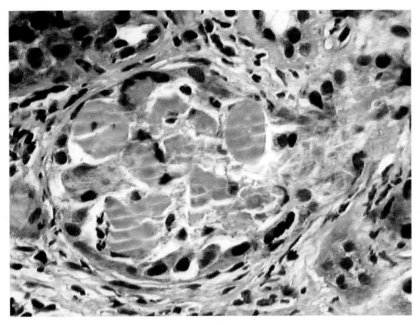

FIG. 3.101 Cast nephropathy. A granulomatous appearance of the cell reaction is seen in this tubule with irregular fractured casts and a cellular reaction (trichrome, ×400).

Key Diagnostic Features of Light Chain Cast Nephropathy

- Angulated, fractured-appearing casts with syncytial cell reaction
- Chronic interstitial nephritis
- May show clonal staining of casts by IF

Note: In the acute phase, casts may be more amorphous and with a more acute inflammatory response. This must be distinguished from acute pyelonephritis (see above).

Monoclonal staining for kappa or lambda light chains helps to confirm the diagnosis, although it should be noted that only about half of casts in proven light chain cast nephropathy stain (Fig. 3.102). Therefore, the absence of monoclonal staining of the casts cannot be taken as definitive evidence ruling out light chain cast nephropathy.

An uncommon form of light chain disease is light chain tubulopathy. Crystalline light chain crystals accumulate within tubular epithelial cells. The parietal epithelium of the glomerular capsule may also be involved. This is often manifested clinically by a Fanconi-like renal tubular acidosis, and is the most common cause of Fanconi syndrome in adults (Fig. 3.103, 3.104). It may also be accompanied by light chain deposition in tubular basements (Fig. 3.105).

Electron microscopy can also be useful in that the tubular epithelium and the tubular casts may have a very distinctive composition of finely granular material of moderate electron density, often forming crystal-like structures (Figs. 3.106-3.110). Because of the distinctive nature of the cast material and the giant cell reaction to it, the differential diagnosis is relatively limited but does include other forms of paraproteinemias, including Waldenström macroglobulinemia. Light chain cast nephropathy may coexist with other manifestations of the monoclonal light chain, with either amyloidosis or light chain deposition disease (see section on Monoclonal Immunoglobulin Deposition Disease).

Text continued on page 448

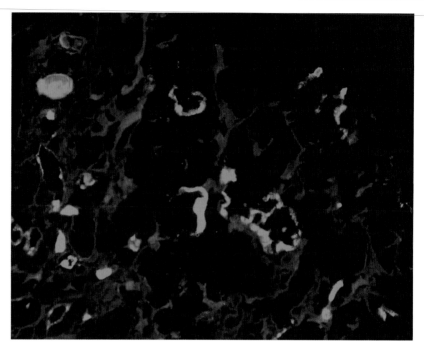

FIG. 3.102 Cast nephropathy. Immunofluorescence reveals the cast material to stain positively in a monoclonal pattern with kappa or lambda light chains (anti-kappa, ×200).

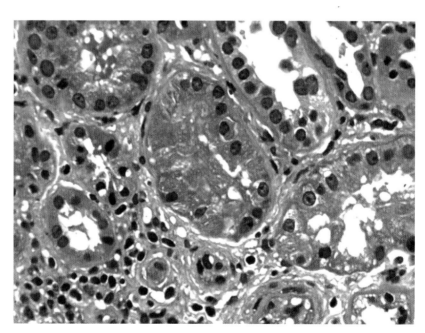

FIG. 3.103 Light chain tubulopathy. Tubular epithelial cells contain crystalline precipitates of reabsorbed light chains (hematoxylin and eosin, ×400).

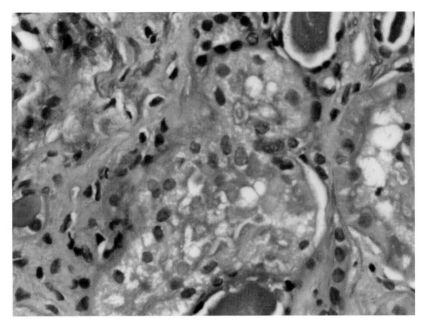

FIG. 3.104 Light chain tubulopathy. Tubules may also show a granular vacuolated appearance (hematoxylin and eosin, ×400).

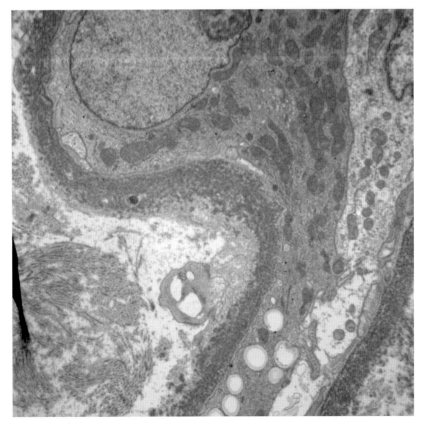

FIG. 3.105 Light chain tubulopathy. Electron microscopy reveals granular light chain deposition in tubular basement membrane (transmission electron microscopy, ×5000).

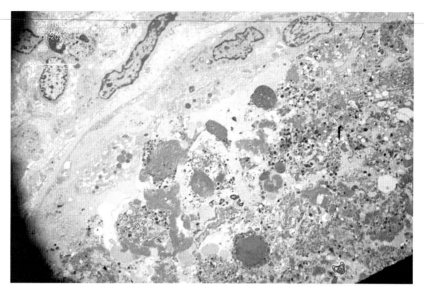

FIG. 3.106 Cast nephropathy. Electron microscopy reveals the tubules to be occluded by a mixture of dense homogenous cast material with fragments of cells and cellular debris (transmission electron microscopy, ×2000).

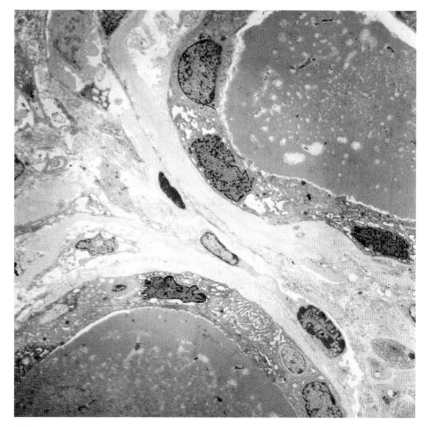

FIG. 3.107 Cast nephropathy. In contrast to other casts which are more homogenous in appearance and have a dark electron-dense appearance, these light chain casts are heterogenous and lighter (transmission electron microscopy, ×2000).

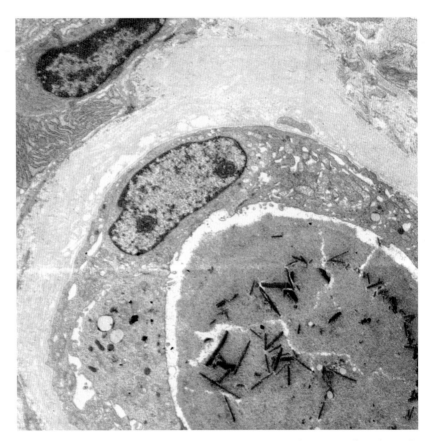

FIG. 3.108 Cast nephropathy. Some cast material also has dense crystalline material surrounded by proteinaceous material (transmission electron microscopy, ×4000).

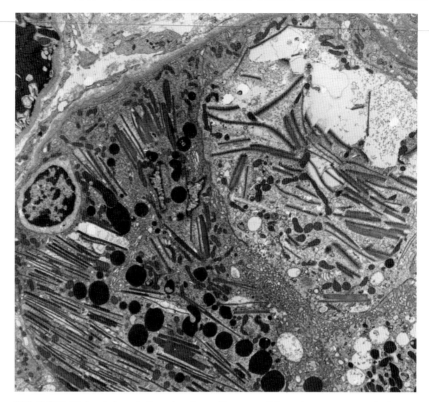

FIG. 3.109 Light chain tubulopathy. Crystalline material can be present in tubular epithelium (transmission electron microscopy, ×4000).

Etiology/Pathogenesis

The mechanism by which urinary light chains lead to renal failure is incompletely understood. Light chains precipitate in the tubules, leading to casts in the distal and collecting tubules. These casts contain Tamm–Horsfall mucoprotein, which is a protein normally secreted by the cells of the thick ascending limb of the loop of Henle and constitute the matrix of all urinary casts. The limitation of obstructing casts to the distal nephron reflects the requirement of the excreted light chains to aggregate with Tamm–Horsfall mucoprotein. Experimental studies have shown that light chains are tubulotoxic depending on the potential of an individual light chain to bind Tamm–Horsfall mucoprotein.

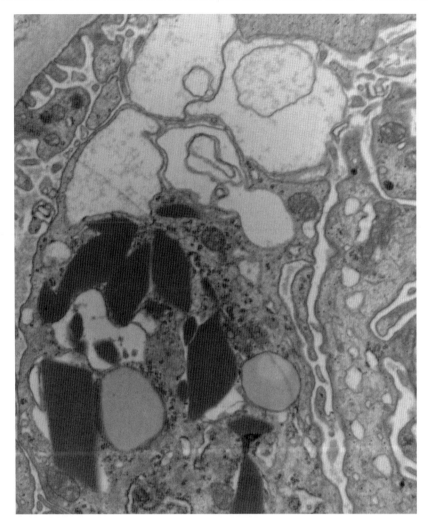

FIG. 3.110 Light chain tubulopathy. Crystalline material is sometimes present in podocytes (transmission electron microscopy, ×4000).

Selected Reading

Kyle, R.A., 1994. Monoclonal proteins and renal disease. Annual Review of Medicine 45, 71-77.

Sanders, P.W., 1993. Renal involvement in plasma cell dyscrasias. Current Opinion in Nephrology and Hypertension 2, 246-252.

Tubular Crystallopathies

CYSTINOSIS

Cystinosis is a lysosomal storage disease with autosomal recessive inheritance, with defect in cystinosin, resulting in lysosomal accumulation of cystine. Cystinosis is divided into an infantile form with frequent kidney manifestations, a juvenile form with intermediate kidney phenotype, and an adult, nonnephropathic form. The incidence is 1 in 100,000-200,000 live births, with a higher incidence seen in the Brittany region of France (1 in 26,000). Patients may have disease manifestations even when they are compound heterozygous. Children present with growth retardation, renal tubular Fanconi syndrome, and chronic kidney disease, and may also show photophobia with corneal crystals, hypothyroidism, neurobehavioral abnormalities, impaired sweating, delayed puberty, and portal hypertension. Fanconi syndrome is nearly invariably present in affected patients with the infantile nephropathic form. Hypothyroidism and photophobia present by age 5-10 years in half of patients. Chronic kidney disease is evident by age 8-12 years in 95% of patients.

Tubular injury results in the clinical findings of polyuria, polydipsia, dehydration, acidosis, hypocalcemia and hypokalemia (Fanconi syndrome), and sometimes hypophosphatemic rickets. Cystinosis is the most common identifiable cause of Fanconi syndrome in children.

Diagnosis may be made by slitlamp examination revealing corneal crystals, and confirmed by leukocyte cystine content measurement, or by genetic studies to show cystinosin mutation.

Patients are treated with cysteamine. Cysteamine enters the lysosome through a transporter and forms disulfide cysteamine-cystine, which can exit the lysosome via the lysine transporter. Glutathione in the cytosol reduces this compound to cystine and cysteamine, and cysteamine can then enter the lysosome again to shuttle out more cystine. When cysteamine therapy is started early, renal deterioration can be slowed down, and crystal accumulation can be prevented in other organs. Ongoing cystine crystal accumulation can also cause disease in the transplant.

In cystinosis, cystine crystals accumulate in the tubular epithelium and in macrophages in the interstitium and may also be free in the interstitium (Fig. 3.111).

Classically, the first part of the proximal tubule is thinned and atrophic, the so-called swan neck deformity. Cystinosis results in patchy tubular atrophy and interstitial fibrosis (Fig. 3.111, 3.112). Glomeruli may show secondary sclerosis and tubular epithelial cells and podocytes may be multinucleated (Fig. 3.113). The latter is not a pathognomonic feature, as multinucleated podocytes may also be seen in other storage diseases, for example, Niemann-Pick or Gaucher disease. The crystals are hexagonal, rhombohedral, or polymorphous and can be visualized under polarized light in alcohol-fixed or frozen tissue (Fig. 3.114). Aqueous

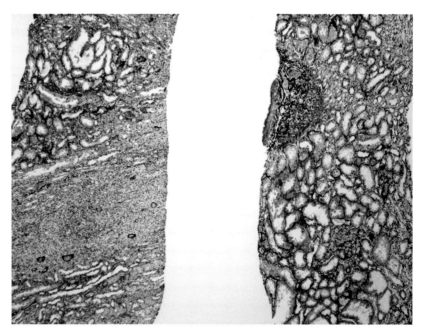

FIG. 3.111 Cystinosis. Cystinosis results in patchy tubular atrophy and interstitial fibrosis (Jones silver stain, ×100).

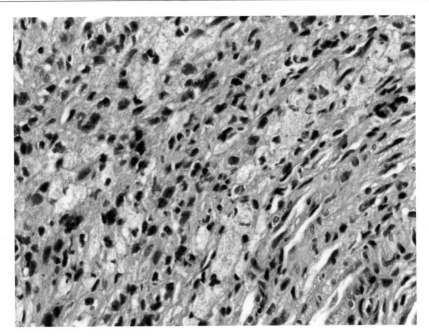

FIG. 3.112 Cystinosis. Cystinosis with interstitial fibrosis and lymphocytic and macrophage infiltrate, with occasional crystals present within the interstitium (hematoxylin and eosin, ×400).

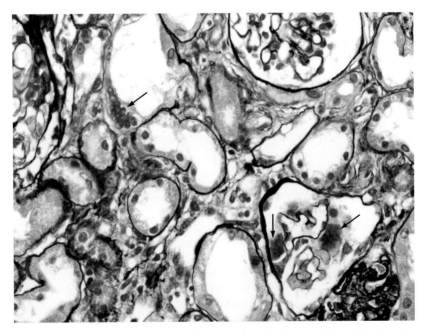

FIG. 3.113 Cystinosis. Cystinosis may show multinucleation of tubular epithelial cells and of podocytes (arrows). Multinucleated podocytes are not pathognomonic of cystinosis, as they may be seen in other storage diseases (Jones silver stain, ×400).

fixatives dissolve crystals, so they may not be readily identifiable in tissue sections. Polarization should, therefore, be done on nonaqueous fixed or frozen sections. Some crystals may also be retained in paraffin-processed hematoxylin and eosin–stained sections (Fig. 3.115). Standard immunofluorescence is negative. Toluidine blue–stained slides and electron microscopy visualize the clear crystals (Figs. 3.116, 3.117).

FIG. 3.114 Cystinosis. Cystinosis with polarizable rectangular, rhomboid crystals are best visualized on polarized frozen sections. As shown here, crystals are present within glomerular epithelial cells and in interstitial macrophages (hematoxylin and eosin frozen section, ×400).

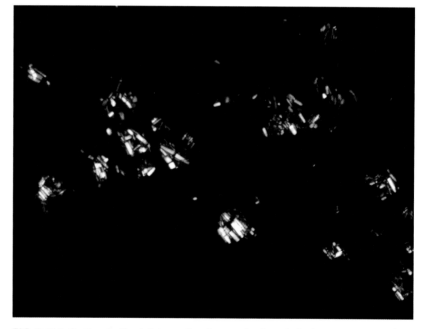

FIG. 3.115 Cystinosis. Crystals in cystinosis may also be relatively more preserved in paraffin-processed tissue on hematoxylin and eosin stains compared to other special stains, as demonstrated here. Numerous rhomboid and rectangular cystine crystals are present in the interstitium (polarized hematoxylin and eosin, ×200).

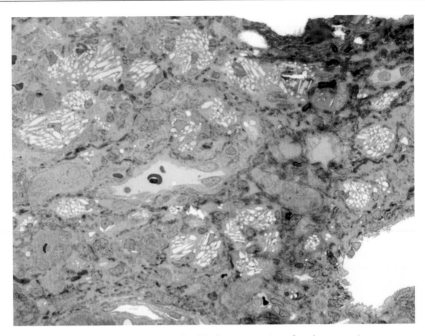

FIG. 3.116 Cystinosis. In plastic-embedded scout sections for electron microscopy, clear spaces of the cystine crystals are readily visualized in macrophages in the tubulointerstitium (toluidine blue stain, ×200).

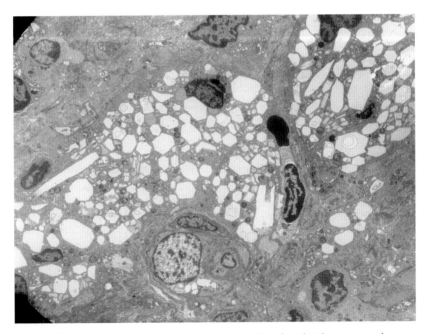

FIG. 3.117 Cystinosis. Cystine crystals are seen as clear rhomboid or rectangular clear spaces in macrophages by electron microscopy (transmission electron microscopy, ×8000).

Etiology/Pathogenesis

Cystinosis is due to mutated cystinosin, a key protein for cystine handling. The cystinosin protein contains seven transmembrane domains. The most common molecular defect removes the first ten exons of cystinosin and is found in 50-75% of cystinotic patients of northern European descent, with a founder effect arising in Germany in AD 500. More than 80 mutations have been identified in different kindreds. The accumulated cystine in cystinosis is derived from degradation of disulfate cysteine-cysteine, due to a gene defect in cystinosin. The GYDQL motif in cystinosin plays a role in targeting. When this region is deleted, cystinosin relocalizes to the plasma membrane, but a signal still remains in the lysosome. Lysosomal cystine efflux by cystinosin is coupled to an efflux of hydrogen ions. Thus, the influx of hydrogen ions by the lysosomal H+-ATPase drives cystinosin-mediated cystine transport toward the cytosol.

Selected Reading

Gahl, W.A., Theone, J.G., Schneider, J.A., 2002. Cystinosis. New England Journal of Medicine 347, 111-121.

Gebrail, F., Knapp, M., Perotta, G., et al., 2002. Crystalline histiocytosis in hereditary cystinosis. Archives of Pathology and Laboratory Medicine 126, 1135-1136.

Kalatzis, V., Antignac, C., 2003. New aspects of the pathogenesis of cystinosis. Pediatric Nephrology 18, 207-215.

Kalatzis, V., Nevo, N., Cherqui, S., et al., 2004. Molecular pathogenesis of cystinosis: effect of CTNS mutations on the transport activity and subcellular localization of cystinosin. Human Molecular Genetics 13, 1361-1371.

Kleta, R., Bernardini, I., Ueda, M., et al., 2004. Long-term follow-up of well-treated nephropathic cystinosis patients. The Journal of Pediatrics 145, 555-560.

Nephrocalcinosis

Nephrocalcinosis is a tubulointerstitial nephropathy that either reflects a primary metabolic process involving calcium or phosphorus metabolism or results from severe tissue injury of any cause, so-called dystrophic calcification. In cases of hyperparathyroidism, calcium salts are typically found along TBMs, as concretions within tubules, and in the interstitium (Fig. 3.118). The calcium-phosphate deposits seen in renal allografts, acute kidney injury, and "acute phosphate nephropathy" (see above) are found primarily in the tubular lumens and the cytoplasm of distal tubular epithelial cells, with rare interstitial deposits (Fig. 3.119). Paradoxically, many patients with nephrocalcinosis detected radiographically may have minimally impaired renal function, whereas nephrocalcinosis seen in association with acute kidney injury is often only detected by kidney biopsy.

Nephrocalcinosis occurs when calcium precipitates in conjunction with either oxalate or phosphate. Calcium is detected by Alizirin Red staining (Fig. 3.120). Phosphates in calcium phosphate deposits are detected with the von Kossa stain. The nature of crystals can help determine their composition. Calcium oxalate and calcium urate are birefringent whereas calcium phosphate is not. Hypercalciuria is a well-established risk factor for calcium crystal deposition, but nephrocalcinosis can occur in the setting of normal calcium excretion, particularly in the presence of primary or secondary hyperoxaluria or hyperphosphaturia as seen in acute phosphate nephropathy.

Etiology/Pathogenesis

Hypercalcemia and hypercalciuria associated with primary hyperparathyroidism or metastatic malignancy are the most common causes, whereas granulomatous disease, immobilization,

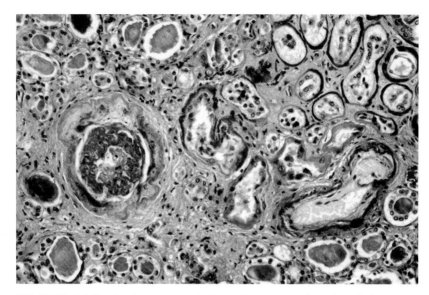

FIG. 3.118 Calcification is present in the interstitium and outlines the tubular basement membranes (hematoxylin and eosin, ×350).

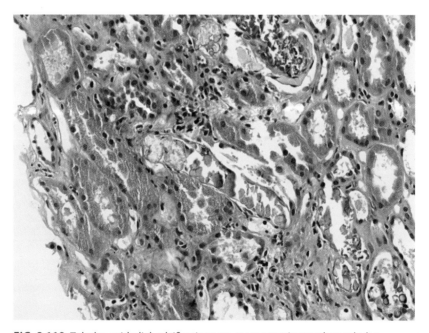

FIG. 3.119 Tubular epithelial calcifications are more prominent when tubular damage is present (hematoxylin and eosin, ×400).

bone disease, vitamin D intoxication, or milk alkali syndrome also have been implicated in the pathogenesis. Hypercalciuria can occur without hypercalcemia through a variety of mechanisms. Distal renal tubular acidosis is associated with nephrocalcinosis, although nephrocalcinosis itself may cause distal acidification defects. Inherited tubulopathies, including Bartter syndrome, hypomagnesemic hypercalciuric nephrocalcinosis, and autosomal dominant hypocalcemia, are manifested by hypercalciuria. In Dent disease and Lowe syndrome, both hypercalciuria and hyperphosphaturia are present. In children, medullary sponge kidney and nephrocalcinosis may coexist.

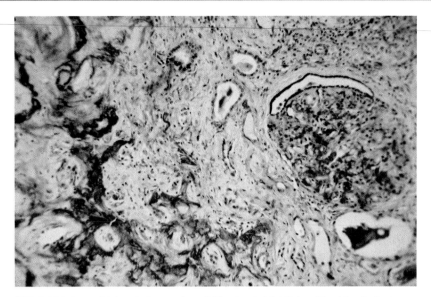

FIG. 3.120 Interstitial and glomerular calcification is highlighted by Alizarin Red staining specific for calcium (×200).

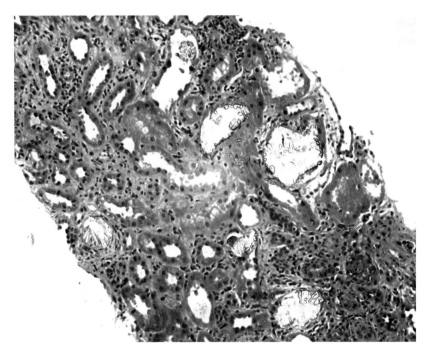

FIG. 3.121 Oxalate nephropathy. There is dilatation of the tubules with crystalline material within the lumen. The crystals have a plate-like appearance (hematoxylin and eosin, ×100).

OXALOSIS

Oxalate crystals within the tubular lumina are frequently present in end-stage kidneys but extensive oxalate crystal deposition is indicative of hyperoxaluric states (Figs. 3.121, 3.122). The histological findings are the nonspecific findings of tubular atrophy and interstitial fibrosis with the distinctive feature being crystal deposition. Calcium oxalate crystals are often fan-shaped and can be seen by light microscopy, but are more readily visualized by their

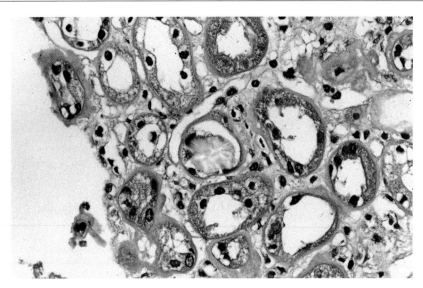

FIG. 3.122 Calcium oxalate. Calcium oxalate crystals are clear and fan-shaped with a plate-like appearance by light microscopy. There is associated acute tubular injury (hematoxylin and eosin, ×200).

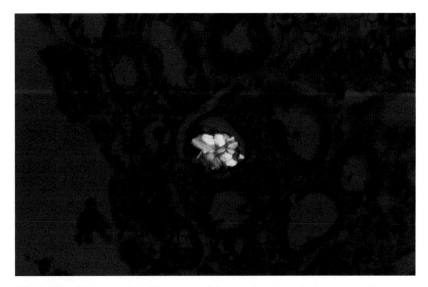

FIG. 3.123 Calcium oxalate. The same calcium oxalate crystals that are barely discernible in Fig. 3.122 are now readily visible under polarized light as birefringent polarizable fan-shaped crystals (polarized hematoxylin and eosin, ×200).

birefringence under polarized light (Figs. 3.122-3.125). Severe fibrosis and inflammation, even with giant cell reaction, can occur when crystals break through the tubular lumina into the interstitium. Calcium oxalate tends to precipitate particularly in proximal tubules, although with extensive disease, all nephron segments may be involved. Calculi are often found in calyces or the pelvis of the kidney. Glomerulosclerosis is proportional to the degree of interstitial injury. Massive crystal deposition occurs in primary hyperoxaluria and ethylene glycol ingestion. Lesser degree of oxalate crystals can occur secondarily, for example, ethylene glycol ingestion, after jejunal-intestinal bypass, or in chronic renal disease due to other causes. Calcium oxalate crystals must be distinguished from the similar fan-shaped, polarizable,

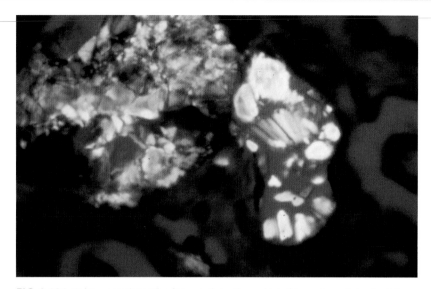

FIG. 3.124 Calcium oxalate. The fan- or plate-shaped birefringent crystals of calcium oxalate are readily apparent (polarized hematoxylin and eosin, ×400).

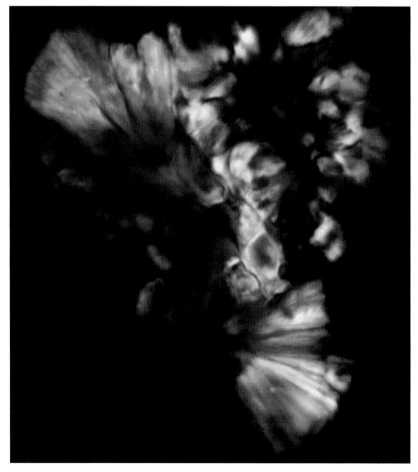

FIG. 3.125 Calcium oxalate. The fan-shaped birefringent crystals of calcium oxalate are readily apparent under oil (polarized hematoxylin and eosin, ×400).

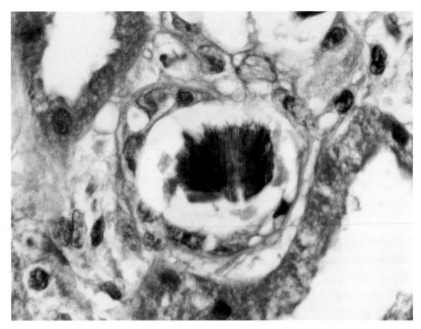

FIG. 3.126 Dihydroxyadeninuria. In 2,8-dihydroxyadeninuria crystalline nephropathy, crystals are present in tubular lumina. There is associated tubular injury. In contrast to calcium oxalate crystals, these are brown on hematoxylin and eosin stain, as shown here (hematoxylin and eosin, ×1000).

Key Diagnostic Findings of Oxalosis

- Fan-shaped polarizable birefringent crystals
- Accompanying acute tubular injury, or chronic tubulointerstitial fibrosis

---

Key Differential Diagnosis of Oxalosis

- Brown polarizable fan-shaped crystals – consider 2,8-dihydroxyadeninuria disease
- Numerous oxalate crystals – consider primary hyperoxaluria (may present in adulthood) vs. ethylene glycol ingestion
- Scattered oxalate crystals – numerous causes, not distinguishable morphologically

---

but brown colored by hematoxylin and eosin crystals of the autosomal recessive 2,8-dihydroxyadeninuria disease (Figs. 3.126, 3.127). These patients have deficiency of the enzyme adenine phosphoribosyltransferase deficiency and develop recurrent nephrolithiasis.

Etiology/Pathogenesis

There are numerous causes of hyperoxaluria. These include ethylene glycol poisoning, excessive ingestion of oxalate-containing foods (cocoa, tea, rhubarb, beet greens, fruit, berries, and spinach), chronic intestinal disease (small bowel resections, malabsorptive states), and primary genetic hyperoxaluria. Type I deficiency is the most common, is inherited as an autosomal recessive disease, and is due to lack of hepatic microsomal alanine glyoxalate aminotransferase. Type II deficiency is very rare, and occurs secondary to a defect in hydroxypyruvate metabolism that has not been defined. Renal disease is less severe than in type I. Type III is due to

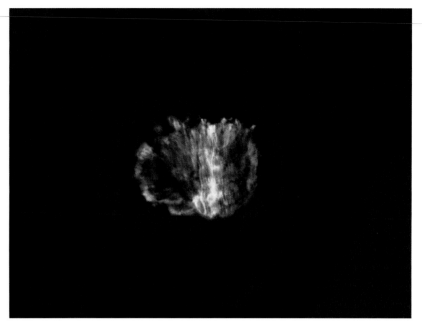

FIG. 3.127 Dihydroxyadeninuria. In 2,8-dihydroxyadeninuria, crystals polarize in similar pattern as calcium oxalate, but their distinct brown appearance by hematoxylin and eosin stain (see Fig. 3.116) allows distinction from calcium oxalate (hematoxylin and eosin polarized, ×1000).

primary intestinal hyperabsorption of oxalate and appears to be very rare. Treatment with pyridoxine, a cofactor for aminotransferase, has been used with some benefit in primary hyperoxaluria. Recent studies have focused on possible benefit of probiotic therapy with *Oxalobacter formigenes* to metabolize oxalate. Kidney transplantation was not successful in early series, with very low graft survival rates due to continued oxalate deposits and mobilization of tissue oxalate pools after surgery. With aggressive supportive therapy with intensive hemodialysis before surgery, pyridoxine, and fluid therapy, results have been better. Combined hepatic and kidney transplantation would be necessary to effect a cure for the underlying defect in patients with primary hyperoxaluria.

Selected Reading

Aponte, G.E., Fetter, T.R., 1954. Familial idiopathic oxalate nephrocalcinosis. American Journal of Clinical Pathology 24, 1363-1373.

Hoppe, B., von Unruh, G., Laube, N., et al., 2005. Oxalate degrading bacteria: new treatment option for patients with primary and secondary hyperoxaluria? Urological Research 33, 372-375.

Morgan, S.H., Watts, R.W.E., 1989. Perspectives in the assessment and management of patients with primary hyperoxaluria Type I. Advances in Nephrology 18, 95-106.

Nasr, S.H., Sethi, S., Cornell, L.D., et al., 2010. Crystalline nephropathy due to 2,8-dihydroxyadeninuria: an under-recognized cause of irreversible renal failure. Nephrology Dialysis Transplantation 25, 1909-1915.

Scheinman, J., 1991. Primary hyperoxaluria: therapeutic strategies for the 90's. Kidney International 40, 389-399.

Williams, A.W., Wilson, D.M., 1990. Dietary intake, absorption, metabolism, and excretion of oxalate. Seminars in Nephrology 10, 2-8.

URATE NEPHROPATHY

There are three different types of urate nephropathy, acute uric acid nephropathy, chronic urate nephropathy, and uric acid nephrolithiasis. Acute urate nephropathy is characterized by acute oliguric or anuric renal failure caused by overproduction of uric acid in patients with lymphoma, leukemia, myeloproliferative diseases, and tumor cell lysis syndrome after chemotherapy. Chronic urate nephropathy can occasionally be found in some patients with tophaceous gout. The combination of secondary focal sclerosis and urate nephropathy is highly suggestive of chronic lead poisoning. Uric acid nephrolithiasis is the more common complication of hyperuricemia in these patients.

Urate nephropathy may be difficult to detect because standard histologic procedures result in dissolution of the intratubular deposits of urate (Fig. 3.128). Routine histology reveals distended collecting ducts, sometimes containing granular casts and focal calcification. There is interstitial fibrosis and foci of interstitial inflammation with occasional foreign body–type giant cells (tophus reaction). Urate crystals with their characteristic needle-like configuration can be identified if the tissue is fixed in alcohol instead of aqueous formalin. Nephrosclerosis is a common feature. Thus, a specific diagnosis of urate nephropathy may not be made, unless specialized fixation is used to detect the crystals.

Etiology/Pathogenesis

The contribution of serum uric acid levels to chronic kidney disease, and the importance of urate nephropathy, have been controversial topics. Epidemiologic studies show correlations of hyperuricemia with chronic kidney disease and hypertension, but it is not known in humans whether this is causal or merely reflects that serum uric acid may be an excellent marker for glomerular filtration. Certainly, direct tissue injury by urate crystals and surrounding tophus reaction contributes to tubulointerstitial fibrosis. Recent animal studies also have demonstrated that elevated serum uric acid can cause tubulointerstitial fibrosis and hypertension.

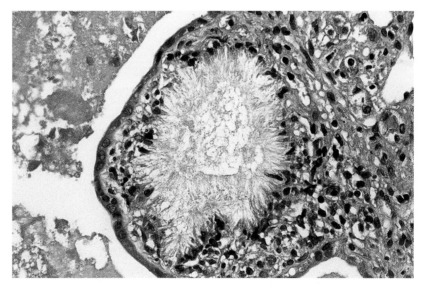

FIG. 3.128 Urate nephropathy. There is an accumulation of needle-like crystals associated with an inflammatory infiltrate in the interstitium typical of a gouty tophus (hematoxylin and eosin, ×400).

Selected Reading

Johnson, R.J., Kivlighn, S.D., Kim, Y.G., et al., 1999. Reappraisal of the pathogenesis and consequences of hyperuricemia in hypertension, cardiovascular disease, and renal disease. American Journal of Kidney Disease 33, 225-234.

Mazzali, M., Hughes, J., Kim, Y.G., et al., 2001. Elevated uric acid increases blood pressure in the rat by a novel crystal-independent mechanism. Hypertension 38, 1101-1106.

Indinavir Nephropathy

The advent of the use of HIV-1 protease inhibitors in the treatment of HIV infection has introduced a new entity of indinavir nephropathy. This can present clinically as acute renal failure and may be diagnosed clinically by the presence of crystalluria. The crystals are needle-like and obstruct the tubules extensively, with surrounding inflammatory reaction (Figs. 3.129, 3.130).

Etiology/Pathogenesis

Indinavir is excreted in the urine. Low solubility is exacerbated by elevated pH, dehydration, high drug levels, and interactions with various other drugs. These factors then together cause crystals to form in the tubules, with direct tubular injury. Indinavir crystals have also been observed in biopsies of patients with more insidious renal insufficiency and tubulointerstitial fibrosis.

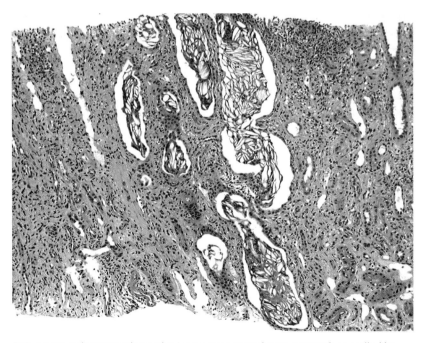

FIG. 3.129 Indinavir nephropathy. Low-power view demonstrates the needle-like crystals surrounded by the desquamated tubular epithelium filling the tubular lumina (hematoxylin and eosin, ×200).

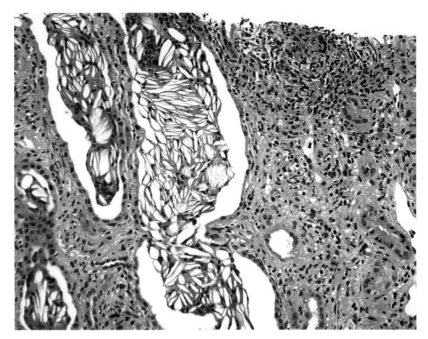

FIG. 3.130 Indinavir nephropathy. Intratubular needle-like crystals are present (hematoxylin and eosin, ×200).

Selected Reading

Famularo, G., Di Toro, S., Moretti, S., et al., 2000. Symptomatic crystalluria associated with indinavir. Ann Pharmacother 34, 1414-1418.

Perazella, M.A., Kashgarian, M., Cooney, E., 1998. Indinavir nephropathy in an AIDS patient with renal insufficiency and pyuria. Clinical Nephrology 50, 194-196.

Lithium Nephropathy

Long-term treatment of patients with bipolar (manic-depressive) illness has been associated with several different forms of renal injury secondary to lithium, the most common of which is a chronic tubulointerstitial nephritis. Lithium appears to act by accumulating in tubule cells, causing cellular injury and initiating a fibrotic response. The degree of interstitial fibrosis on renal biopsy may be directly related to the duration and cumulative dose of lithium. The histology is generally nonspecific, but there is a predominance of tubular lesions with dilatation of tubules in the distal segments and collecting ducts and interstitial fibrosis. Glomerulosclerosis appears to be secondary process to the fibrotic process.

Key Diagnostic Finding of Lithium Nephropathy

- Tubular dilatation, interstitial fibrosis

Note: The findings are nonspecific, and other causes of tubular dilation should be ruled out before suggesting lithium nephropathy.

Selected Reading

Hansen, H.E., Hestbech, J., Sorensen, J.L., et al., 1979. Chronic interstitial nephropathy in patients on long-term lithium treatment. Quarterly Journal of Medicine 48, 577-591.

Markowitz, G.S., Radhakrishnan, J., Kambham, N., et al., 2000. Lithium nephrotoxicity: A progressive combined glomerular and tubulointerstitial nephropathy. Journal of the American Society of Nephrology 2000 11, 1439-1448.

Aristolochic Acid Nephropathy

Chinese herbal medicines that contain aristolochic acid have been associated with acute, often near end-stage renal disease. A chronic interstitial nephritis located principally in the cortex is present with extensive interstitial fibrosis and tubular atrophy. Cellular infiltration of the interstitium is scarce. Thickening of the walls of the interlobular and afferent arterioles result from endothelial cell swelling. The glomeruli are relatively spared and immune deposits are not observed. These findings suggest that the primary lesions may be centered in the vessel walls, thereby leading to ischemia and interstitial fibrosis. An extremely high incidence of cellular atypia and urothelial (transitional cell) carcinoma of the renal pelvis, ureter, and bladder has also been associated with aristolochic acid herbal nephropathy.

Selected Reading

Depierreux, M., Van Damme, B., Vanden Houte, K., et al., 1994. Pathologic aspects of a newly described nephropathy related to the prolonged use of Chinese herbs. American Journal of Kidney Disease 24:172-180.

Yang, C.S., Lin, C.H., Chang, S.H., et al., 2000 Rapidly progressive fibrosing interstitial nephritis associated with Chinese herbal drugs. American Journal of Kidney Disease 35:330-332.

Chronic Kidney Disease

Introduction

Chronic or end-stage kidney disease can result from widely divergent causes: glomerular, vascular, and tubulointerstitial diseases. The use of the formulaic estimation of glomerular filtration rate (eGFR) is now a standard practice, and this has resulted in the identification of patients at risk of end-stage disease at an early stage. A system of staging of chronic kidney disease related to eGFR is routinely applied. A direct correlation of eGFR with the severity of interstitial fibrosis is difficult, but an approximation of the degree of functional impairment can often be made in an adequate sample of tissue. Chronic interstitial nephritis in which the histologic lesion is interstitial fibrosis and tubular atrophy with little or no significant active inflammatory infiltrate can be due to the wide variety of causes described in Chapter 3 (Figs. 4.1, 4.2). It is often difficult to identify a specific etiologic agent, and although an association of a particular agent with chronic renal failure or hypertension suggests the possibility of a cause-and-effect relationship, a strict relationship is often difficult to prove. Even identification of a potential suspect agent may not be sufficient evidence because increased levels could be due to lack of excretion in a patient with renal insufficiency rather than indicative of increased exposure. Chronic interstitial nephritis is therefore often designated as idiopathic. The histologic findings consist of diffuse interstitial fibrosis and tubular atrophy with a variable degree of an interstitial infiltrate of lymphocytes. The findings are nonspecific and are accompanied by vascular changes of arterial and arteriolar sclerosis (Figs. 4.3, 4.4).

Age-Related Sclerosis

Vascular sclerosis and glomerulosclerosis increase in normal populations with aging (Fig. 4.5). The overall young adult U.S. population under age 50 years has less global sclerosis (1-3%); however, it increases up to 30% by age 80 years. However, sclerosis rates vary in different populations. The native Mexican population has less aortic fibroplasia and renal sclerosis at all ages compared to the U.S. population. Furthermore, renal vascular sclerosis was more severe in first- and second-generation Hispanic immigrants than in Mexico City natives, but remained less than that in other U.S. residents. These findings support the interplay of genetic and environmental factors in the determination of vascular sclerosis. In similar morphologic

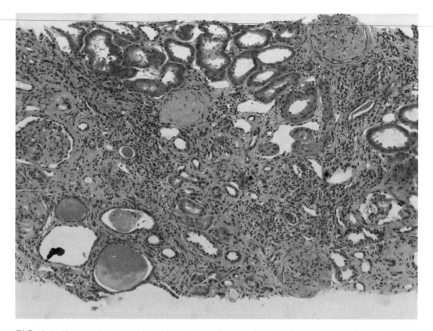

FIG. 4.1 Chronic interstitial nephritis in end-stage kidney disease. There is diffuse interstitial scarring with a nonspecific mononuclear infiltrate (hematoxylin and eosin, ×200).

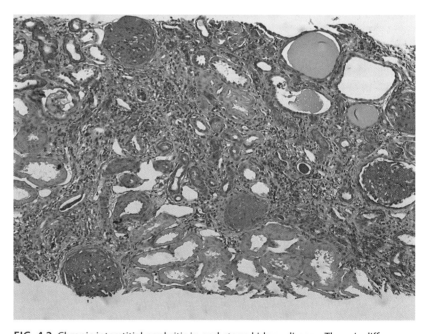

FIG. 4.2 Chronic interstitial nephritis in end-stage kidney disease. There is diffuse interstitial scarring and globally sclerotic glomeruli (trichrome, ×200).

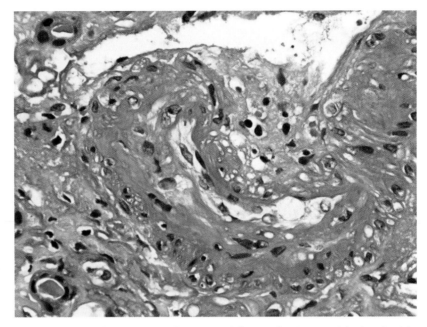

FIG. 4.3 Interlobular artery in end-stage renal disease showing arterial sclerosis with myointimal proliferation and luminal narrowing (hematoxylin and eosin, ×400).

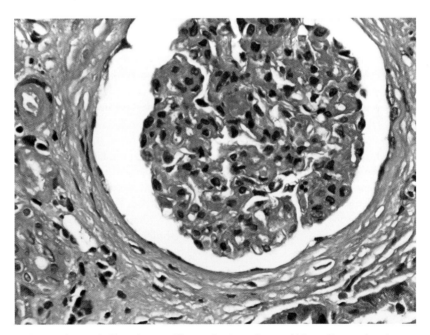

FIG. 4.4 Chronic kidney disease. Glomerulus in end-stage kidney disease showing capillary ischemic retraction without epithelial cell proliferation secondary to hyaline arteriolar sclerosis.

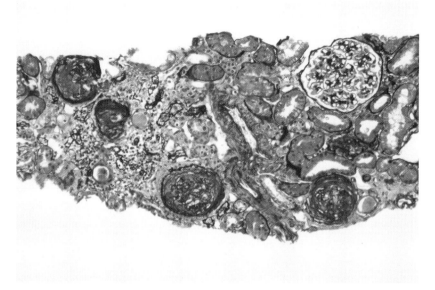

FIG. 4.5 Age-related sclerosis. In aging kidneys, there is increased global sclerosis of obsolescent type, with patchy interstitial fibrosis and tubular atrophy with vascular sclerosis (Jones silver stain, ×200).

studies of Bolivian Indians and elderly Japanese subjects, only minimal vascular sclerosis was present, even at advanced age, much less than expected in older U.S. residents.

Within the United States, vascular sclerosis increases even more with aging in normal African Americans than in the Caucasians. These advanced vascular changes in African Americans correlated with higher screening clinic blood pressures versus Caucasians as measured in a different population-based cohort from the same New Orleans region. However, the blood pressure differences (if indeed representative of the autopsied patients in that area) would not completely account for the greater vascular sclerosis in the African American population (see above). These findings suggest possible differences in injury set point and rates and mechanisms of vascular lesions between these varying populations, both in "normal" aging and in response to injury. In our retrospective patient-based study of African Americans and Caucasians, we observed that aging was associated with an increase of the obsolescent type of globally sclerosed glomeruli but not of the solidified type. This suggests different mechanisms leading to the varying phenotypes of sclerosis in different populations and may support different antihypertensive medications based on ethnicity.

Selected Reading

Marcantoni, C., Ma, L.J., Federspiel, C., et al, 2002. Hypertensive nephrosclerosis in African-Americans vs Caucasians. Kidney International 62, 172-180.

Smith, S.M., Hoy, W.E., Cobb, L., 1989. Low incidence of glomerulosclerosis in normal kidneys. Archives of Pathology & Laboratory Medicine 113, 1253-1256.

Tamura, T., 1966. Histologic features of renal biopsies from patients with essential hypertension and from the aged. Japanese Circulation Journal 30, 829-862.

Tracy, R.E., 1996. Renovasculopathies of hypertension and the rise of blood pressure with age in blacks and whites. Seminars in Nephrology 16, 126-133.

Tracy, R.E., Guileyardo, J.M., 1999. Renovasculopathies of hypertension in Hispanic residents of Dallas, Texas. Archives of Medical Research 30, 40-48.

Tracy, R.E., Rios-Dalenz, J.L., 1994. Rarity of hypertensive stigmata in aging renocortical arteries of Bolivians. Virchows Archiv 424, 307-314.

Tracy, R.E., Berenson, G.S., Cueto-Garcia, L., et al, 1992. Nephrosclerosis and aortic atherosclerosis from age 6 to 70 years in the United States and Mexico. Virchows Archive A: Pathological Anatomy and Histopathology 420, 479-488.

Tracy, R.E., Guzman, M.A., Oalmann, M.C., et al, 1993. Nephrosclerosis in three cohorts of black and white men born 1925 to 1944, 1934 to 1953, and 1943 to 1962. American Journal of Hypertension 6, 185-192.

Glomerular vs. Tubulointerstitial vs. Vascular Disease

Chronic or end-stage kidney disease can result from widely divergent causes: glomerular, vascular, and tubulointerstitial diseases. The use of the formulaic eGFR is now a standard practice, and this has resulted in the identification of patients at risk of end-stage disease at an early stage. A system of staging of chronic kidney disease related to eGFR is routinely applied. A direct correlation of eGFR with the severity of interstitial fibrosis is difficult, but an approximation of the degree of functional impairment can often be made in an adequate sample of tissue, although accurate assessment of degree or quality of fibrosis is also challenging.

Specific immune complex glomerular diseases are diagnosed by immunofluorescence and electron microscopic findings. Non–immune complex glomerular sclerosing processes can be diagnosed when these lesions are dominant, with proportional interstitial fibrosis and vascular sclerosis, as outlined in the section on Primary vs Secondary Segmental Glomerulosclerosis. When vascular lesions dominate, as may be seen in arterionephrosclerosis, there usually is accompanying dominant obsolescent or solidified appearance of the glomerulosclerosis (see Arterionephrosclerosis), or disease-specific findings of, for example, malignant hypertension, scleroderma, or thrombotic microangiopathy. In the absence of such glomerular or vascular lesions, we turn our attention to the tubules and interstitium. Chronic interstitial nephritis in which the histologic lesion is interstitial fibrosis and tubular atrophy with little or no significant active inflammatory infiltrate can be due to the wide variety of causes described in specific sections in Chapter 3. When there is disproportionate inflammatory infiltrate associated with the fibrosis, we consider a diagnosis of chronic interstitial nephritis and search for specific causes, such as crystals, pathogenic casts, virus, heavy metals, or even immune injury (e.g., granular TBM deposits, or anti-TBM injury). It is often difficult to identify a specific etiologic agent and although an association of a particular agent with chronic renal failure or hypertension suggests the possibility of a cause-and-effect relationship, a strict relationship is often difficult to prove. Even identification of a potential suspect agent may not be sufficient evidence because increased levels could be due to lack of excretion in a patient with renal insufficiency rather than indicative of increased exposure. Chronic interstitial nephritis is therefore often designated as idiopathic. The histologic findings consist of diffuse interstitial fibrosis and tubular atrophy with a variable degree of an interstitial infiltrate of lymphocytes. The findings are nonspecific and are accompanied by vascular changes of arterial and arteriolar sclerosis.

Selected Reading

Coresh, J., Selvin, E., Stevens, L.A., et al, 2007. Prevalence of chronic kidney disease in the United States. Journal of the American Medical Association 298, 2038-2047.

Fogo, A.B., Alpers, C.E., 2010. Navigating the challenges of fibrosis assessment – land in sight? Journal of the American Society of Nephrology. in press.

Hallan, S.I., Ritz, E., Lydersen, S., et al, 2009. Combining GFR and albuminuria to classify CKD improves prediction of ESRD. Journal of the American Society of Nephrology 20, 1069-1077.

Segmental Glomerulosclerosis: Primary vs. Secondary

Focal and segmental glomerulosclerosis (FSGS) is a common endpoint in a variety of settings, including idiopathic FSGS, or scarring secondary to other glomerular disease or systemic abnormalities, such as immune complex–mediated injury, hypertension, obesity, diabetes, reflux nephropathy, chronic interstitial nephritis, and HIV infection. These different etiologies contribute to the diverse clinical outcomes and morphologic appearances of histologic focal sclerosis. The diagnosis and distinction of variants of primary FSGS are discussed in Chapter 1. We will here consider an approach to distinction of secondary causes of FSGS lesions from primary FSGS.

Secondary sclerosis may occur as a superimposed, nonspecific scarring lesion in many immune complex diseases. Immune complex entities underlying FSGS lesions can be easily differentiated from primary FSGS by full examination with immunofluorescence and electron microscopy, using diagnostic criteria outlined in specific sections on immune complex diseases.

Secondary sclerosis without immune deposits may be due to healed crescentic lesions, podocyte injury, be related to hypertension or chronic pyelonephritis, occur in the transplant, or result from adaptive processes due to loss of nephrons from another primary disease process.

Pauci-immune crescentic glomerulonephritis can demonstrate characteristic segmental areas of sclerosis with adhesion and retraction of Bowman's capsule, with a "tethered" appearance: important clues to the past proliferative, destructive lesion.

FSGS lesions with a collapsing phenotype, that is, collapse of the tuft with podocyte hyperplasia, may result from, for example, virus (HIV, parvovirus B19, SV40) and drugs (heroin, pamidronate, calcineurin inhibitors). However, foot process effacement, visceral cell hypertrophy, and hyperplasia may be less frequent in secondary forms as compared to primary FSGS, and subtotal foot process effacement favors secondary etiology. Additional lesions, such as reticular aggregates in HIV-associated nephropathy, immunostaining positivity for parvovirus, and other features of calcineurin inhibitor toxicity, may all aid in distinction from primary FSGS lesions.

Lesions of segmental sclerosis in the renal transplant may be due to recurrence of primary FSGS (see FSGS, Chapter 1) or due to injury related to chronic allograft nephropathy or chronic transplant glomerulopathy. Chronic transplant glomerulopathy demonstrates glomerular basement membrane splitting with increased lamina rara interna by electron microscopy, a finding not typical of recurrent idiopathic FSGS. When chronic allograft nephropathy is contributed to by cyclosporin toxicity, interstitial fibrosis in a striped pattern with concentric nodular arteriolar hyalinosis involving the media may be present and provide further clues for correct diagnosis. Nonspecific secondary sclerosis may also occur in this setting, frequently with contracted, small glomeruli, glomerular basement membrane corrugation, periglomerular fibrosis, and subtotal foot process effacement. Clinical history is also important because FSGS usually recurs in the first months after the transplant, whereas secondary sclerosis related to chronic allograft nephropathy and chronic transplant glomerulopathy are later events.

FSGS can also be observed secondary to arterionephrosclerosis. Usually sclerosis and hyalinosis are located at the vascular pole when sclerotic lesions are associated with arterionephrosclerosis. The biopsy usually shows predominance of small, shrunken, globally sclerotic glomeruli, the presence of periglomerular fibrosis, glomerular basement membrane corrugation, increased lucency of the lamina rara interna, and subtotal foot process effacement by electron microscopy, and disproportionately severe vascular lesions relative to sclerosis. Of course, the clinical course is crucial, with proteinuria developing *after* a long history of hypertension in this setting.

In FSGS secondary to reflux nephropathy, there is typically glomerulomegaly, frequently with prominent periglomerular fibrosis and thickening of Bowman's capsule. The interstitium shows patchy, so-called geographical areas of fibrosis with disproportionate tubulointerstitial injury, in addition to the heterogeneous glomerulosclerosis. The term *geographical* is used to describe the jigsaw puzzle–like, sharply delineated patches of fibrosis, alternating with intact parenchyma.

Lastly, adaptive secondary sclerosis occurs following significant loss of nephrons, likely through structural–functional adaptations contributed to by a complex array of compensatory changes, including but not limited to altered hemodynamics, growth factors, and reactive oxygen species. These lesions often show a hilar-type FSGS, with glomerulomegaly, and limited foot process effacement.

Selected Reading

D'Agati, V., 1994. The many masks of focal segmental glomerulosclerosis. Kidney International 46, 1223-1241.

D'Agati, V.D., Fogo, A.B., Bruijn, J.A., et al, 2004. Pathologic classification of focal segmental glomerulosclerosis: a working proposal. American Journal of Kidney Disease 43, 368-382.

Howie, A.J., Lee, S.J., Green, N.J., et al, 1993. Different clinicopathological types of segmental sclerosing glomerular lesions in adults. Nephrology Dialysis Transplantation 8, 590-599.

Marcantoni, C., Ma, L.J., Federspiel, C., et al, 2002. Hypertensive nephrosclerosis in African Americans versus Caucasians. Kidney International 62, 172-180.

Rennke, H., Klein, P.S., 1989. Pathogenesis and significance of non-primary focal and segmental glomerulosclerosis. American Journal of Kidney Disease 13, 443-455.

Rossini, M., Fogo, A.B., 2004. Interpreting segmental glomerular sclerosis. Current Diagnostic Pathology 10, 1-10.

Schwartz, M.M., Korbet, S.M., Rydell, J., et al, 1995. Primary focal segmental glomerular sclerosis in adults: prognostic value of histologic variants. American Journal of Kidney Disease 25, 845-852.

Renal Transplantation

Introduction

Evaluation of the renal morphology in allograft patients is used to answer two major questions. Is the failure of the graft caused by rejection or some other unrelated lesion? And if rejection is present, is the lesion potentially reversible using available therapeutic approaches? In the absence of rejection, it should be ascertained whether the graft failure results from acute tubular injury, acute infectious pyelonephritis, obstruction of the vasculature or urinary outflow tract, presence of recurrent or de novo glomerular disease, or toxicity associated with the therapeutic agents used to modulate the immune response. In assessing whether rejection lesions are potentially reversible, it is necessary to evaluate not only the intensity but also the nature of the rejection episode.

The Banff working classification of renal allograft pathology modified in 1997 is now an internationally agreed upon standardized classification of the morphologic changes associated with various types of rejection (Table 5.1). It was updated in 2007 and 2009 to include peritubular capillaritis grading, C4d scoring, and interpretation and introduction of a new scoring for interstitial scarring and tubular atrophy. This newer version of the Banff system was influenced by data from several clinical trials using the Banff 94 Schema and the results of clinical correlations of the Cooperative Clinical Trials in Transplantation (CCTT). Interstitial infiltration of activated lymphocytes with tubulitis characteristic of cellular rejection (Type I) and intimal arteritis characteristic of vascular rejection (Type II) are considered the main lesions indicative of acute rejection episodes (Table 5.2). The goal of the use of this classification is to be able to give a diagnostic biopsy grading that will provide both a prognostic and therapeutic tool (Tables 5.3, 5.4). The standardized classification also promotes international uniformity in reporting of renal allograft pathology and is useful to facilitate the performance of multicenter trials of new therapeutic modalities.

TABLE 5-1 Banff 97 Diagnostic Categories for Renal Allograft Biopsies – Banff '07 Update

1. **Normal**
2. **Antibody-mediated changes** (may coincide with categories 3, 4 and 5 and 6)
   Due to documentation of circulating antidonor antibody, and C4d positivity or allograft pathology
   C4d deposition without morphologic evidence of active rejection
   C4d+, presence of circulating antidonor antibodies, no signs of acute or chronic TCMR or ABMR (i.e. g0, cg0, ptc0, no ptc lamination). Cases with simulatenous borderline changes or AT1 are considered as indeterminate
   Acute antibody-mediated rejection4*
   C4d+, presence of circulation antidonor antibodies, morphologic evidence of acute tissue injury, such as (Type/Grade):
   I.   ATI-like minimal inflammation
   II. Capillary and/or glomerular inflammation (ptc/g >0) and/or thromboses
   III. Arterial v3 changes
   Chronic active antibody-mediated rejection*
   C4d+, presence of circulating antidonor antibodies, morphologic evidence of chronic tissue injury, such as glomerular double contours and/or peritubular capillary basement membrane multilayering and/or interstitial fibrosis/tubular atrophy and/or fibrous intimal thickening in arteries
3. **Borderline changes:** "Suspicious" for acute TCMR (may coincide with categories 2 and 5 and 6)
   This category is used when no intimal arteritis is present, but there are foci of tubulitis (t1, t2 or t3) with minor interstitial infiltration (i0 or i1) or interstitial infiltration (i2, i3) with mild (t1) tubulitis
4. **T-cell-mediated rejection** (TCMR, may coincide with categories 2 and 5 and 6)
   Acute TCMR (Type/Grage):
   IA. Cases with significant interstitial infiltration (>25% of parenchyma affected, i2 or i3) and foci of moderate tubulitis (t2)
   IB. Cases with significant interstitial infiltration (>25% of parenchyma affected, i2 or i3) and foci of severe tubulitis (t3)
   IIA. Cases with mild-to-moderate intimal arteritis (v1)
   IIB. Cases with severe intimal arteritis comprising >25% of the luminal area (v2)
   III. Cases with "transmural" arteritis and/or arterial fibrinoid change and necrosis of medial smooth muscle cells with accompanying lymphocytic inflammation (v3)
   Chronic active T-cell-mediated rejection
   "Chronic allograft arteriopathy" (arterial initmal fibrosis with mononuclear cell infiltration in fibrosis, formation of neo-intima)
5. Interstitial fibrosis and tubular atrophy, no evidence of any specific etiology (may include nonspecific vascular and glomerular sclerosis, but severity graded by tubulointerstitial features)
   Grade
   I.   Mild interstitial fibrosis and tubular atrophy (<25% of cortical area)
   II. Moderate interstitial fibrosis and tubular atrophy (26-50% of cortical area)
   III. Severe interstitial fibrosis and tubular atrophy/loss (>50% of cortical area)
6. **Other:** Changes not considered to be due to rejection–acute and/or chronic (e.g., hypertensive changes, calcineurin inhibitor toxicity, obstruction, bacterial pyelonephritis, viral infection)

ABMR, antibody-mediated rejection; *ATI,* acute tubular injury; *PTC,* peritubular capillary; *TCMR,* T cell-mediated rejection.
*Suspicious for ABMR if C4d (in the presence of antibody) or alloantibody (C4d+) note demonstrated in the presence of morphologic evidence of tissue injury.

TABLE 5-2 Overview of Acute Rejection

Banff 97	Banff 93-95	CCTT
Suspicious for acute rejection, borderline	Borderline	Type I[a]
Type 1A (tubulointerstitial with t2 and at least i2)	Grade I	Type I[a]
Type 1B (tubulointerstitial with t3 and at least i2)	Grade IIA	Type I[a]
Type IIA (vascular with v1)	Grade IIB	Type II
Type IIB (vascular with v2)	Grade III	
Type III v3 (fibrinoid change/transmural arteritis)	Grade III	Type III

[a]A semiquantitative scoring system has been developed to produce an acute or chronic numerical index for purposes of evaluation of severity.

TABLE 5-3 Quantitative Criteria for Tubulitis ('t') Score[a]

t0	No mononuclear cells in tubules
t1	Foci with 1-4 cells/tubular cross section (or 10 tubular cells)
t2	Foci with 5-10 cells/tubular cross section
t3	Foci with >10 cells/tubular cross section, or the presence of at least two areas of tubular basement membrane destruction accompanied by i2/i3 inflammation and t2 tubulitis elsewhere in the biopsy

[a]Applies to tubules no more than mildly atrophic.

TABLE 5-4 Quantitative Criteria for Intimal Arteritis ("v")

v0	No arteritis
v1	Mild to moderate intimal arteritis in at least one arterial cross section
v2	Severe intimal arteritis with at least 25% luminal area lost in at least one arterial cross section
v3	Transmural arteritis and/or arterial fibrinoid change and medial smooth muscle necrosis with lymphocytic infiltrate in vessel

Note number of arteries present and number affected. Indicate infarction and/or interstitial hemorrhage by an asterisk (with any level v score).

Etiology/Pathogenesis

The mechanisms involved in allograft rejection are complex and involve both cellular and humoral immunity. Efforts to reduce the immune response to alloantigens include cross-matching human leukocyte antigens (HLAs) as closely as possible and blocking of the presentation and recognition of these antigens. The status of the graft at time of transplant is also important because outcomes are poorer with prolonged cold ischemia times.

Antibody-Mediated Rejection

This category is divided into immediate (hyperacute) and delayed (accelerated acute). Hyperacute rejection refers to allograft failure that occurs within minutes or hours after transplantation. It is thought to be the result of preexisting circulating antibodies of the recipient that are directed against donor-specific HLA class 1 or ABH antigens present in the grafted endothelium. Presensitization of the recipient is often related to previous pregnancies, blood transfusions, or other previous antigenic stimuli. However, hyperacute rejections may also be related to endothelial damage that is not immunologic in nature. A separate form of acute graft failure that is not immunologic has been termed acute imminent transplant nephropathy and has been related to injury occurring in the graft during the preservation phase. Delayed or accelerated acute rejection refers to situations where sudden graft loss occurs due to the development of antidonor antibodies. Both types have a similar histologic appearance.

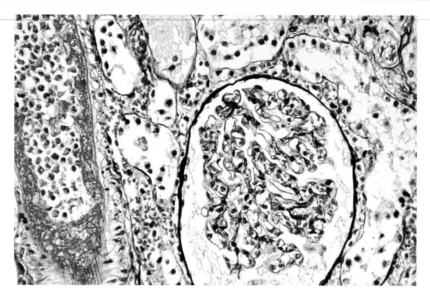

FIG. 5.1 Hyperacute rejection. The artery is occluded by a fibrin thrombus and there is evidence of congestion in the peritubular capillaries. Focal tubular necrosis is also seen in this silver methenamine Masson stain (×200).

TABLE 5-5 Antibody-Mediated Rejection (Meeting Criteria of C4d+ and with Circulating Antidonor Antibody)

1. Acute tubular necrosis–like
2. Capillary-glomerulitis, polymorphonuclear, and/or mononuclear leukocytes in peritubular capillaries
3. Arterial–transmural inflammation/fibrinoid change

Key Diagnostic Features of Antibody-Mediated Rejection

- Peritubular capillary leukocytes
- C4d staining

Microscopically, fibrin thrombi are seen in all renal vessels (Fig. 5.1), including the glomerular capillaries and peritubular venules. The vascular thrombosis is associated with infarction and tubular necrosis. There is prominent polymorphonuclear leukocyte infiltration in peritubular capillaries. Immunofluorescence may show linear staining for immunoglobulins along the capillary walls of the peritubular venules, but this is not a constant finding. Electron microscopy demonstrates platelets, fibrin-sludged red blood cells, and necrosis of glomerular capillaries and other vascular structures.

An addition to the Banff 97 classification proposes to replace category 2 described above with a special categorization for antibody-mediated rejection (Table 5.5). It takes into account that antibody-mediated rejection is being recognized more frequently and not always in the early posttransplant period. This, combined with the identification of some relatively specific markers such as peritubular capillary staining of C4d, has given rise to a more precise classification (Table 5.5). The criteria for acute antibody-mediated rejection have three cardinal features: evidence of acute renal tissue injury, including tubular injury, inflammatory cells in the peritubular capillaries, or vascular necrosis (Fig. 5.2). Immunopathologic evidence of antibody-mediated disease includes C4d staining of peritubular capillaries (Fig. 5.3) or, less

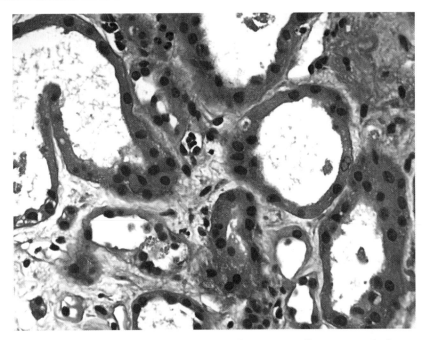

FIG. 5.2 Acute antibody-mediated rejection. Inflammatory cells are present in the peritubular capillaries associated with interstitial edema. Tubulitis and an interstitial infiltrate are not present. These findings are typical of acute antibody-mediated rejection (hematoxylin and eosin, ×400).

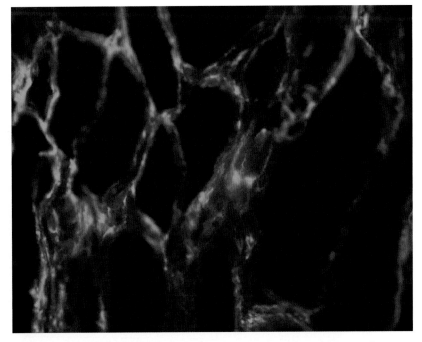

FIG. 5.3 Acute antibody-mediated rejection. Immunopathologic evidence of antibody-mediated rejection is confirmed by the presence of staining for C4d in peritubular capillaries shown here by indirect immunofluorescence (anti-C4d immunofluorescence, ×400).

specifically, immunoglobulin or complement deposition in vessels or serologic evidence of antidonor antibodies. This classification also recognizes that antibody-mediated rejection may accompany Banff Type I or Type II rejection as described in the following sections.

Chronic Active Antibody-Mediated Rejection and Transplant Glomerulopathy

The hallmark of chronic active antibody-mediated rejection is the glomerular lesion of transplant glomerulopathy. Glomeruli show varying degrees of lobular accentuation with an increase in mesangial matrix, mesangial interposition, and irregular thickening of basement membrane (Figs. 5.4, 5.5). This lesion is associated with significant proteinuria. By electron microscopy, there is separation of the endothelial cells from the basement membrane with the accumulation of a granular material in the subendothelial space. The exact mechanisms involved are still unknown, but humoral immunity directed against donor-specific or vascular endothelial antigens has been suggested as a likely possibility. In addition, many factors involved with progressive fibrosis in the native kidney may play a role in the transplant, such as hypertension, abnormal lipids, and reactive oxygen species, all of which can activate endothelial cells. A method of scoring was presented at the meeting in 2009, including the following modified criteria, which take into account the fraction of involved glomeruli (Table 5.6).

Key Diagnostic Feature of Chronic Active Antibody-Mediated Rejection and Transplant Glomerulopathy

- Glomerular basement membrane reduplication

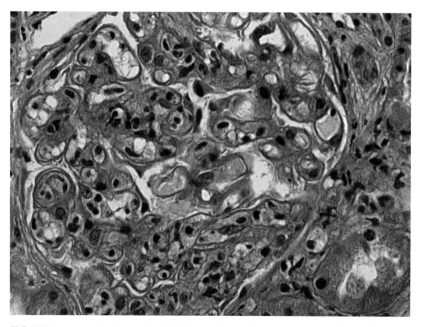

FIG 5.4 Acute antibody-mediated rejection. Transplant glomerulitis. Glomerulus showing lobular accentuation with an increase in mesangial matrix, mesangial interposition, and irregular thickening of basement membrane (periodic acid Schiff, ×400).

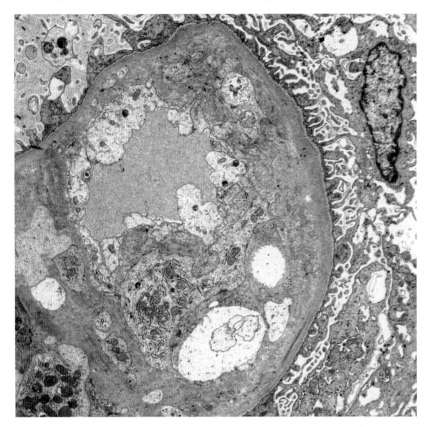

FIG. 5.5 Acute antibody-mediated rejection. Transplant glomerulitis. By electron microscopy, there is endothelial cell swelling with separation of the endothelial cells from the basement membrane with the accumulation of a granular material in the subendothelial space.

TABLE 5-6 Scoring of Transplant Glomerulopathy	
cg0	No glomeruli with double contours in 10% or more of peripheral capillary loops
cg1	Double contours in up to 25% of glomeruli, with double contours in ≥10% of capillary loops in at least 1 glomerulus
cg2	Double contours in 26-50% of glomeruli, with double contours in ≥10% of capillary loops in at least 1 glomerulus
cg3	Double contours in >50% of glomeruli, with double contours in ≥10% of capillary loops in at least 1 glomerulus

Acute T Cell–Mediated Rejection

Acute rejection, despite its terminology, can occur at any time during the course of the life of the allograft. It is most frequently seen during the initial months after grafting but can also be seen later in graft life, particularly when disturbances of graft therapy are incurred. In the Banff classification, the severity is determined by the degree of tubulitis and the presence or absence of intimal arteritis.

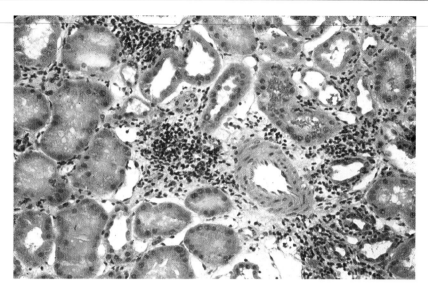

FIG. 5.6 Acute rejection, Banff type, borderline, suspicious for acute rejection. Changes suspicious for acute rejection are seen here as a minimal focal interstitial infiltrate with minimal evidence of tubulitis. Less than four lymphocytes are seen in a single tubule cross section in this image (hematoxylin and eosin, ×200).

Key Diagnostic Features of Acute Cellular Rejection

- Tubulitis
- Interstitial lymphoplasmacytic inflammation

Note: Threshold criteria vary for Banff and CCTT (Cooperative Clinical Trials in Transplantation) classifications.

BORDERLINE CHANGES: "SUSPICIOUS FOR ACUTE REJECTION"

This category is used to describe very mild, acute interstitial cellular rejection. No intimal arteritis is present and only mild focal mononuclear cell infiltrates with rare foci of mild tubulitis defined as 1-4 mononuclear cells per tubular cross section present (Fig. 5.6). This degree of rejection is frequently encountered and probably does not reflect a degree of rejection that needs modification by additional therapy. Some investigators have suggested that such mild persistent infiltrates may contribute to the progression to chronic rejection.

BANFF TYPE I ACUTE REJECTION

Type I or acute interstitial cellular rejection is characterized by edema and infiltration of the interstitium by immunoblasts, lymphocytes, plasma cells, macrophages, and a scattering of polymorphonuclear leukocytes in the eosinophils. The infiltrate is generally diffuse but appears somewhat more concentrated around vessels in glomeruli. In Type IA, greater than 25% of the parenchyma is affected and foci of moderate tubulitis with more than 4 mononuclear cells per tubular cross section or group of 10 tubular cells is considered characteristic (Fig. 5.7). In Type IB, greater than 25% of the parenchyma is affected and numerous foci of severe tubulitis with more than 10 mononuclear cells per tubular cross section or group of 10 tubular

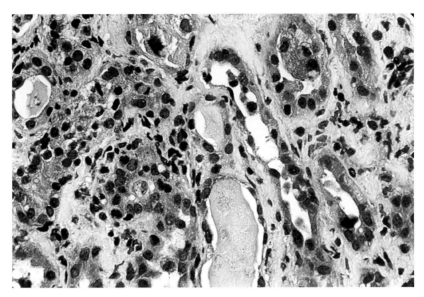

FIG. 5.7 Acute rejection, Banff Type IA. This category is defined by the presence of an interstitial infiltrate of lymphocytes with moderate tubulitis with greater than four mononuclear cells per tubular cross section. The interstitial infiltrate consists of lymphocytes and is patchy, involving less than 25% of the biopsy (hematoxylin and eosin, ×400).

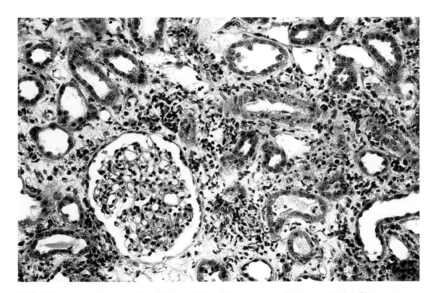

FIG. 5.8 Acute rejection, Banff Type IB. In this category, the interstitial infiltrate is more extensive, involving greater than 25% of the biopsy with numerous foci of severe tubulitis with greater than 10 mononuclear cells per tubular cross section. The vessels show no evidence of involvement (hematoxylin and eosin, ×200).

cells is considered characteristic (Fig. 5.8). Identification of the lymphocytes in the infiltrate demonstrates a large population of T cells identifiable by the CD3 antigen (Fig. 5.9) and a greater number of cytotoxic T cells identified by the antigen CD8 than helper inducer T cells identified by the presence of the antigen CD4. The ratio of activation antigens RO and RA is also of use in identifying the activity of the rejection. This degree of rejection generally has a good response to antirejection therapy.

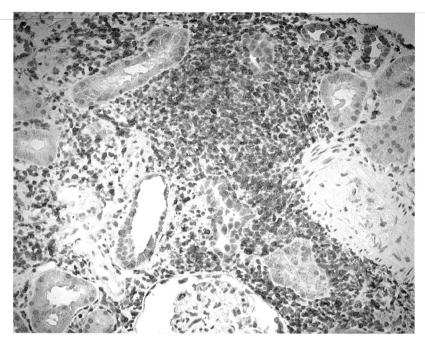

FIG. 5.9 Acute rejection. The interstitial infiltrate consists of a mixed population of T cells. The large population of T cells is identifiable by the presence of the CD3 antigen here shown by immunohistochemistry (anti-C3 immunostaining, ×200).

Key Differential Diagnosis of Acute Cellular Rejection

Acute Cellular Rejection
- Interstitial inflammation and tubulitis may be seen in numerous conditions, such as drug hypersensitivity reaction, injury related to pyelonephritis, and viral infections.
- Specific studies to rule out viral infection and search for viral cytopathic change distinguish viral infection from acute cellular rejection.
- Numerous eosinophils and nonnecrotizing granulomas suggest hypersensitivity reaction, although eosinophils may be part of eosinophil-rich acute cellular rejection.
- Eosinophilic tubulitis may be more common with hypersensitivity reaction.

Acute Vascular Rejection
- Endothelialitis may very rarely be seen in other entities causing vascular injury, such as cryoglobulinemic glomerulonephritis in the transplant.

BANFF TYPE II ACUTE REJECTION

Type II or acute rejection with a vascular component consists of cases with mild to moderate intimal arteritis Type IIA in addition to any degree of interstitial cellular rejection. Intimal arteritis is defined as intimal thickening with inflammation of the arterial subendothelial space ranging from rare intimal inflammatory cells to necrosis of the endothelium with deposition of fibrin, platelets, and inflammatory cells (Figs. 5.10, 5.11). Type IIB describes cases with intimal arteritis compromising greater than 25% of the luminal area. The cellular infiltrate is composed of lymphocytes and monocytes. Severity is determined by the number of vessels affected as well as the intensity of the individual lesions (Fig. 5.12). The finding of intimal arteritis as seen in these categories is often focal. Response to therapy is more variable in this group.

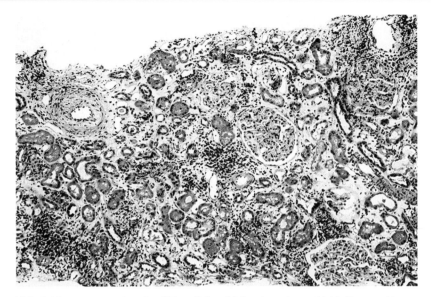

FIG. 5.10 Acute rejection, Banff Type II. In addition to an interstitial infiltrate with tubulitis, there is evidence of vascular involvement. The artery in this low-power image demonstrates marked myointimal proliferation associated with lymphocytic infiltration underneath the endothelium (hematoxylin and eosin, ×100).

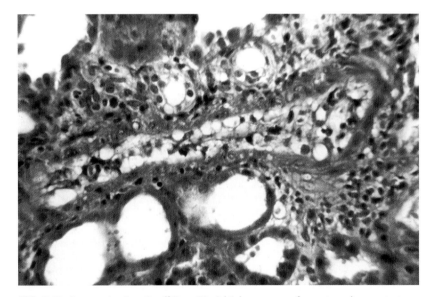

FIG. 5.11 Acute rejection, Banff Type IIA. A higher power of an artery demonstrates marked endothelial cell swelling and numerous lymphocytes just beneath the endothelium. This is a mild but definite form of endothelial activation (hematoxylin and eosin, ×400).

BANFF TYPE III ACUTE REJECTION

Grade III consists of severe acute vascular rejection. These are cases with severe intimal arteritis and transmural arteritis as defined by injury and inflammation of the whole arterial wall, including the media, necrosis of medial smooth muscles, fibrin deposition, and cellular infiltration with mononuclear as well as polymorphonuclear leukocytes (Fig. 5.13). Focal infarction and interstitial hemorrhage without other obvious cause can be assumed to be associated

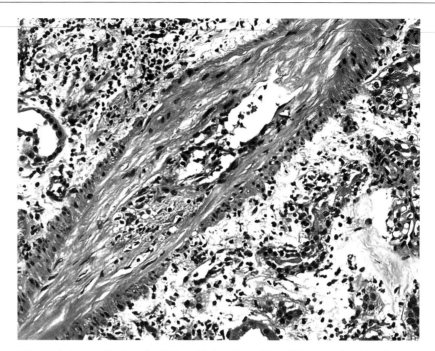

FIG. 5.12 Acute rejection, Banff Type IIB. Severity of Type II is determined by the number of vessels involved as well as the intensity of the individual lesions. In this artery, there is evidence of more severe infiltration with lymphocytes that involves not only the endothelium but also the media. Myointimal proliferation is prominent (hematoxylin and eosin, ×200).

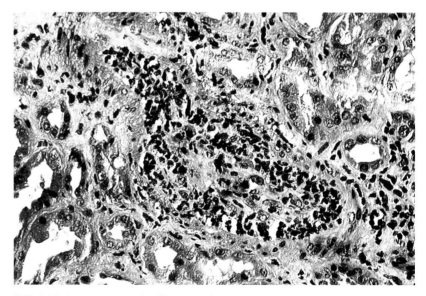

FIG. 5.13 Acute rejection, Banff Type III. This category consists of severe acute vascular rejection, which may be mediated in part by humoral mechanisms. Severe intimal and transmural arteritis with medial necrosis that typify this category are present in this artery (hematoxylin and eosin, ×200).

with vascular lesions consistent with this degree of rejection. Rejection episodes of this severity are often associated with graft loss.

Chronic Allograft Failure (Chronic Allograft Nephropathy)

In 2005, the Banff Conference eliminated the term *chronic allograft nephropathy*. This was due to the fact that this was a generic term, summarizing all disease processes including hypertension, hyperlipidemia, and viral infection associated with chronic allograft failure. It had become an entity explaining kidney allograft failures regardless of the etiology. Since 2005, pathologists have been urged to assign a specific diagnosis instead of using the nonspecific term *chronic allograft nephropathy*.

Chronic allograft failure occurs anywhere from several months to several years after transplantation. Clinically, it is associated with a slow and gradual decrease in renal function in contrast to the more acute explosive loss of renal function seen in acute rejection. Microscopically, the picture is similar to that of nephrosclerosis (Fig. 5.14). There is arterial and arteriolar narrowing of the interlobular arcuate and radial arteries by myointimal proliferation and medial hypertrophy (Fig. 5.15). The vascular lesions are associated with a diffuse interstitial fibrosis and tubular atrophy. The glomerular lesions of chronic allograft failure consist of ischemic glomerular capillary collapse, thickening of the capillary walls and segmental and global sclerosis (Fig. 5.16). Chronic changes designated as IF/TA (interstitial fibrosis/tubular atrophy) are now graded as mild, moderate, and severe in the Banff schema. Interstitial fibrosis and tubular atrophy are independently graded depending on the amount of cortical area that is involved. However, this designation does not include the chronic lesions affecting the

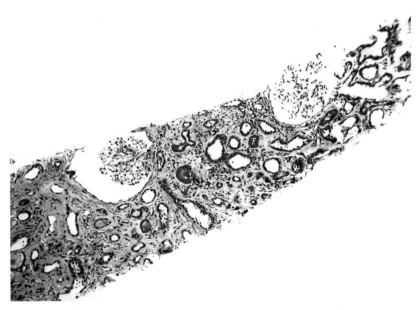

FIG. 5.14 Chronic/sclerosing allograft nephropathy. An example of Grade II–III is characterized by a diffuse increase in interstitial tissue and marked tubular atrophy as seen on this trichrome stain. Grade I has mild focal interstitial fibrosis and tubular atrophy. Grade II and III are defined as moderate and severe interstitial fibrosis. Microscopically, the picture is relatively nonspecific and similar to that seen in nephrosclerosis (trichrome, ×100).

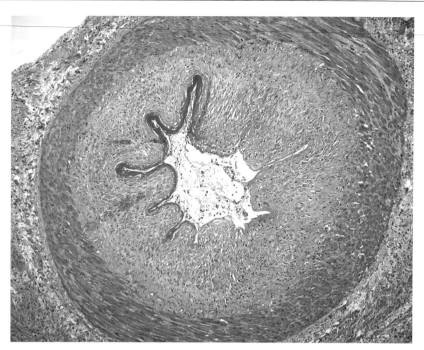

FIG. 5.15 Chronic/sclerosing allograft nephropathy. The classical lesion of chronic transplant vasculopathy is a circumferential proliferation of myointimal cells with an intact internal elastic lamina (hematoxylin and eosin, ×200).

Key Diagnostic Features of Calcineurin Inhibitor Nephrotoxicity

- Nodular hyalin extending to media of arterioles/arteries
- Striped interstitial fibrosis
- Thrombotic microangiopathy

Note: None of these findings are pathognomonic, although the nodular arteriolar hyalin is most closely associated with calcineurin inhibitor toxicity.

---

vasculature, which should then be scored separately. The Banff conference in 2009 further attacked the questions of the nature of fibrosis and the reproducibility of its assessment. The discussion included the type of stain used and how and when morphometry should be used. It has also been suggested that correlation of IF/TA score with antibody status and genomic analysis can better identify the specific etiology in individual patients.

Cyclosporin/FK506 Nephrotoxicity

The toxic effects of immunosuppressant drugs also are to be considered in the evaluation of the allograft biopsy. The toxic effects of calcineurin inhibitors including both cyclosporin and tacrolimus have fairly characteristic histologic findings. Importantly, cyclosporine toxicity on a functional basis, that is, vasoconstriction-related, should be considered when serum creatinine has risen quickly and the biopsy is morphologically normal. Characteristic findings include tubular vacuolization, isometric expansion of tubular epithelial cells, and evidence of microvascular damage as characterized by the presence of nodular hyaline sclerosis of arterioles (Fig. 5.17). With severe toxic injury, arteriolar myocyte vacuolization can be seen associated with endothelial swelling, mucoid intimal thickening, and accumulation of proteins within

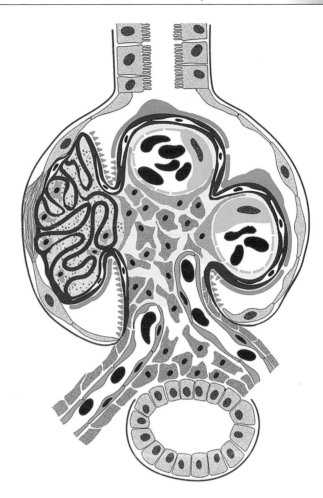

FIG. 5.16 Transplant glomerulopathy. There is segmental sclerosis and duplication of the GBM due to increased lamina rara interna without deposits.

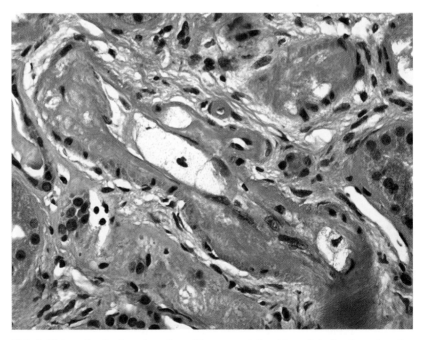

FIG. 5.17 Longitudinal section of an afferent arteriole with nodular hyaline sclerosis typical of calcineurin inhibitor toxicity effect (hematoxylin and eosin, ×400).

the vessel wall. Chronic calcineurin inhibitor toxicity is manifested by the ischemic changes that accompany these vascular changes. The most characteristic is that of striped fibrosis (Fig. 5.18). In some instances, thrombotic microangiopathic changes may also be seen and these must be distinguished from acute humoral rejection (Figs. 5.19, 5.20).

Etiology/Pathogenesis

Cyclosporin induces elaboration of several vasoconstrictors, including endothelin, and is also directly toxic to renal parenchymal cells. The striped pattern of fibrosis reflects this ischemic injury along medullary rays.

Posttransplant Lymphoproliferative Disease

Patients typically show systemic signs of hematopoietic illness when disease is more advanced, with hepatosplenomegaly and lymphadenopathy. However, early in the course, these findings may not be present. Renal biopsies show a uniform dense plasma cell infiltrate, which appears

---

Key Differential Diagnosis of PTLD

- Numerous plasma cells may suggest the possibility of polyoma virus nephropathy, plasma cell–rich acute cellular rejection, or posttransplant lymphoproliferative disease. Immunostaining may help with this differential diagnosis.
- The presence of viral changes suggests polyoma virus nephropathy.
- Clonal expansion of atypical B cells, serpiginous necrosis, and mass effect all suggest PTLD.
- Epstein–Barr virus is often positive in PTLD.

PTLD, posttransplant lymphoproliferative disease.

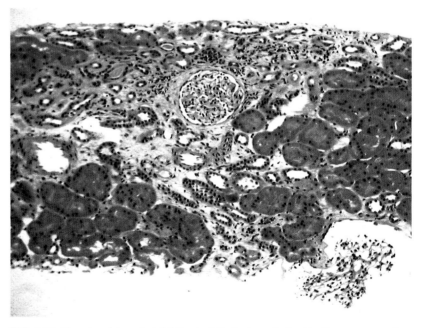

FIG. 5.18 Chronic calcineurin inhibitor toxicity is characterized by the presence of stripes of fibrosis as seen here in this low-power micrograph (hematoxylin and eosin, ×100).

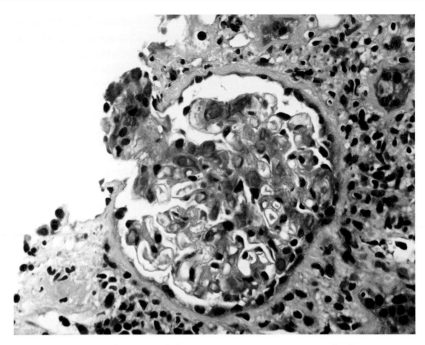

FIG. 5.19 Chronic calcineurin inhibitor toxicity. In some instances of calcineurin inhibitor toxicity, endothelial activation results in a thrombotic microangiopathy seen here by the presence of intracapillary thrombi (hematoxylin, phloxine, and saffron, ×400).

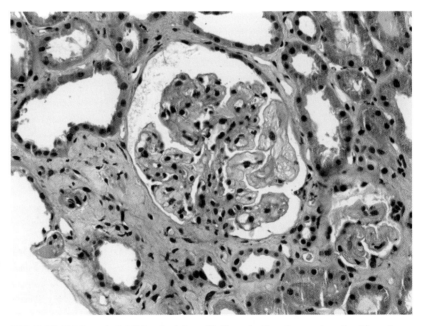

FIG. 5.20 Calcineurin inhibitor toxicity with thrombotic microangiopathy. There is endothelial cell swelling and focal denudation of the capillary basement membrane (toluidine blue, ×400).

to expand between tubules. Cells may have an atypical immunoblastic appearance, or there may be serpiginous necrosis, in which case the diagnosis of posttransplant lymphoproliferative disease (PTLD) may be obvious (Figs. 5.21-5.23). More often, the findings by light microscopy are more subtle. Use of immunohistochemical staining for the presence of monoclonal B (more commonly) or T (rarely) cells in the infiltrate is a helpful adjunct in the evaluation of such biopsies.

If PTLD is seriously considered, the presence of Epstein–Barr virus can be determined by in situ hybridization. The differential diagnosis includes plasma cell–rich acute rejection.

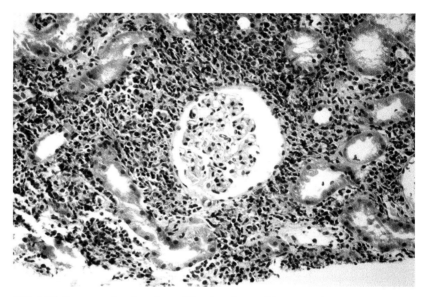

FIG. 5.21 Posttransplant lymphoproliferative disease. Most transplant lymphoproliferative disorders may also mimic the findings of acute allograft rejection. The major difference is the absence of tubulitis and the presence of a space-occupying infiltrate without damage to the tubular epithelial cells (hematoxylin and eosin, ×200).

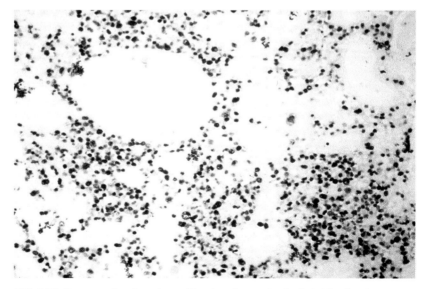

FIG. 5.22 Posttransplant lymphoproliferative disease. In situ hybridization for Epstein–Barr virus confirms the presence of posttransplant lymphoproliferative disease (in situ hybridization, ×200).

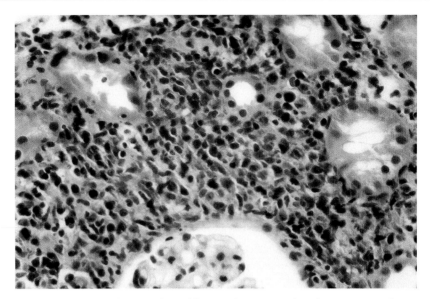

FIG. 5.23 Posttransplant lymphoproliferative disease. Another characteristic is the atypia seen in the lymphocytic infiltrate in the interstitium (hematoxylin and eosin, ×400).

Etiology/pathogenesis

PTLD arises in the setting of abnormal T cell regulation of B cells, with the resulting PTLD most often being of B cell origin. Epstein–Barr virus infection is present in nearly all cases but may not be detected in all cases. Some PTLD are polyclonal. Typically, the process regresses when immunosuppression is decreased or removed.

Selected Reading

Hanto, D.W., 1995. Classification of Epstein–Barr virus-associated posttransplant lympho-proliferative diseases: implications for understanding their pathogenesis and developing rational treatment strategies. Annual Review of Medicine 46, 381-394.

Viral Infections

It must be remembered that a variety of different processes can involve the allograft other than those associated with an acute or chronic rejection. These processes may present as graft failure, and biopsy diagnosis must differentiate these disease entities from those related to rejection. An important example is acute bacterial infection (Fig. 5.24). This entity can be distinguished by the presence of polymorphonuclear leukocytes in tubular lumens and in the interstitium (Fig. 5.25). Viral infections must also be considered. Cytomegalovirus, polyoma virus, and adenovirus all may infect the allograft.

The biopsy must be examined for the signs of viral infection, including nuclear and cyto-plasmic inclusions (Fig. 5.26), the presence of cytomegalic cells (Figs. 5.26-5.29), and strati-fication of the epithelium (Figs. 5.30-5.33). Viral infections may be particularly difficult to differentiate from acute rejection as they are frequently associated with a lymphocytic infiltrate and significant tubulitis may be present. Furthermore, the cytologic features of regeneration can mimic those of viral infection. The presence of plasma cells also poses a diagnostic dilemma, as they can be a prominent component of the interstitial infiltrate in patients who have been noncompliant with their therapy.

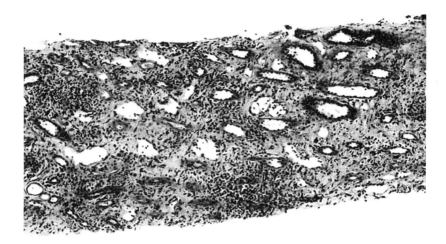

FIG. 5.24 Acute pyelonephritis. Infection of the allograft can mimic acute rejection by the presence of a diffuse interstitial infiltrate with tubulitis (hematoxylin and eosin, ×100).

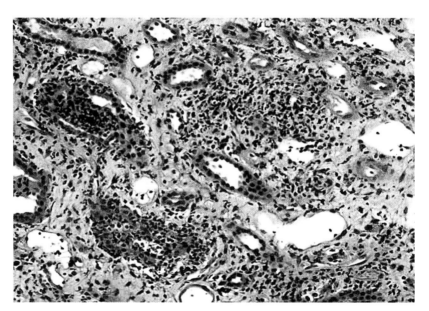

FIG. 5.25 Acute pyelonephritis. The major distinguishing feature is the presence of polymorphonuclear leukocytes in both the tubular lumina and in the interstitium (hematoxylin and eosin, ×200).

Key Diagnostic Features of Polyoma Virus Nephropathy

- Pleomorphic interstitial infiltrate
- Viral cytopathic changes
- Positive SV40 staining in tubular epithelial cells

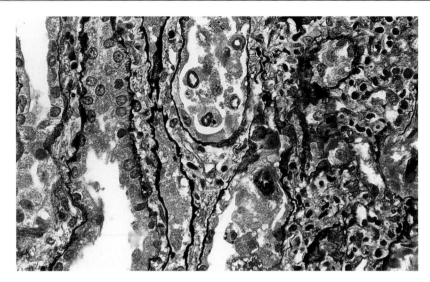

FIG. 5.26 Viral infection. Graft failure may be the result of infection by viruses associated with immunosuppression. They can be identified by the presence of nuclear inclusions. Epithelial necrosis and tubulitis may mimic acute rejection (hematoxylin and eosin/silver, ×400).

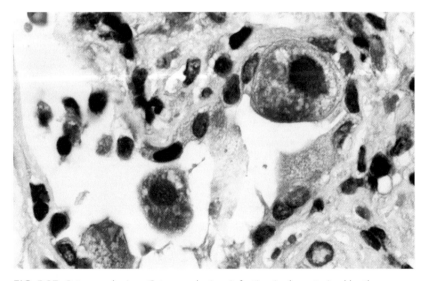

FIG. 5.27 Cytomegalovirus. Cytomegalovirus infection is characterized by the presence of large cytomegalic cells and a homogeneous ground glass nucleus (hematoxylin and eosin, ×600).

The principal finding associated with polyoma virus infection among renal transplant patients is a viral interstitial nephritis. Intranuclear basophilic viral inclusions without a surrounding halo are present. Cytomegalovirus has both intranuclear and cytoplasmic inclusions. With electron microscopy, intranuclear viral inclusions (with a particle diameter size of 30-50 nm) and tubular damage characterized by tubular cell necrosis, prominent lysosomal inclusions, and luminal cellular casts can be seen. It has been suggested that viral infection should be staged as A, Early; B, Fully Developed; or C, Fibrosing (Table 5.7).

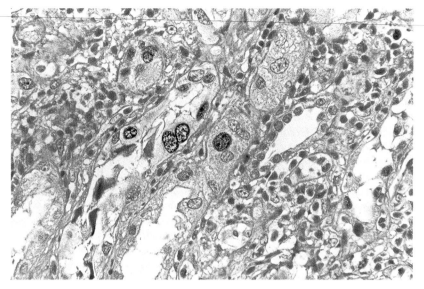

FIG. 5.28 Cytomegalovirus. The presence of cytomegalovirus infection can be confirmed by histochemical staining specific for the viral antigen (anti-CMV, ×200).

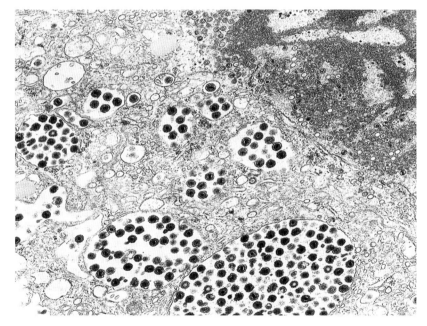

FIG. 5.29 Cytomegalovirus. Electron microscopy may also be helpful demonstrating viral particles in the nucleus (transmission electron microscopy, ×16,000).

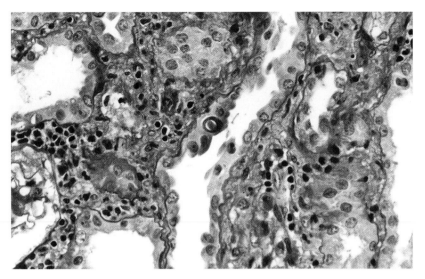

FIG. 5.30 Viral infection. Polyoma virus infection characterized by stratification of irregular epithelium associated with pleomorphic nuclei with amphophilic inclusions (hematoxylin and eosin, ×400).

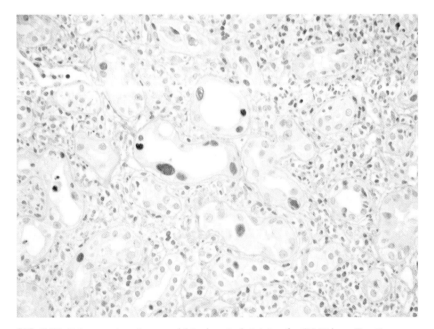

FIG. 5.31 Polyoma virus. Immunohistochemical staining for SV-40 large T antigen confirms polyoma virus infection in tubular epithelial cells, with tubulointerstitial pleomorphic infiltrate and tubulitis, and enlarged nuclei with viral cytopathic change (anti-SV40 immunostain, ×200).

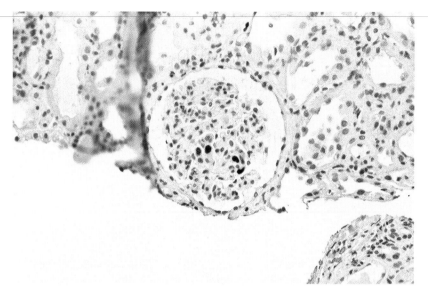

FIG. 5.32 Polyoma virus. This is best confirmed by histochemical staining for the large T antigen of SV40 seen here in glomerular cells (anti-SV40 immunostaining, ×200).

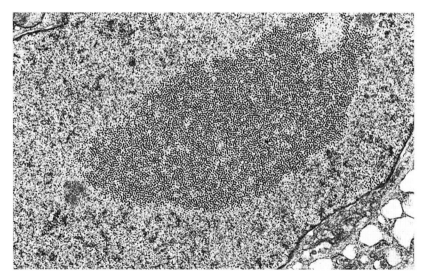

FIG. 5.33 Polyoma virus. Electron microscopy is also helpful by the demonstration of intranuclear viral particles (transmission electron microscopy, ×16,000).

TABLE 5-7 Viral Infection Staging

Stage A (early phase)

- Viral activation in cortex and/or medulla with intranuclear inclusion bodies and/or positive immunohistochemical or in situ hybridization signals with no or minimal tubular epithelial cell necrosis/lysis or inflammation.

Stage B (fully developed phase)

- Pronounced viral activation in cortex and/or medulla with marked virally induced tubular epithelial cell lysis, denudation of tubular basement membranes, interstitial inflammation (mild to marked), and interstitial fibrosis and tubular atrophy.

Stage C (fibrosing phase)

- Viral activation in cortex and medulla (minimal to marked) with interstitial fibrosis and tubular atrophy >50% of sample with interstitial inflammation but minimal cell lysis.

Although these standard histologic markers are satisfactory for current evaluation, it is anticipated that newer molecular biological techniques and more specific characterization of the lymphocytic infiltrate will aid the diagnosis and evaluation of renal allograft biopsies in the future.

Selected Reading

Sis, B., Mengel, M., Haas, M., et al, 2010. Banff '09 Meeting report: antibody mediated graft deterioration and implementation of Banff Working Groups. American Journal of Transplantation 10, 464-471.

Solez, K., Colvin, R.B., Racusen, L.C., et al, 2008. Banff 07 classification of renal allograft pathology: updates and future directions. American Journal of Transplantation 8, 753-760.

Cystic Diseases of the Kidney

Introduction

Although single simple cysts of the kidney are relatively common and have little clinical implication, there are a group of hereditary cystic diseases that are of importance because of their contribution to the development of end-stage renal disease. Each of the diseases has its own genetic abnormality, and each of the diseases has its own characteristic clinical presentation. The exact mechanisms by which the genetic abnormalities result in the physiologic and pathologic abnormalities are still incompletely identified. Cystic diseases are classified according to the genetic presentation and according to the regions of the kidney that are involved. This is summarized in Table 6.1.

Autosomal Dominant Polycystic Kidney Disease

Autosomal dominant polycystic kidney disease affects between 1 in 500 and 1 in 1000 individuals. It is found in all racial and ethnic groups and is seen throughout the world. It is the most common of genetic polycystic kidney disorders. As its name implies, autosomal dominant polycystic kidney disease is inherited in autosomal dominant pattern with complete penetrance. Thus, a child of an affected parent has a 50% chance of inheriting the abnormal gene. About half the patients affected are unable to give a family history consistent with autosomal dominant polycystic kidney disease. Autosomal dominant polycystic kidney disease was previously termed adult form of polycystic kidney disease because it may not become clinically apparent until the third or fourth decade of life. Although 100% of gene carriers will show evidence of the disease, only about 50% progress on to renal failure.

Pathology

Autosomal dominant polycystic kidney disease results in kidneys that are enlarged and diffusely cystic (Figs. 6.1-6.4). It is important to note that whereas the cysts appear to involve the entire kidney, only a portion of the total number of nephrons in the kidney is cystic

TABLE 6-1 Classifications of Cystic Diseases

1. Autosomal dominant polycystic kidney disease (adult)
2. Autosomal recessive polycystic kidney disease (infantile)
3. Medullary cystic disease
4. Medullary sponge kidney
5. Cystic renal dysplasia
6. Acquired polycystic disease

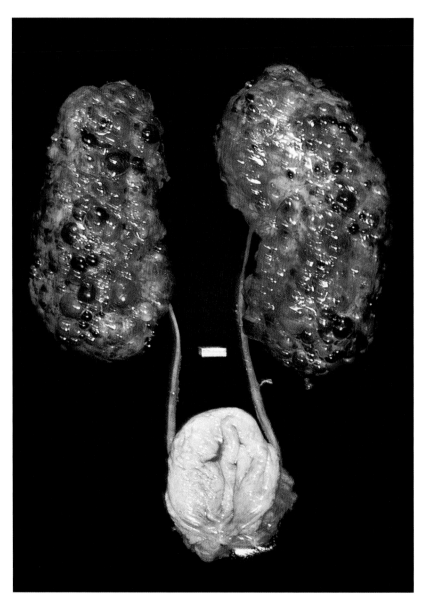

FIG. 6.1 Autosomal dominant polycystic kidney disease. The kidneys are markedly enlarged and consist of numerous cystic structures bulging throughout the surface. Many of the cysts contain dark material.

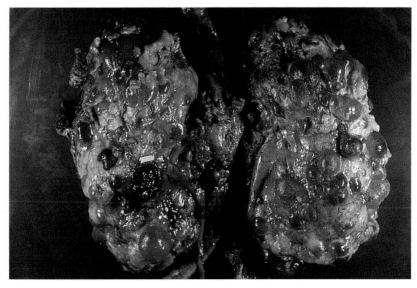

FIG. 6.2 Autosomal dominant polycystic kidney disease.

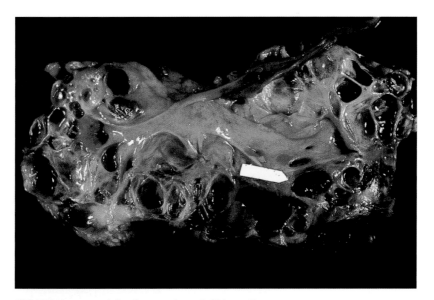

FIG. 6.3 Autosomal dominant polycystic kidney disease.

(Figs. 6.5-6.8). The cysts range in size from barely visible to several centimeters in diameter. Microdissection studies have demonstrated the cyst to be spherical dilatations or outpouchings from existing renal tubules (Fig. 6.9). As the cysts enlarge, they appear to become detached from their tubule of origin. In the early stages of the disease, the noncystic parenchymal elements remain normal, but as cysts increase in number and grow in size, the residual normal tissue becomes atrophic and nonfunctional and results in the development of end-stage renal disease. The disease is a systemic one and can produce cysts in other organs, including liver, pancreas, and lung.

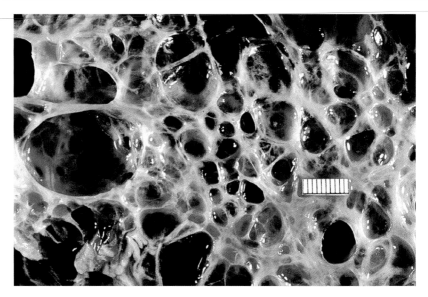

FIG. 6.4 Autosomal dominant polycystic kidney disease. Cut surface shows that the cysts are interspersed by fibrous tissue.

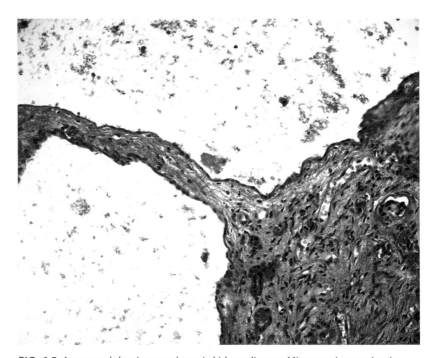

FIG. 6.5 Autosomal dominant polycystic kidney disease. Microscopic examination reveals the cysts to be lined by flattened epithelium and the interstitial tissue to consist predominately of fibrous tissue with small capillaries and atrophic tubules (hematoxylin and eosin, ×400).

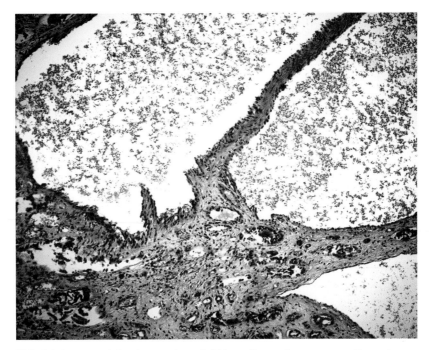

FIG. 6.6 Autosomal dominant polycystic kidney disease. In some areas, the cysts can be seen to displace normal tubular structures (hematoxylin and eosin, ×200).

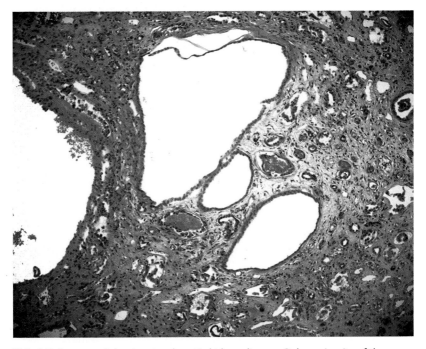

FIG. 6.7 Autosomal dominant polycystic kidney disease. Only a minority of the nephrons are involved by cystic formation. Normal tubular structures are scattered throughout the interstitial fibrous tissue (hematoxylin and eosin, ×200).

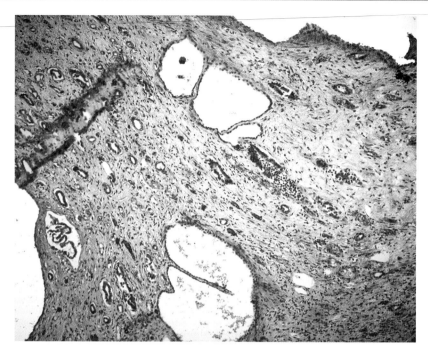

FIG. 6.8 Autosomal dominant polycystic kidney disease. Cysts involve both cortex and medulla and are seen extending into the inner medullary region (hematoxylin and eosin, ×200).

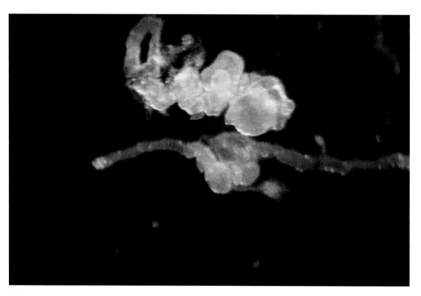

FIG. 6.9 Autosomal dominant polycystic kidney disease. The cysts initially begin as saccular aneurysmal dilatations of the tubule that then separate from the tubule itself as is seen here in a microdissected specimen.

Autosomal Recessive Polycystic Kidney Disease

Autosomal recessive polycystic kidney disease is a rare disorder that occurs in 1 in 6000 to 55,000 live births. It was previously termed infantile polycystic disease in that it manifests itself at birth and results in significant perinatal mortality. In approximately three quarters of the cases, autosomal recessive polycystic disease results in death within a few days of birth. Occasional patients have survived through adolescence.

Pathology

Autosomal recessive polycystic kidney disease (ARPKD) affects both the kidneys and liver in approximately equal proportions. The kidneys are grossly enlarged and may fill the entire abdomen at the time of birth (Figs. 6.10, 6.11). They are markedly enlarged and demonstrate numerous elongated fusiform cylindrical cysts that occupy the entire kidney. The cysts are lined by a flattened cuboidal epithelium, and histochemical and specific binding studies have demonstrated that they appear to be dilated terminal branches of the collecting ducts. The kidneys in these disorders have a similar morphologic pattern (Figs. 6.12, 6.13).

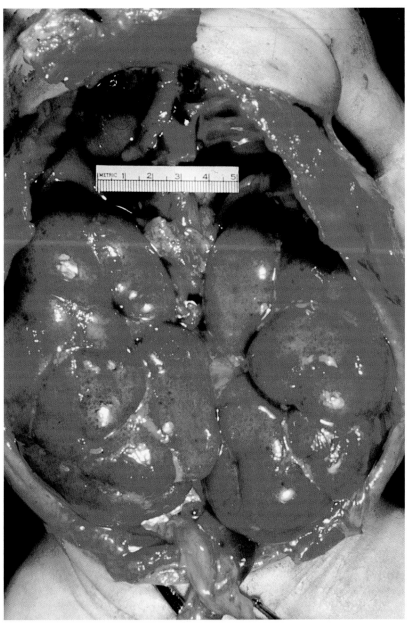

FIG. 6.10 Autosomal recessive polycystic kidney disease. The kidneys are shown in situ occupying almost the complete abdominal cavity of a newborn infant.

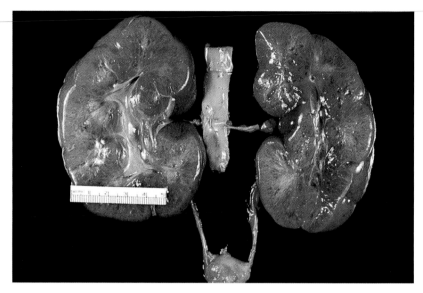

FIG. 6.11 Autosomal recessive polycystic kidney disease. Cut surface of the kidney demonstrates that both the cortex and medulla are completely replaced by a sponge-like appearance.

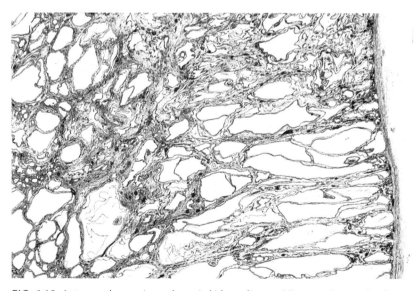

FIG. 6.12 Autosomal recessive polycystic kidney disease. Microscopic examination shows the cysts to be elongated tubular structures, which reach from the cortical surface and extend into the medulla (hematoxylin and eosin, ×200).

Medullary Cystic Disease/Nephronophthisis

This is a group of three distinct genetic disorders that have similar morphologic findings but with different clinical presentations. Juvenile nephronophthisis is an autosomal recessive disorder mapped to nine different genes that usually presents in childhood. Uremic medullary cystic disease on the other hand is an autosomal dominant disorder that usually presents in teens and adults. Medullary cystic disease of Type 1 has been linked to chromosome 1q21 and Medullary cystic disease of Type 2 is associated with mutations in the uromodulin gene.

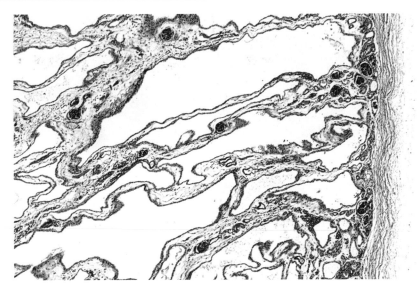

FIG. 6.13 Autosomal recessive polycystic kidney disease. The dilated tubular structures are separated by loose connective tissue with glomerular structures interspersed.

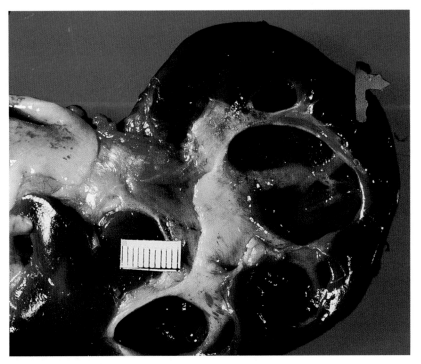

FIG. 6.14 Medullary cystic disease. The cortex is preserved and the medulla appears somewhat blunted. Cysts are present at the junction of the cortex and medulla and in this example measure up to 4 cm in diameter.

Aside from the hereditary features and ages of presentation, the conditions appear essentially similar morphologically.

In longitudinal sections of the kidney, the cysts are present at the cortical medullary junction (Figs. 6.14-6.16). The cysts can vary in size from microscopic to 1-2 cm in diameter. The cortex is spared from cyst formation but nonspecific glomerular hyalinosis and interstitial

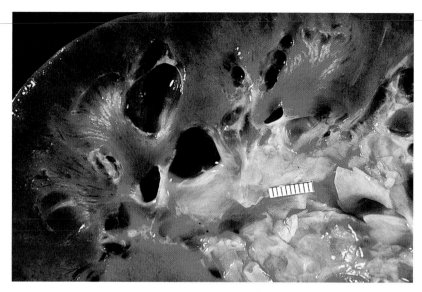

FIG. 6.15 Medullary cystic disease. Another example demonstrates the presence of cysts at the cortical medullary junction. In this example, cysts vary in size from less than 1 mm to more than 1 cm in diameter.

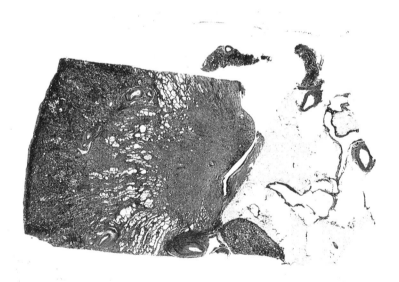

FIG. 6.16 Medullary cystic disease. The cysts are confined to the cortical medullary junction and the cortex appears atrophic (hematoxylin and eosin, ×1).

fibrosis with tubular atrophy is present (Figs. 6.17-6.19). The microdissection studies have shown that the nephrons are altered by numerous small diverticula, highly variable in size involving the late distal tubule and collecting duct.

Medullary Sponge Kidney

Medullary sponge kidney is usually not recognized until late in life when secondary calcification of the medulla is associated with recurrent infection. The incidence of this disease is approximately 1 in 5000.

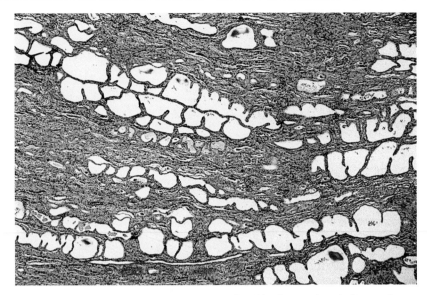

FIG. 6.17 Medullary cystic disease. The cyst is lined by flattened epithelium and surrounded by some relatively normal-appearing tubular structures (hematoxylin and eosin, ×200).

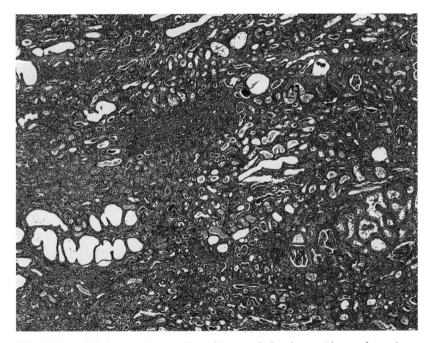

FIG. 6.18 Medullary cystic disease. The adjacent tubules show evidence of atrophy, and there is the presence of interstitial fibrosis. There is no significant interstitial infiltrate (hematoxylin and eosin, ×100).

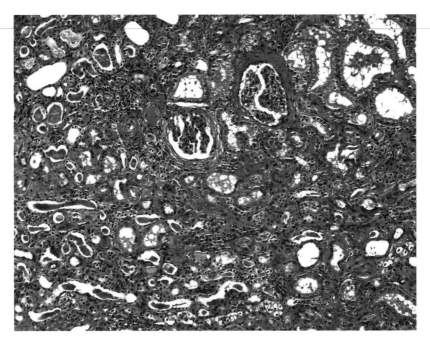

FIG. 6.19 Medullary cystic disease. End-stage disease. The cortex proximal to the cysts shows marked atrophy with interstitial scarring and glomerulosclerosis. There is also marked hyalin and arteriolosclerosis (hematoxylin and eosin, ×200).

The only visible abnormality in this disease is the presence of irregular enlargement of the medullary and inner papillary portion of the collecting duct. The papillary are often calcified and shed to form renal calcinosis. Obstruction and infection are common secondary changes (Fig. 6.20).

Etiology/Pathogenesis

Autosomal dominant polycystic kidney disease (PKD) is caused by genetic mutations in chromosome 16 for PKD1 and chromosome 4 in PKD2. PKD1 and PKD2 encode proteins called polycystins. Polycystins are a family of eight-transmembrane proteins united by sequence homology. Polycystins appear to play key roles during development. In mature organs, their roles in primary cilia, shear stress sensation, alteration of intracellular calcium, and planar cell polarity that regulates tubular diameter have been shown. PKD is a ciliopathy that arises from abnormalities in the primary cilium. Numerous mutations including deletions, substitutions, and frame shifts have been identified in the genes encoding the polycystins, all of which, however, appear to diminish cellular function and alter cellular physiology and cell proliferation/ cell/matrix interaction leading to cyst formation. The phenotype produced by these abnormal proteins is essentially identical in morphology and the clinical presentation is similar, except that PKD2, the less common genotype, progresses to end-stage renal failure at a slower rate. ARPKD is caused by mutation in PKHD1, and two truncating mutations are associated with neonatal lethality. The ARPKD protein, fibrocystin, is localized to cilia/basal body and complexes with polycystin-2. Juvenile nephronophthisis is mapped to a gene defect on chromosome 2P. Positional cloning and candidate gene approaches led to the identification of eight causative genes (NPHP1, 3, 4, 5, 6, 7, 8, and 9) responsible for the juvenile NPH and one gene NPHP2 for the infantile form. NPH and associated disorders are considered as ciliopathies, as all NPHP gene products are expressed in the primary cilia, similarly to the

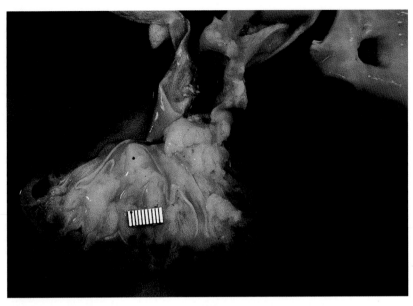

FIG. 6.20 End stage of medullary sponge kidney. The cortex is grossly atrophic and the prominent finding is the presence of shortened papillae with foci of calcification.

PKD proteins. Uremic medullary cystic disease type 1 has been mapped to a defect on chromosome 1Q21. Medullary cystic disease of Type 2 is associated with mutations in the uromodulin gene.

Selected Reading

Dahan, K., Fuchshuber, A., Adamis, S., et al., 2001. Familial juvenile hyperuricemic nephropathy and autosomal dominant medullary cystic kidney disease type 2: Two facets of the same disease? Journal of the American Society of Nephrology 12, 2348-2357.

Harris, P.C., Torres, V.E., 2009. Polycystic kidney disease. Annual Review of Medicine 60, 321-337.

Hildebrandt, F., Attanasio, M., Otto, E., 2009. Nephronophthisis: disease mechanisms of a ciliopathy. Journal of the American Society of Nephrology 20, 23-35.

Wolf, M.T., Mucha, B.E., Hennies, H.C., et al., 2006. Medullary cystic kidney disease type 1: mutational analysis in 37 genes based on haplotype sharing. Human Genetics 119, 649-658.

Zhou, J., 2009. Polycystins and primary cilia: primers for cell cycle progression. Annual Review of Physiology 71, 83-113.

Acquired Cystic Disease

With the advent of long-term renal maintenance therapy, it has been observed that individuals on relatively long periods of dialysis develop multiple cysts in their remnant kidneys. This phenomenon is known as acquired cystic disease. An additional feature in acquired cystic disease is the occurrence of renal tumors. Papillary adenocarcinomas of small size are common, and larger tumors have a definite propensity for metastases.

The pathology of the kidneys is variable (Figs. 6.21, 6.22). On section, the kidneys demonstrate cysts involving the cortex and medulla of the kidney in an irregular fashion. The cysts vary in size and are sometimes as large as those seen in adult polycystic kidney disease.

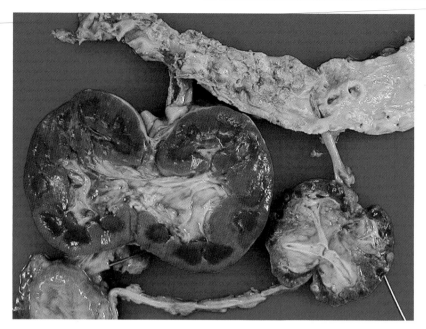

FIG. 6.21 Acquired cystic disease. This image demonstrates both end-stage native kidney and transplanted kidney from a patient with longstanding renal failure. The native kidney is atrophic and demonstrates acquired cystic disease involving the cortex.

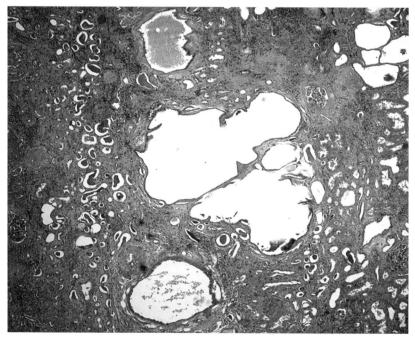

FIG. 6.22 Acquired cystic disease. There are randomly distributed cysts of irregular shape lined by flattened epithelium (hematoxylin and eosin, ×100).

Selected Reading

Tantravahi, J., Steinman, T.I., 2000. Acquired cystic kidney disease. Seminars in Dialysis 13, 330-334.

Cystic Renal Dysplasia

The term *cystic renal dysplasia* implicates a developmental disorder that occurs during the development of the embryo and its maturation. Renal dysplasia includes a spectrum of renal defects, which are often associated with abnormal collecting systems.

Dysplastic kidneys are grossly deformed in an irregular fashion. Histologically, they have a characteristic of having irregular cysts of varying size surrounded by primitive mesenchyme, which in some instances is variably differentiated (Figs. 6.23-6.28).

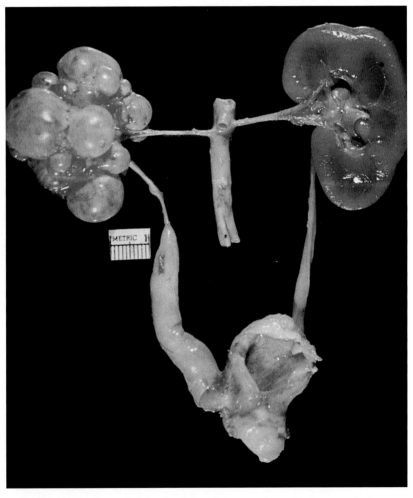

FIG. 6.23 Unilateral renal cystic dysplasia. This image demonstrates a cystically altered kidney with multiple cysts proximal to the kidney. There is evidence of obstruction of the ureter. The distal ureter is dilated suggesting ureterovesical obstruction as well.

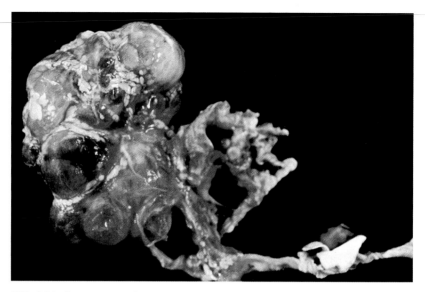

FIG. 6.24 The cysts in multicystic dysplasia are irregular in size and are distributed throughout the parenchyma.

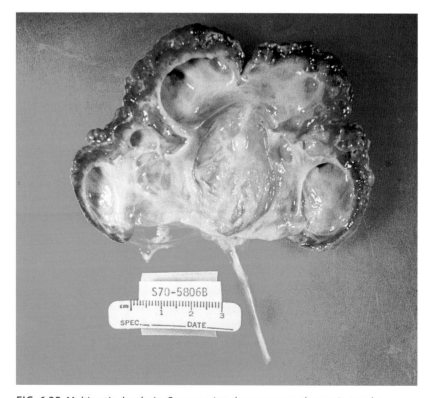

FIG. 6.25 Multicystic dysplasia. Cross section demonstrates obstruction at the ureteral pelvic junction with dilatation of the pelvis and multiple cysts involving the residual cortex.

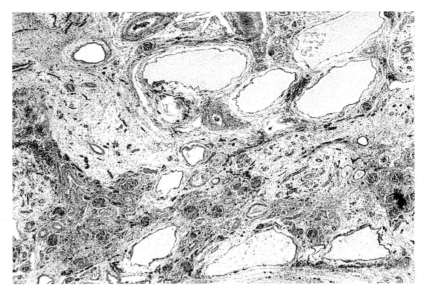

FIG. 6.26 Renal dysplasia. There is immature mesenchyme in the interstitium, and cysts of varying sizes are distributed randomly throughout the parenchyma. Glomeruli are seen scattered in the interstitium (hematoxylin and eosin, ×200).

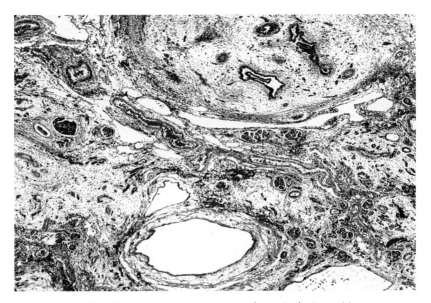

FIG. 6.27 Renal dysplasia. Loose primitive mesenchyme in the interstitium sometimes resembling cartilage is present (hematoxylin and eosin, ×200).

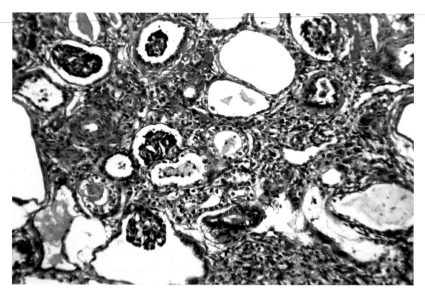

FIG. 6.28 Renal dysplasia. Cysts may also involve the glomeruli, and abortive glomerular structures are seen here with cystic dilatation of Bowman's space (hematoxylin and eosin, ×400).

Etiology/Pathogenesis

Cystic renal dysplasia may be syndromal or nonsyndromal and has multiple possible etiologies, all due to abnormal development of the kidney and urinary tract during development.

Selected Reading

Woolf, A.S., Price, K.L., Scambler, P.J., et al., 2009. Evolving concepts in human renal dysplasia. Journal of the American Society of Nephrology 15, 998-1007.

Renal Neoplasia

chapter

7

Introduction

Primary neoplastic lesions of the kidney can be divided according to the age group that is affected. Renal tumors in children in general resemble the nephrogenic tissues of embryogenesis and include Wilms tumor and clear cell sarcoma. Renal cell carcinomas are the major neoplasia of the kidney in adults. They have been classified on the basis of the histologic appearance, but recent studies have determined that they also can be stratified according to cytogenetic characteristics. These are summarized in Table 7.1. In addition to the tumors involving the renal parenchyma, the collecting system is also subject to neoplasia, which histologically fit into the same categories as those involving the ureters and bladder and are variants of transitional cell carcinoma.

Renal Cell Carcinomas

Renal cell carcinomas range widely in size ranging from one to two centimeters to several to massive tumors weighing several times the weight of the normal kidney. They are typically solid, ovulated masses that bulge into the renal parenchyma. Although they may appear circumscribed, they frequently have infiltration of the perinephric tissues and invade the vasculature, predominately the venous structures. The orange-yellow coloration is typical of the clear cell type, which often has foci of necrosis and scattered areas of hemorrhage. Chromophilic tumors may give a more friable, crumbling appearance. Microscopically, renal cell carcinomas have a great diversity of patterns (Table 7.2). They may be diffuse, tubular, cystic, papillary, or sarcomatoid. As the kidney is derived from mesenchyme, the sarcomatoid tumors have features that resemble leiomyo- or fibrosarcomas. Ultrastructurally, clear cell renal carcinoma contains abundant lipid and glycogen whereas chromophobe renal cell carcinoma is characterized by the presence of abundant intracytoplasmic vesicles (Figs. 7.1-7.16).

The College of American Pathologists has provided standards for the reporting of the surgical resections of renal tumors that provides a synopsis of cancer pathology staging and prognostic and predictive parameters (Table 7.3). These can be obtained from the website of the College. It includes macroscopic and microscopic grading and staging in a standard format. It also includes a specific section for description of the pathology of the nonneoplastic kidney

TABLE 7-1 Pathologic Classification of Renal Neoplasms

Carcinoma	Growth pattern	Cell of origin	Cytogenetic characteristics		Incidence (%)
			Major	**Minor**	
Clear cell	Acinar or sarcomatoid	Proximal tubule	3p 25-26	+5, +7, +12, −6q, −8p, −9, −14q, −Y	75-85
Chromophilic	Papillary or sarcomatoid	Proximal tubule	+7, +17, −Y	+12, +16, +20, −14	12-24
Chromophobic	Solid, tubular, or sarcomatoid	Intercalated cell of cortical collecting duct	Hypodiploidy	–	4-6
Oncocytic	Typified by tumor nests	Intercalated cell of cortical collecting duct	LOH 1p,14q	–	2-4
Collecting duct	Papillary or sarcomatoid	Medullary collecting	LOH 8p,13q	–	1

TABLE 7-2 WHO/AFIP Classification of Histologic Types

RENAL CELL TUMORS

Clear cell renal cell carcinoma
Multilocular clear cell renal cell carcinoma
Papillary renal cell carcinoma (type 1 or type 2)
Chromophobe renal cell carcinoma (classic or eosinophilic)
Carcinoma of the collecting ducts of Bellini
Renal medullary carcinoma
Xp11 translocation carcinomas/TFE3 gene
Carcinoma associated with neuroblastoma
Mucinous tubular and spindle cell carcinoma
Renal cell carcinoma unclassified
Benign
Papillary adenoma
Oncocytoma

METANEPHRIC TUMORS

Metanephric adenoma
Metanephric adenofibroma
Metanephric stromal tumors

MIXED MESENCHYMAL AND EPITHELIAL TUMORS

Cystic nephroma
Mixed epithelial and stromal tumor
Synovial sarcoma

NEPHROBLASTIC TUMORS

Nephrogenic rests
Nephroblastoma
Cystic partially differentiated nephroblastoma

TABLE 7-3 Fuhrman Nuclear Grade Classification for Renal Cell Carcinomas (used as Prognostic Indicators)

Grade	Nuclei Size and Shape	Nucleoli
Grade 1	10 µm Round, uniform	Inconspicuous or absent
Grade 2	15 µm Slightly irregular	Evident at 400× magnification
Grade 3	20 µm Obviously irregular	Prominent at 100× magnification
Grade 4	20+ µm Bizarre, multilobed	Heavy clumped chromatin

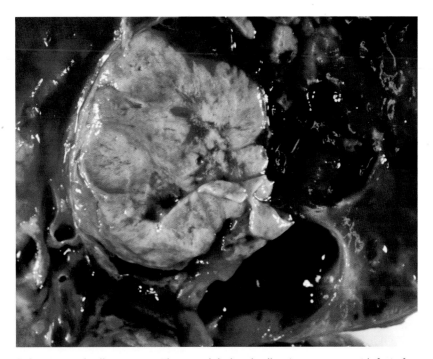

FIG. 7.1 Renal cell carcinoma. There is a lobulated yellow/orange mass with foci of hemorrhage typical of conventional (clear cell) renal cell carcinoma.

that should identify evidence of medical renal disease involvement. Glomerular, tubulointerstitial, and vascular changes should be described and interpreted.

Other Renal Epithelial Tumors

A rare form of renal cell carcinoma is that which arises in the collecting ducts and has been termed collecting duct carcinoma. Histologically, this has a pattern of branching tubules surrounded by an abundant stroma. Another important variant of renal cell tumors is the so-called renal oncocytoma. This is of importance in that the prognosis of oncocytomas is much more favorable than that of renal cell carcinoma. Renal oncocytomas have a homogeneous dark-brown appearance and histologically cells have a finely granular eosinophilic cytoplasm. Electron microscopy reveals abundant mitochondria (Figs. 7.17-7.20).

Etiology/Pathogenesis

Inactivation of the von Hippel Lindau tumor suppressor protein has been shown to play a critical role in clear cell renal carcinoma. Inactivation of the von Hippel Lindau protein leads

Text continued on page 527

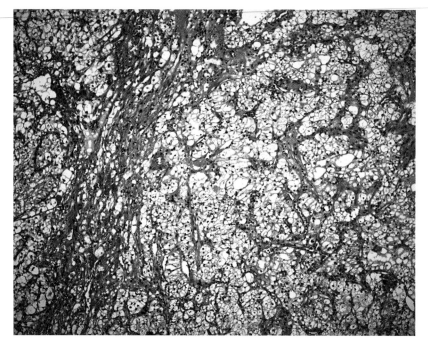

FIG. 7.2 Renal cell carcinoma. There is a prominent delicate vasculature throughout the tumor with strands of fibrosis. The cells are clear with dark central nuclei (hematoxylin and eosin, ×100).

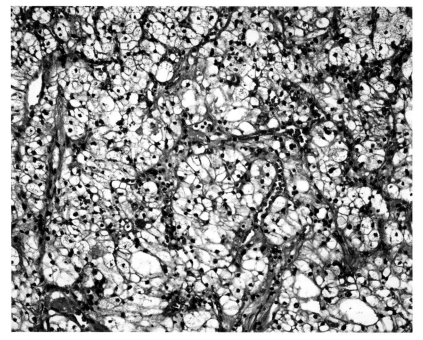

FIG. 7.3 Renal cell carcinoma. Higher power demonstrates the fibrovascular core and the nature of the clear cells (hematoxylin and eosin, ×200).

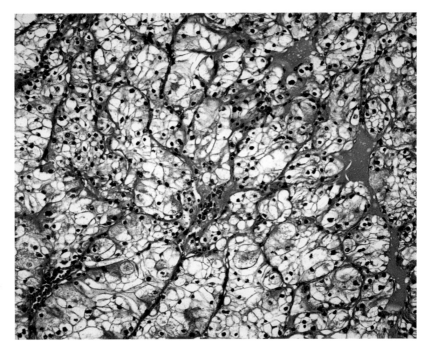

FIG. 7.4 Renal cell carcinoma. Delicate fibrovascular stroma surrounds cells with clear cytoplasm and eccentric dark nuclei (hematoxylin and eosin, ×400).

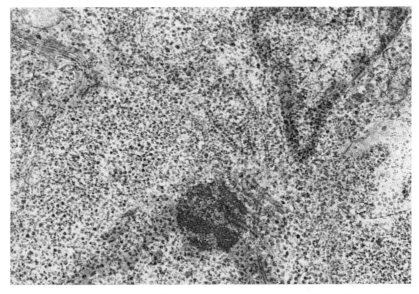

FIG. 7.5 Renal cell carcinoma. Electron microscopy reveals cytoplasm of clear cell tumors containing abundant glycogen (transmission electron microscopy, ×8000).

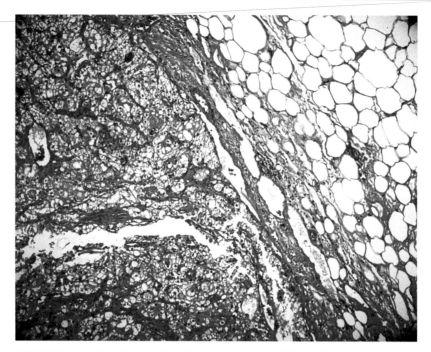

FIG. 7.6 Renal cell carcinoma. Periphery of conventional (clear cell) carcinoma demonstrates invasion of the perinephric adipose tissue (hematoxylin and eosin, ×100).

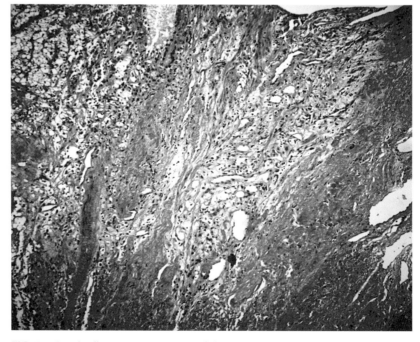

FIG. 7.7 Renal cell carcinoma. Invasion of the capsule is also evident with abundant vascular formation (hematoxylin and eosin, ×100).

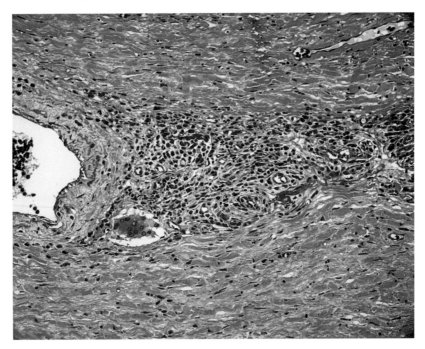

FIG. 7.8 Renal cell carcinoma. The invasive component sometimes has a sarcomatous appearance with elongated fibroblast-like tumor cells with irregular hyperchromatic nuclei (hematoxylin and eosin, ×200).

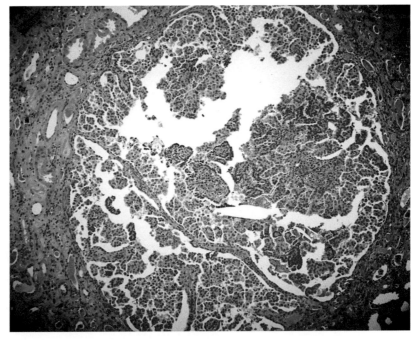

FIG. 7.9 Chromophilic carcinoma of the eosinophilic type. The cells are arranged in a pseudopapillary pattern in this islet of tumor, which has eosinophilic cytoplasm and central nuclei (hematoxylin and eosin, ×100).

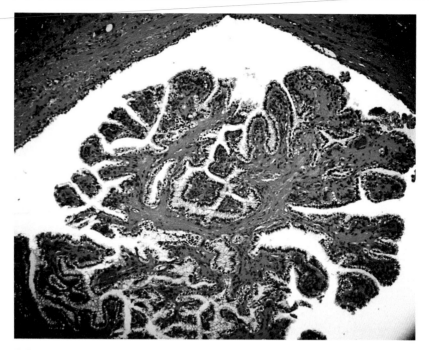

FIG. 7.10 Chromophilic (papillary) renal cell carcinoma. There is an obvious papillary pattern with papillae with a central fibrovascular core and surface lining of tumor cells (hematoxylin and eosin, ×200).

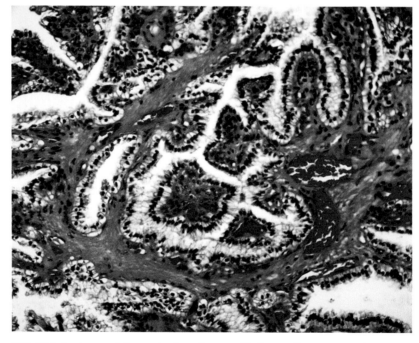

FIG. 7.11 In chromophilic renal cell carcinoma with the papillary pattern, the tumor cells contain basally located nuclei with an eosinophilic cytoplasm (hematoxylin and eosin, ×400).

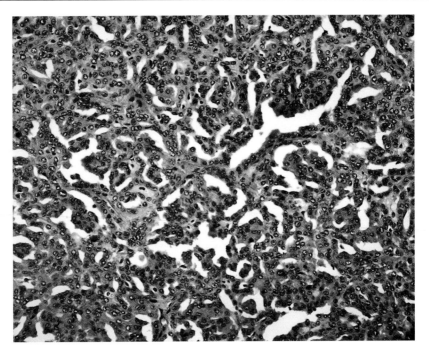

FIG. 7.12 Basophilic renal cell carcinoma can present in a more solid pattern. The cells have a scant cytoplasm and prominent nuclei that appears to give a basophilic appearance (hematoxylin and eosin, ×400).

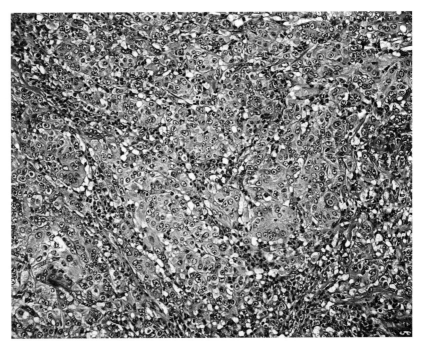

FIG. 7.13 Chromophobe carcinoma. The tumor consists of sheets of cells, with a thin fibrovascular stroma. The cytoplasm is prominent and has a pale staining pattern (hematoxylin and eosin, ×100).

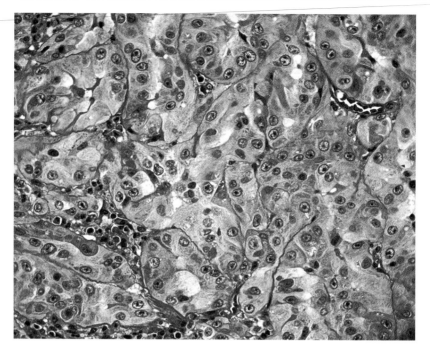

FIG. 7.14 Chromophobe carcinoma. The cytoplasm of the cells contains large numbers of minute intracytoplasmic vesicles, which gives a pale reticular or flocculent appearance to the cytoplasm (hematoxylin and eosin, ×400).

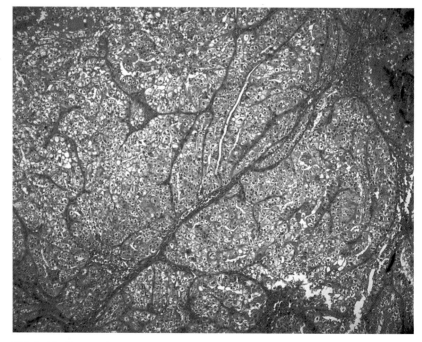

FIG. 7.15 Chromophobe renal carcinoma. Some solid variants of the chromophobe type have a more eosinophilic appearance than typical chromophobe carcinoma cells (hematoxylin and eosin, ×100).

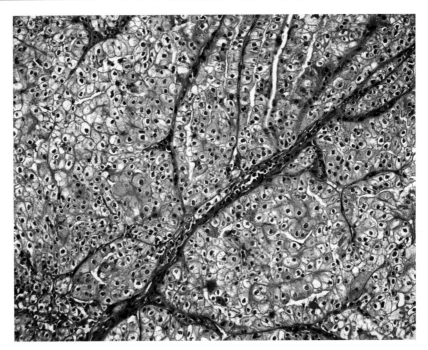

FIG. 7.16 Chromophobe renal carcinoma. The fibrovascular stroma surrounding islets of tightly packed tumor cells with slightly eosinophilic cytoplasm is shown (hematoxylin and eosin, ×100).

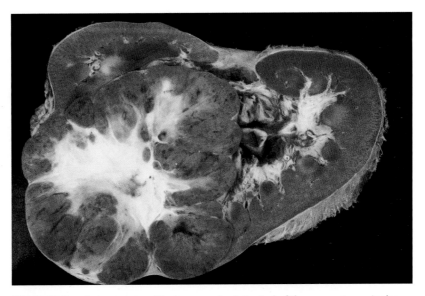

FIG. 7.17 Renal oncocytoma. The brown color is typical of the oncocytoma. It also demonstrates a central fibrous core.

to the increased accumulation of a transcription factor called hypoxia-inducible factor. Hypoxia-inducible factor in turn drives the overexpression of a number of genes, including the gene encoding for vascular endothelial growth factor, and overexpression of vascular endothelial growth factor is a hallmark of clear cell carcinoma and is consistent with the angiogenic nature of these tumors. Numerous other chromosomal abnormalities have been identified and have been associated with specific tumor histologies.

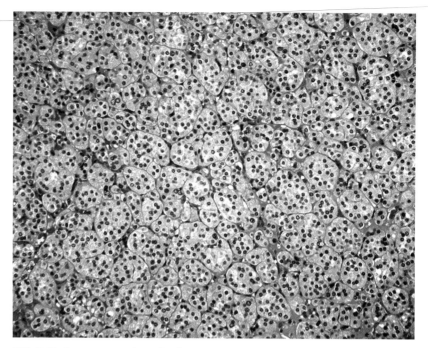

FIG. 7.18 Oncocytoma. The cells of the oncocytoma are arranged in diffuse sheets or islands of tumor cells with a background of edematous connective tissue (hematoxylin and eosin, ×100).

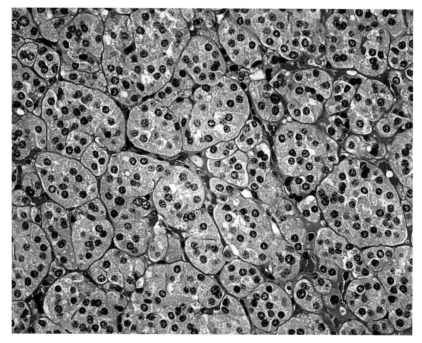

FIG. 7.19 Oncocytoma. There is a relatively even pattern of cells with uniform nuclei and granular eosinophilic appearance of the cytoplasm (hematoxylin and eosin, ×400).

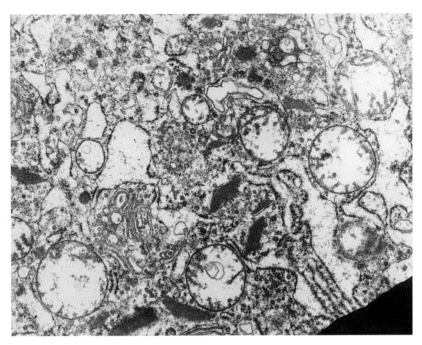

FIG. 7.20 Oncocytoma. There are abundant mitochondria, which gives a granular appearance by light microscopy (transmission electron microscopy, ×8000).

Selected Reading

Kennedy, S.M., Merino, M.J., Linehan, W.M., et al., 1990. Collecting duct carcinoma of the kidney. Human Pathology 21, 449-456.

Morra, M.N., Das, S., 1993. Renal oncocytoma: A review of histogenesis, histopathology, diagnosis and treatment. Journal of Urology 150, 295-302.

Rathmell, W.K., Chen, S., 2008. VHL inactivation in renal cell carcinoma: implications for diagnosis, prognosis and treatment. Expert Review of Anticancer Therapy 8, 63-73.

Thoenes, W., Storkel, S., Rumpelt, H.J., 1986. Histopathology and classification of renal cell tumors (adenomas, oncocytomas and carcinomas): The basic cytological and histopathological elements and their use for diagnostics. Pathology, Research and Practice 181, 125-143.

Wiesener, M.S., Münchenhagen, P.M., Berger, I., et al., 2001. Constitutive activation of hypoxia-inducible genes related to overexpression of hypoxia-inducible factor-1alpha in clear cell renal carcinomas. Cancer Research 61, 5215-5222.

Wilms Tumor

Wilms tumors comprise more than 80% of renal tumors of childhood. They are mostly identified in children 2-4 years of age and are often associated with congenital anomalies, which fall into syndromic patterns. Of these, the so-called Denys–Drash syndrome is of particular interest in that it is associated with the presence of focal and segmental glomerulosclerosis in the nonneoplastic renal tissue (see Chapter 1). Histologically, Wilms tumor consists of sheets of small cells with inconspicuous cytoplasmic hyperchromatic nuclei and frequent mitotic figures. The cells may be present in a variety of patterns – sometimes showing abortive glomerulogenesis and, in other areas, showing tubular structures (Figs 7.21-7.26).

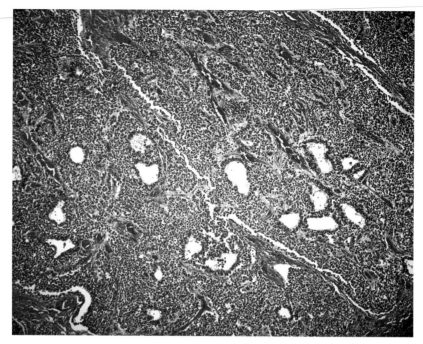

FIG. 7.21 Wilms tumor. Histologically, Wilms tumors are composed of various mixtures of primitive renal blastema, epithelium, and stroma. Blastema here appears as sheets of uniform small blue cells, which surround abortive tubular structures composed of epithelium and supported by a dense fibrovascular stroma (hematoxylin and eosin, ×100).

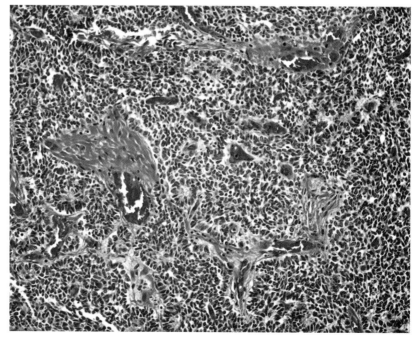

FIG. 7.22 Wilms tumor. The blastema consists of randomly arranged densely packed small cells with dark blue nuclei with frequent mitotic figures and a relatively inconspicuous cytoplasm (hematoxylin and eosin, ×200).

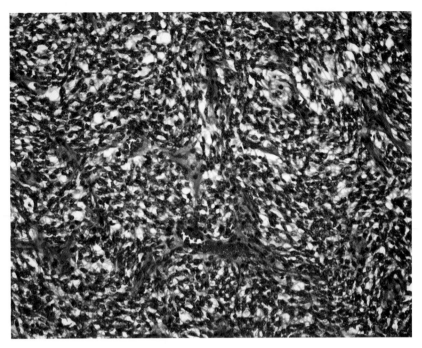

FIG. 7.23 Wilms tumor. In some areas, the blastema has a serpentine appearance with an elongated spindle cell pattern (hematoxylin and eosin, ×200).

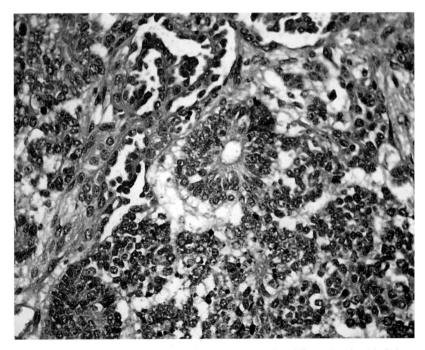

FIG. 7.24 Wilms tumor. Abortive tubular structures with a differentiated epithelial lining can be found surrounded by more primitive blastema (hematoxylin and eosin, ×400).

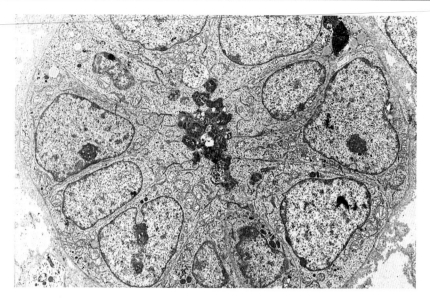

FIG. 7.25 Wilms tumor. Electron micrograph demonstrates a primitive tubule made up of blastema epithelial cells forming a lumen (transmission electron microscopy, ×2000).

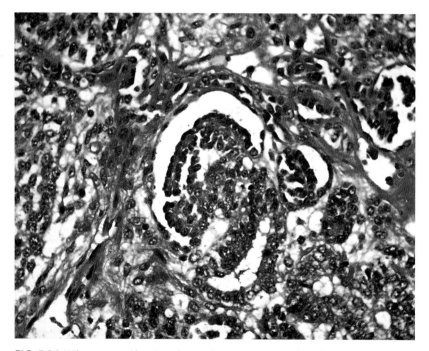

FIG. 7.26 Wilms tumor. Abortive glomerular structures are also identified within the mass of blastema. True capillary lumina are not present (hematoxylin and eosin, ×400).

Etiology/Pathogenesis

Wilms tumor is thought to be the result of abnormal proliferation of metanephric blastema, without normal differentiation into tubules and glomeruli. A number of genetic aberrations have been implicated in the pathogenesis of Wilms tumor. The chromosomal deletion of the WT1 gene located within the short arm of chromosome 11p13 often leads to the combination of Wilms tumor and aniridia, genitourinary malformation, and mental retardation (i.e., WAGR syndrome). Other Wilms tumor genes include WT2 at 11p15.5 linked to Beckwith–Wiedemann syndrome, deletion of chromosome 16, and duplication of chromosome 12.

Interestingly, in nonsyndromal Wilms tumor, the WT-1 gene itself is only rarely mutated. Rather, abnormalities of, for example, imprinting affecting WT-1 function are thought to be involved.

Selected Reading

Skolarikos, A.A., Papatsoris, A.G., Alivizatos, G., et al., 2006. Molecular pathogenetics of renal cancer. American Journal of Nephrology 218-231.

Ritchey, M.L., Azizkhan, R.G., Beckwith, J.B., et al., 1995. Neonatal Wilms' tumor. Journal of Pediatric Surgery 30, 856-859.

Scott, R.H., Douglas, J., Baskcomb, L., et al., 2008. Constitutional 11p15 abnormalities, including heritable imprinting center mutations, cause nonsyndromic Wilms tumor. Nature Genetics 40, 1329-1334.

Transitional Cell Carcinoma of the Renal Pelvis

Primary transitional cell carcinoma (TCC) of the renal pelvis or ureter accounts for less than 5% of all renal tumors. Tumors of the upper urinary tract are twice as common in men, and the peak incidence occurs between age 50 and 60 years. Transitional tumors of the renal pelvis and ureter are histologically identical to bladder epithelial tumors. Morphologically, these tumors can be papillary or solid in configuration, and they may have associated carcinoma in situ (Figs. 7.27, 7.28).

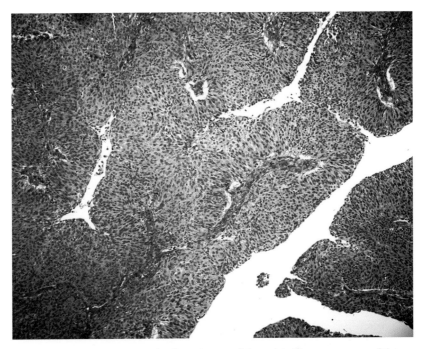

FIG. 7.27 Papillary transitional cell carcinoma of the pelvis. The appearance of the tumor is similar to that seen in papillary transitional cell carcinoma of the bladder. There are fibrovascular cores surrounded by a stratified transitional epithelium (hematoxylin and eosin, ×100).

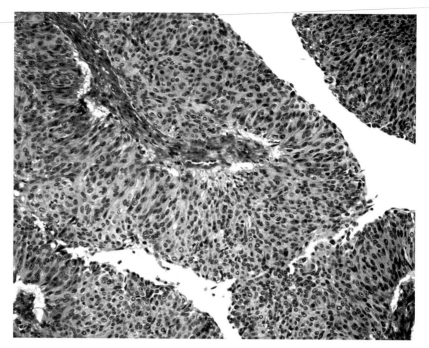

FIG. 7.28 Papillary transitional cell carcinoma. The epithelium has pleomorphic nuclei, which vary in size and shape and vary in degree of differentiation (hematoxylin and eosin, ×200).

Etiology/Pathogenesis

The surface epithelium (urothelium) that lines the mucosal surfaces of the entire urinary tract is exposed to potential carcinogens that may be excreted in the urine, or activated in the urine by hydrolyzing enzymes. Environmental exposures are thought to account for most cases of urothelial cancer. Cigarette smoking, occupational carcinogen exposure, and Chinese herbs that contain aristolochic acid have all been implicated in the pathogenesis.

Selected Reading

Munoz, J.J., Ellison, L.M., 2000. Upper tract urothelial neoplasms: incidence and survival during the last 2 decades. Journal of Urology 164, 1523-1525.

Index

Page numbers followed by f indicate figure(s); t, table(s); b, box(es).